WIDE AWAKE
HAND SURGERY

AND THERAPY TIPS

WIDE AWAKE HAND SURGERY

AND THERAPY TIPS

EDITED BY

DONALD H. LALONDE, BSc (HONS), MD, MSc, FRCSC
PROFESSOR, DIVISION OF PLASTIC
AND RECONSTRUCTIVE SURGERY, DEPARTMENT
OF SURGERY, DALHOUSIE UNIVERSITY,
SAINT JOHN, NEW BRUNSWICK, CANADA

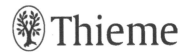

Library of Congress Cataloging-in-Publication Data
is available from the publisher

Thieme Medical Publishers, Inc.
333 Seventh Avenue, 18th Floor,
New York, NY 10001, USA
www.thieme.com
+1 800 782 3488, customerservice@thieme.com

Illustrations: Tiffany Slaybaugh Davanzo
Cover design: © Thieme
Cover images source: © Thieme
Typesetting by Thomson Digital, India

Printed in Germany by Beltz Grafische Betriebe 5 4 3 2 1

ISBN: 978-1-68420-230-0
Also available as an e-book
eISBN: 978-1-68420-231-7

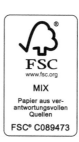

FSC
www.fsc.org
MIX
Papier aus ver-
antwortungsvollen
Quellen
FSC® C089473

CONTENTS

SECTION I   ATLAS OF TUMESCENT LOCAL ANESTHESIA ELBOW, FOREARM, WRIST, HAND, AND FINGER INJECTIONS

SECTION II   GENERAL PRINCIPLES OF WIDE AWAKE HAND SURGERY

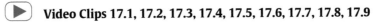

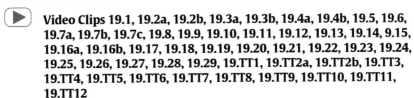

VIDEO CONTENTS

PART E TENDON SURGERY: TENDON GRAFTS AND PULLEY RECONSTRUCTION

25 Tendon Grafts and Pulley Reconstruction   217

Donald H. Lalonde, Egemen Ayhan, Alison Wong, Chao Chen, Nikolas Alan Jagodzinski, Alistair Phillips, Kamal Rafiqi, Thomas Apard, and Ian Maxwell

PART F NERVE SURGERY

26 Carpal Tunnel Decompression of the Median Nerve   225
*Donald H. Lalonde, Andrew W. Gurman, Xavier Gueffier, Shu Guo Xing,
Jin Bo Tang, Amir Adham Ahmad, and Thomas Apard*

PART H   JOINT AND ARTHRITIS SURGERY: PIP AND MP

36   Finger Joint Arthroplasty, Fusion, and Ligament Repair   285
Donald H. Lalonde, Amanda Higgins, Jason Wong, Chye Yew Ng, Xavier Gueffier, Thomas Apard, and Asif Ilyas

37   Thumb Metacarpophalangeal Joint Fusion and Ulnar Collateral Ligament Repair   291
Donald H. Lalonde, Elisabet Hagert, Jean Paul Brutus, Paul Sibley, Amir Adham Ahmad, Xavier Gueffier, and Thomas Apard

(see Chapter 10 for evidence on safety of field sterility for K-wire insertion).[1,2,3,4,5]

Video 42.9 Operative reduction of fourth and fifth metacarpal fractures in the patient injected with local anesthetic seen in Video 42.2 (Xing, China).

Video 42.10 Simple distraction method for transverse fractures (Gueffier, France).

Video 42.11 Testing stability of open compression screw fixation (Escobar, Columbia).

Video 42.12 Two metacarpal shaft fractures headless compression screw (Sibley, USA).

Video 42.13 Suture fixation of metacarpal fracture with testing of stability of suture (Apard, France).

Video 42.14 Check scissoring correction after dynamic compression bone clamp reduction of transverse metacarpal fracture before plating (Lalonde, Canada).[6]

Video 42.15 Plating after correction of metacarpal malunion fracture (Lalonde, Canada).

Video 42.16 Plating after correction of metacarpal malunion fracture (Jagodzinski England).

Video 42.17 Verifying no scissoring of plate metacarpal (Ahmad, Malaysia).

Video 42.TT1 Early protected movement after open reduction and K-wire fixation of maluniting fracture at 4 weeks post injury (includes detailed surgery) (Kean, Canada).[7]

43 Wrist Fracture and Ligament Injuries   325
Celso R. Folberg, Xavier Gueffier, Carlos Ramos de Pina, Donald H. Lalonde, Nikolas Alan Jagodzinski, Elisabet Hagert, Thomas Apard, and Amir Adham Ahmad

Video 43.1 Injection of local anesthesia for major wrist trauma such as perilunate dislocation (de Pina, Portugal).[1,2]

Video 43.2 Scaphoid screw local anesthesia, preoperative ultrasound, and surgery (Gueffier, France).

Video 43.3 Local anesthesia injection for volar percutaneous screw scaphoid fracture (Jagodzinski, England).

Video 43.4 Local anesthesia injection for volar percutaneous screw scaphoid fracture (Folberg, Brazil).

Video 43.5a Local injection and surgery for dorsal screw scaphoid fracture (Ahmad, Malaysia).

Video 43.5b Open dorsal screw for scaphoid fracture (Apard, France).

Video 43.6 Local anesthesia injection and dorsal percutaneous screw for scaphoid fracture (Folberg, Brazil).

Video 43.7 Studying active movement of the carpus after reduction of the lunate in perilunate dislocation (de Pina, Portugal).

Video 43.8 Studying active movement after triangular fibrocartilage complex (TFCC) repair (Hagert, Sweden).[3]

Video 43.9 Surgery for scaphoid lunate separation (de Pina, Portugal).

Video 43.10 Volar percutaneous screw fixation for scaphoid fracture (de Pina, Portugal).

PREFACE

The purpose of this book is to provide a recipe-type "How to do it" wide awake hand (and the rest of the upper and lower limbs) surgery approach for surgeons and hand therapists. The goals are to: (1) improve surgical outcomes by seeing active movement during the surgery and educating awake patients on how to decrease complications, (2) decrease the unnecessary risks and costs of sedation, (3) decrease medical trash in landfills, and (4) increase the access of surgical care in developing nations by decreasing costs and improving safety by avoiding sedation and unnecessary sterility.

This second edition of *Wide Awake Hand Surgery (and Therapy Tips)* is MUCH more extensive than the first edition. The video count has more than tripled to over 500—most of them new. Video is the best learning tool for surgeons and therapists. There is more to learn in this book than most people have the capacity to absorb.

There are new chapters on WALANT upper and lower limb fracture treatment (wrist, forearm, elbow, acromion, clavicle, patella, tibia, fibula, ankle, and foot). Many chapters have new therapy tip sections to help surgeons and therapists decrease the all-too-common, postoperative finger stiffness that happens after fracture and tendon surgery.

There is a new chapter to help surgeons and therapists treat hand pain and finger stiffness with the pencil test and relative motion splinting.

New chapters on nerve decompression are there for radial and peroneal compressions as well as a new chapter specifically designed to help with simultaneous multiple nerve decompression procedures (e.g., cubital and carpal tunnel decompression in the same operation).

We have added more than 8 hours of video education on hand ultrasound diagnosis and ultrasound-guided surgery to give you a solid foundation in starting ultrasound in hand surgery and therapy.

We show new ways to decrease pain with local anesthesia injection.

We share with you several new strategies in implementing WALANT in your hospital.

We bring you the latest science of evidence-based sterility.

We have more than doubled the number of authors, now representing 15 countries. So many surgeons from all over the world have started using wide awake hand surgery that it is difficult to put all in one book. I have spent hundreds of hours doing this to the best of my ability. I hope this book and its videos are helpful for you and your patients.

Donald H. Lalonde, BSc (Hons), MD, MSc, FRCSC

Acknowledgments

Above all and most importantly, I give my deepest gratitude to Jan Lalonde. She truly is the wind beneath the wings of wide awake surgery. The whole WALANT movement, let alone this book and its 500+ videos, would not exist if it were not for Jan. She is my truly amazing wife, soul mate, surgery center manager, operating room nurse, research coordinator, and so much more. She has kept our lives on track for 25+ years in our work at the office, on the road, and at home during the countless hours of writing, video editing, travel, international surgeon hosting, presentation, and webinar preparation that allowed the creation of both the editions of *Wide Awake Hand Surgery*. She did it all with humor, clever perception, balance, and love.

I thank all the surgeons, hand therapists, and patients who were so generous with their time and their stories to contribute to the making of this amazing collection of wisdom in the art and science of wide awake extremity surgery with sedation-free local anesthesia.

I want to acknowledge and thank Tiffany Slaybaugh Davanzo for drawing most of the illustrations in both the first and second editions of the *Wide Awake Hand Surgery* book. She has been a pleasure to work with (https://www.medillsb.com/artist.aspx?AID=4124).

I would like to thank the Thieme team members who contributed the most to the creation and evolution of both editions of *Wide Awake Hand Surgery*; Sue Hodgson (England), Stephan Konnry (Germany), Shipra Sehgal (India), Apoorva Goel (India), and Karen Edmonson (USA).

I also greatly appreciate the help of Susan MacMichael who works with Jan and I in Saint John. She cheerfully and skillfully accomplished any task she was given to facilitate the progress of the WALANT movement.

Donald H. Lalonde, BSc (Hons), MD, MSc, FRCSC

CONTRIBUTORS

Julie E. Adams, MD, MS
Professor of Orthopedic Surgery, University of Tennessee College of Medicine, Chattanooga, Tennessee, USA

Amir Adham Ahmad, MBBS, Dr Orth & Tr
Consultant, Orthopaedic Surgeon (Hand & Microsurgery), Prince Court Medical Centre, Kuala Lumpur, Malaysia

Gökhan Tolga Akbulut, MD
Orthopedic Surgeon, İrmet Hospital, Tekirdağ, Turkey

Ahsan Akhtar, MBChB, FRCS (Tr & Orth)
Upper Limb Fellow, Trauma & Orthopaedics, Wrightington Hospital, England, UK

Peter C. Amadio, MD
Dean for Research Academic Affairs, Workforce, and Digital Technology; Lloyd A. and Barbara A. Amundson Professor of Orthopedics; Professor of Biomedical Engineering, Mayo Clinic, Rochester, Minnesota, USA

Thomas Apard, MD, FEBHS
Ultrasound Guided Hand Surgery Center, Versailles, France

Egemen Ayhan, MD, FEBHS
Associate Professor, Division of Hand Surgery, Department of Orthopedics and Traumatology, Diskapi YB Training and Research Hospital, University of Health Sciences, Ankara, Turkey

Mark Baratz, MD
Clinical Professor and Vice Chairman; Program Director Hand and Upper Extremity Fellowship, Department of Orthopaedics, University of Pittsburgh Medical Center, Pittsburgh, PA, USA

Jean Paul Brutus, MD
Plastic Surgeon; Hand and Wrist Surgeon, Exception MD, Montreal, Canada

Kevin T. K. Chan, MD
Clinical Assistant Professor, Spectrum Health/Michigan State University College of Human Medicine, Grand Rapids, Michigan, USA

Chao Chen, MD, PhD
Attending Surgeon, Hand and Microsurgery, Shandong Provincial Hospital affiliated to Shandong University, Jinan, China

Chris Chun-Yu Chen, MD
Assistant Professor, Department of Orthopaedics, Kaohsiung Veterans General Hospital, Taiwan

Geoffrey Cook, MD, FRCSC
Assistant Professor, Division of Plastic and Reconstructive Surgery, Department of
Surgery, Dalhousie University, Saint John, New Brunswick, Canada

Carlos Ramos de Pina, MD
Assistant Orthopedic Surgeon; Coordinator, Hand and Arthroscopy Unity, Ortopedia 2,
Centro Hospitalar de Leiria, Leiria, Portugal

Lisa Flewelling, OTReg (NB)
Occupational Therapist, Saint John Regional Hospital, Saint John, Canada

Celso Folberg, Celso R. Folberg MD, MSc
Chief, Hand Surgery Group, Department of Orthopedics, Hospital de Clinicas de Porto
Alegre, Porto Alegre/RS, Brazil

Günter Germann, MD, PhD
Prof. Dr. Med; Medical Director/CEO; Board Certified Plastic & Hand Surgeon –
Aesthetic Surgeon; President, American Society for Reconstructive Microsurgery
(ASRM) Ethianum Clinic, Heidelberg, Germany

Xavier Gueffier, MD
European Board of Hand Surgery – FESSH; Member of French Society of Hand Surgery
(SFCM); International Member, American Society for Surgery of the Hand (ASSH),
Artezieux Center, Isère, France

Andrew W. Gurman, MD
Altoona Hand and Wrist Surgery, Altoona, Pennsylvania, USA

Elisabet Hagert, MD, PhD
Associate Professor of Orthopedics, Karolinska Institutet, Department of Clinical
Science and Education and Sophiahemmet University, Department of Musculoskeletal
& Sports Injury Epidemiology Center, Stockholm, Sweden

Daniel Hess, MD
Department of Orthopedic Surgery, Spectrum Health System, Grand Rapids, Michigan,
USA

Amanda Higgins, BSc OT
Horizon Health Network, Rothesay, New Brunswick, Canada

Levi L. Hinkelman, MD
Section Chief Hand Surgery, Department of Orthopedic Surgery, Spectrum Health
System, Grand Rapids, MI; Assistant Professor, Michigan State University College of
Human Medicine, Grand Rapids, Michigan, USA

Chung-Chen Hsu, MD
Associate Professor, Trauma Division, Department of Plastic and Reconstructive
Surgery, Linkou Medical Center, Chang Gung Memorial Hospital, Chang Gung
University, Taiwan

Yin Ming Huang, MD
Department of Orthopaedics, Kaohsiung Veterans General Hospital, Taiwan

Asif Ilyas, MD, MBA, FACS
Program Director of Hand Surgery Fellowship, Rothman Orthopaedic Institute;
President, Rothman Opioid Foundation; Professor of Orthopaedic Surgery,
Thomas Jefferson University Philadelphia, Philadelphia, PA, USA

**Nikolas Alan Jagodzinski, MBChB, FHEM, FRCS (Tr & Orth), Dip Hand Surg
(BSSH)**
Consultant, Trauma, Orthopaedics, and Hand Surgery, North Devon District Hospital,
Barnstaple, UK

Peter J. L. Jebson, MD
Lakewood Ranch, Florida, USA

Brian Jurbala, MD, FAAOS, CAQSM, CAQSH, RMSK
Lakeland, Florida, USA

Susan Kean, PT, CHT
Rothesay, New Brunswick, Canada

Steven Koehler, MD, FAAOS
Director of Hand and Microsurgery; Assistant Professor, Department of Orthopedic
Surgery, SUNY Downstate Health Sciences University, New York, USA

Donald H. Lalonde, BSc (Hons), MD, MSc, FRCSC
Professor, Division of Plastic and Reconstructive Surgery, Department of Surgery,
Dalhousie University, Saint John, New Brunswick, Canada

Yin Lu, PhD
The First Hand and Microsurgery Ward, Tianjin Hospital, Tianjin, China

Luke MacNeill, PhD
Postdoctoral Fellow, Centre for Research in Integrated Care, University of New
Brunswick, Saint John, New Brunswick, Canada

Ian Maxwell, MD, FRCSC
Assistant Professor, Division of Plastic Surgery, Dalhousie and Memorial Universities,
Saint John Regional Hospital, Saint John, New Brunswick, Canada

D. Joshua Mayich, MSc, MD, FRCSC
Adult Trauma & Foot and Ankle Reconstructive Surgery, Division of Orthopaedic
Surgery, Stanton General Hospital, Yellowknife, NWT, Canada

Duncan Angus McGrouther, MD, FRCS
Senior Consultant, Hand Surgeon, Department of Hand Surgery, Singapore General
Hospital; Professor, Duke-NUS Medical School, Singapore

Daniel McKee, MD, FRCSC
Division of Plastic Surgery, University of British Columbia, Vancouver, British Columbia,
Canada

Chye Yew Ng, MBChB (Hons), FRCS (Tr & Orth), Dip Hand Surg
Consultant; Hand & Peripheral Nerve Surgeon, Wrightington Hospital, England, UK

Michael W. Neumeister, MD, FRCSC, FACS
Professor and Chairman, Department of Surgery, Southern Illinois University of Medicine, Springfield, Illinois, USA

Alistair Phillips, FRCS (Tr & Orth)
Consultant, Hand and Trauma Surgeon, University Hospital Southampton NHS Foundation Trust, Southampton, Hampshire, UK

Kamal Rafiqi, MD
Assistant Professor, Orthopedic Surgery, Faculty of Medicine, Ibn Zohr University, Agadir, Morocco

Julian A. Escobar Rincon, MD
Orthopedic Hand Surgeon, University Hospital of Caldas, Manizales, Colombia

Michael Sauerbier, MD, PhD
Professor Sauerbier; Private Practice for Hand and Plastic Surgery, Bad Homburg vor der Höhe; Professor for Plastic Surgery, Goethe University Frankfurt am Main, Frankfurt, Germany

Xiao Fang Shen, MD
Department of Pediatric Orthopedics, Wuxi 9th People's Hospital, Wuxi, China

Paul A. Sibley, DO, FAOAO
Assistant Clinical Professor, USF College of Medicine – SELECT, Department of Orthopedics and Sports Medicine, Lehigh Valley Health Network, Allentown, Pennsylvania, USA

Jin Bo Tang, MD
Professor and Chair, Department of Hand Surgery, Affiliated Hospital of Nantong University, Nantong, Jiangsu, China

Leigh-Anne Tu, MD
Orthopaedic Hand and Upper Extremity Surgery, Illinois Bone and Joint Institute, Morton Grove, Illinois, USA

Robert E. Van Demark, Jr., MD
Clinical Professor and Section Head, Department of Orthopedic Surgery, Sanford School of Medicine, The University of South Dakota Vermillion, South Dakota, USA

Alison Wong, MD, MSE, FRCSC
Plastic and Hand Surgeon, Roth | McFarlane Hand and Upper Limb Centre (HULC); Adjunct Professor, Western University, London, Ontario, Canada

Jason Wong, MBChB, FHEA, PhD, FRCS (Plast)
Academic Consultant and Senior Clinical Lecturer, Plastic Surgery, University of Manchester and Manchester Academic Health Science Centre, King James IV Professor Royal College of Surgeons of Edinburgh, Manchester, UK

Shu Guo Xing, MD
Attending Surgeon, Department of Hand Surgery, Affiliated Hospital of Nantong University, Nantong, Jiangsu, China

Lei Zhu, MD
Director, Department of Hand Surgery; Director, Department of Foot and Ankle Surgery, Qilu Hospital of Shandong University; Vice Professor, Shandong University, Jinan, China

Section I

ATLAS OF TUMESCENT LOCAL ANESTHESIA ELBOW, FOREARM, WRIST, HAND, AND FINGER INJECTIONS

CHAPTER 1

FINGER BLOCKS AND ATLAS OF IMAGES OF TUMESCENT LOCAL ANESTHETIC DIFFUSION ANATOMY

Donald H. Lalonde

FINGER BLOCK: SINGLE SUBCUTANEOUS INJECTION IN THE MIDLINE PROXIMAL PHALANX WITH LIDOCAINE AND EPINEPHRINE (SIMPLE BLOCK)

SIMPLE is the acronym for single subcutaneous injection in the midline proximal phalanx with lidocaine and epinephrine.

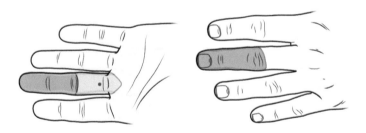

When you inject 2 mL of buffered 1% lidocaine with 1:100,000 epinephrine in subcutaneous fat in the red injection point just under the skin without moving the needle, local anesthetic can be seen and palpated in the blue area in an unscarred patient. The two digital nerves always get numb. You numb the distal green area by nerve block, but this area has no epinephrine vasoconstriction and may bleed more because of the sympathectomy of the nerve block. This block can be helpful in frostbite of the fingertip.[1]

- Only 2 mL is required for a good digital block. Use a 30-gauge needle on a 3-mL Luer-lock syringe.

- There is level II evidence that patients prefer this block to the two dorsal injections block.[2]

- There is level I evidence that needle penetration of the palmar skin is not more painful than needle penetration of web space skin.[3]

- There is level II evidence that this block hurts less if you inject it over 60 seconds than if you inject it over 10 seconds.[4]

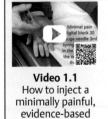

Video 1.1
How to inject a minimally painful, evidence-based SIMPLE digital block.

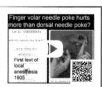

Video 1.2
How the two
dorsal injections
web space block
got replaced by
the single-injection
SIMPLE digital
block.

- There is level II evidence that lidocaine without epinephrine digital blocks lasts 5 hours, whereas lidocaine with epinephrine blocks lasts 10 hours.[5]

- There is level I evidence that the pain-relieving effect of bupivacaine blocks lasts 15 hours, whereas the annoying numbness to touch and pressure lasts more than 30 hours with these blocks.[1]

"SIMPLE" FINGER BLOCK WITH DORSAL BLOCK AUGMENTATION

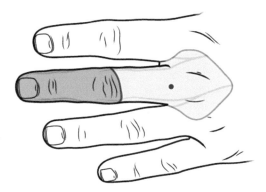

When you inject 2 mL of buffered 1% lidocaine with 1:100,000 epinephrine in subcutaneous fat in the red injection point just under the dorsal skin without moving the needle, local anesthetic can be seen and palpated to diffuse in the blue area in an unscarred patient. In some patients, the SIMPLE block does not numb this dorsal area and it needs to be augmented with this second injection if you are applying a tourniquet at the base of the finger.

"SIMPLE" THUMB BLOCK (SEE ► VIDEO 17.7)

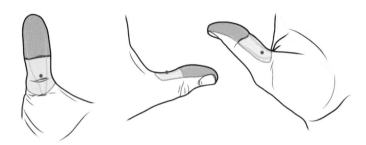

When you inject 2 mL of buffered 1% lidocaine with 1:100,000 epinephrine in subcutaneous fat in the red injection point just under the skin without moving the needle, local anesthetic can be seen and palpated to diffuse in the blue area in an unscarred patient. The two digital nerves always get numb.

DORSAL THUMB PROXIMAL PHALANX BLOCK

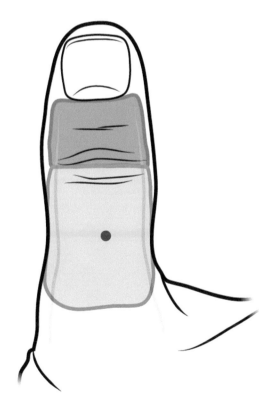

When you inject 2 mL of buffered 1% lidocaine with 1:100,000 epinephrine in subcutaneous fat in the red injection point just under the skin without moving the needle, local anesthetic can be seen and palpated to diffuse in the blue area in an unscarred patient.

GUIDE TO THE ATLAS

- We drew the images in this atlas from photographs of live human volunteers injected with tumescent local anesthesia to determine where the solution naturally diffuses when you inject it in one subcutaneous spot marked in red without moving the needle.
- The *blue areas* show the diffusion of visible and palpable lidocaine with epinephrine that usually takes place within **30 minutes after injection** in most patients. These blue areas will be both numbed and vasoconstricted.
- The *green areas* are blocked by nerve block. It can take longer for the green areas to get numb than the blue areas because the affected nerves are larger. These green areas will not be vasoconstricted. Bleeding in the green areas may be more than in normal skin because of the sympathectomy effect of the nerve blocks. To avoid bleeding in the green areas, simply inject more local anesthetic wherever you will dissect, as described in Chapter 4.
- As in any anatomy, different patients will have small differences. Not all patients will get the green distal nerve blocks.

THUMB MIDMETACARPAL VOLAR

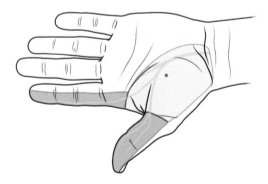

When you inject 10 mL of buffered 1% lidocaine with 1:100,000 epinephrine in the volar aspect of the midmetacarpal thumb red injection point just under the skin without moving the needle, local anesthetic can be seen and palpated to diffuse in the blue area in an unscarred patient. Note that the ligaments at the glabrous/nonglabrous skin junction act as a diffusion barrier to dorsal distribution of the local anesthetic. The thenar eminence creases in the palm also act as a barrier to local anesthetic diffusion.

THUMB MIDMETACARPAL DORSAL

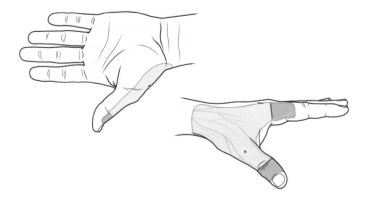

When you inject 10 mL of buffered 1% lidocaine with 1:100,000 epinephrine in the dorsum of the midmetacarpal thumb in the red injection point just under the skin without moving the needle, local anesthetic can be seen and palpated to diffuse in the blue area in an unscarred patient. Note that the ligaments at the glabrous/nonglabrous skin junction act as a natural diffusion barrier to volar distribution of the local anesthetic. The interphalangeal thumb crease also acts as a natural barrier to local anesthetic diffusion.

MIDPALMAR HAND

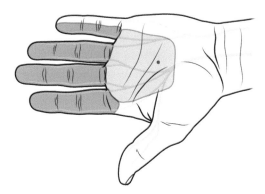

When you inject 10 mL of buffered 1% lidocaine with 1:100,000 epinephrine in the midpalm in the red injection point just under the skin without moving the needle, local anesthetic can be seen and palpated to diffuse in the blue area in an unscarred patient.

MIDDORSAL HAND

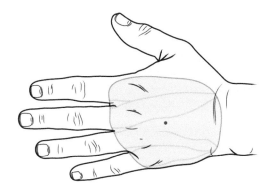

When you inject 10 mL of buffered 1% lidocaine with 1:100,000 epinephrine in the dorsum of the midhand in the red injection point just under the skin without moving the needle, local anesthetic can be seen and palpated to diffuse in the blue area in an unscarred patient. The proximal phalanx dorsal skin may not be blocked past the web space.

ULNAR HAND

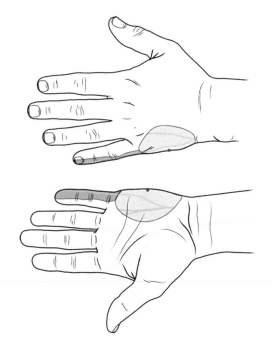

When you inject 10 mL of buffered 1% lidocaine with 1:100,000 epinephrine in the ulnar midhand in the red injection point just under the skin without moving the needle, local anesthetic can be seen and palpated to diffuse in the blue area in an unscarred patient.

MIDLINE ULNAR WRIST

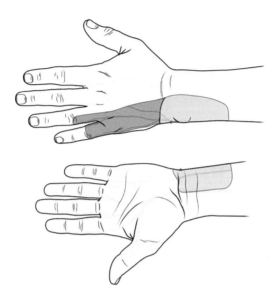

When you inject 10 mL of buffered 1% lidocaine with 1:100,000 epinephrine in the midulnar wrist in the red injection point just under the skin without moving the needle, local anesthetic can be seen and palpated to diffuse in the blue area in an unscarred patient.

MIDLINE ANTERIOR WRIST

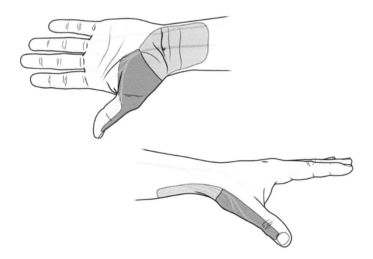

When you inject 10 mL of buffered 1% lidocaine with 1:100,000 epinephrine in the midvolar wrist in the red injection point just under the skin without moving the needle, local anesthetic can be seen and palpated to diffuse in the blue area in an unscarred patient. When the injection is under the skin and not below the forearm fascia, you may not achieve a median or ulnar nerve block, since the deep forearm fascia can act as a natural diffusion barrier to local anesthetic diffusion. More of the local anesthetic tracks proximally, because the wrist crease acts as a natural barrier to local anesthetic diffusion into the palm.

MIDLINE DORSAL WRIST

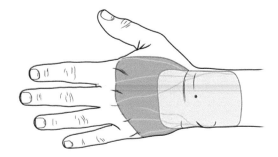

When you inject 10 mL of buffered 1% lidocaine with 1:100,000 epinephrine in the middorsal wrist in the red injection point just under the skin without moving the needle, local anesthetic can be seen and palpated to diffuse in the blue area in an unscarred patient.

MIDLINE RADIAL WRIST

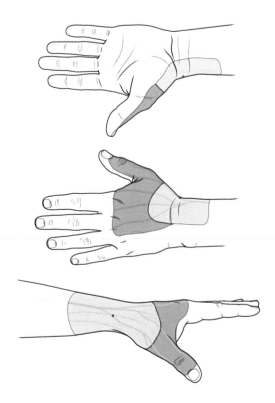

When you inject 10 mL of buffered 1% lidocaine with 1:100,000 epinephrine in the midradial wrist in the red injection point just under the skin
without moving the needle, local anesthetic can be seen and palpated to
diffuse in the blue area in an unscarred patient.

MIDLINE RADIAL FOREARM 10 CM PROXIMAL TO WRIST CREASE

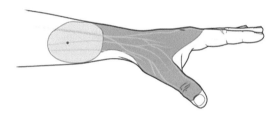

When you inject 20 mL of buffered 1% lidocaine with 1:100,000 epinephrine 10 cm proximal to the wrist crease in the radial forearm midline in the
red injection point just under the skin without moving the needle, local
anesthetic can be seen and palpated to diffuse in the blue area in an unscarred patient.

MIDLINE ANTERIOR FOREARM 10 CM PROXIMAL TO WRIST CREASE

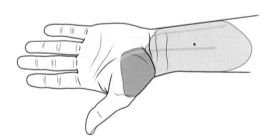

When you inject 20 mL of buffered 1% lidocaine with 1:100,000 epinephrine 10 cm proximal to the wrist crease in the volar forearm midline in the
red injection point just under the skin without moving the needle, local
anesthetic can be seen and palpated to diffuse in the blue area in an unscarred patient. The median and ulnar nerves may not be blocked unless the
needle gets beneath the deep forearm fascia, since the wrist crease can act
as a natural barrier to local anesthetic diffusion.

MIDLINE ULNAR FOREARM 10 CM PROXIMAL TO WRIST CREASE

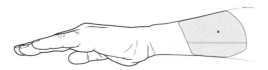

When you inject 20 mL of buffered 1% lidocaine with 1:100,000 epinephrine 10 cm proximal to the wrist crease in the ulnar forearm midline in the red injection point just under the skin without moving the needle, local anesthetic can be seen and palpated to diffuse in the blue area in an unscarred patient.

MIDLINE DORSAL FOREARM 10 CM PROXIMAL TO WRIST CREASE

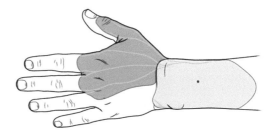

When you inject 20 mL of buffered 1% lidocaine with 1:100,000 epinephrine (at a ratio of 10 mL of lidocaine/epinephrine to 1 mL of 8.4% sodium bicarbonate) 10 cm proximal to the wrist crease in the dorsal forearm midline in the red injection point just under the skin without moving the needle, local anesthetic can be seen and palpated to diffuse in the blue area in an unscarred patient.

ANTERIOR ELBOW

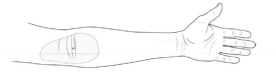

When you inject 20 mL of buffered 1% lidocaine with 1:100,000 epinephrine in the middle of the elbow crease in the red injection point just under the skin without moving the needle, local anesthetic can be seen and palpated to diffuse in the blue area in an unscarred patient.

MEDIAL ELBOW

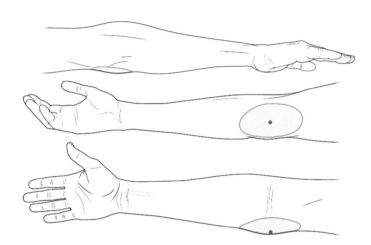

When you inject 20 mL of buffered 1% lidocaine with 1:100,000 epineph-rine in the most medial part of the elbow crease in the red injection point just under the skin without moving the needle, local anesthetic can be seen and palpated to diffuse in the blue area in an unscarred patient.

LATERAL ELBOW

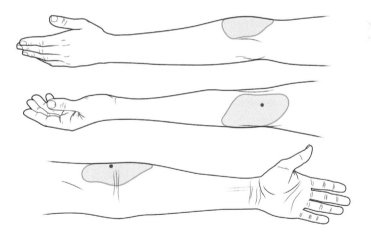

When you inject 20 mL of buffered 1% lidocaine with 1:100,000 epineph-rine in the most lateral part of the elbow crease in the red injection point just under the skin without moving the needle, local anesthetic can be seen and palpated to diffuse in the blue area in an unscarred patient.

References

1. Calder K, Chung B, O'Brien C, Lalonde DH. Bupivacaine digital blocks: how long is the pain relief and temperature elevation? Plast Reconstr Surg 2013;131(5):1098–1104
2. Williams JG, Lalonde DH. Randomized comparison of the single-injection volar subcutaneous block and the two-injection dorsal block for digital anesthesia. Plast Reconstr Surg 2006;118(5):1195–1200
3. Wheelock ME, Leblanc M, Chung B, Williams J, Lalonde DH. Is it true that injecting palmar finger skin hurts more than dorsal skin? New level 1 evidence. Hand (N Y) 2011;6(1):47–49
4. Hamelin ND, St-Amand H, Lalonde DH, Harris PG, Brutus JP. Decreasing the pain of finger block injection: level II evidence. Hand (N Y) 2013;8(1):67–70
5. Thomson CJ, Lalonde DH. Randomized double-blind comparison of duration of anesthesia among three commonly used agents in digital nerve block. Plast Reconstr Surg 2006;118(2):429–432

Section II

CHAPTER 2

ADVANTAGES OF WALANT FOR PATIENTS, SURGEONS, AND ANESTHESIOLOGISTS

Alistair Phillips, Nikolas Alan Jagodzinski, Yin-Ming Huang, and Donald H. Lalonde

WHAT IS WALANT?

- Wide awake hand surgery is well described by its other name, **WALANT, which stands for Wide Awake Local Anesthesia No Tourniquet**.

- The only two medications most patients are given for wide awake hand surgery are tumescent lidocaine for anesthesia and epinephrine for hemostasis.

- Tumescent local anesthesia means large volumes of low concentration lidocaine and epinephrine. We inject enough volume that it is visible and palpable 1 to 2 cm beyond wherever we will insert sharp objects or cause pain by fracture manipulation. This is a form of extravascular Bier block injected only where you need it, but without a painful tourniquet.

- Lidocaine and epinephrine are probably two of the safest and most widely tested injectable drugs that we inject in humans (see Chapter 3 and Chapter 6). American dentists have injected billions of doses of these two medications in their offices since 1950 with no preoperative testing, no monitoring, no intravenous insertion, and very few adverse events.

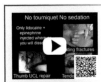

Video 2.1 An introduction to wide awake hand surgery.

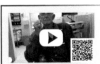

Video 2.2 Safer surgery without sedation in an oxygenated patient who could not sleep before surgery because of carpal tunnel pain. He had surgery sitting up on his oxygen like going to the dentist and then went home. He was able to sleep better for the last 6 months of his life when he died of pulmonary disease.

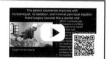

Video 2.3 Patient's perspective of wide awake hand surgery.

- Like dental procedures, we can perform WALANT with no preoperative testing, no insertion of an intravenous line, and no monitoring, because the only medications we inject are very safe doses of lidocaine and epinephrine. After the procedure, the patient simply gets up and goes home.

- There are many advantages of WALANT over the traditional tourniquet and sedation approach.

ADVANTAGES FOR PATIENTS

- Patients who have both hands operated on prefer the WALANT hand experience over the intravenous regional anesthetic tourniquet experience.[1]

- They have no nausea, no vomiting, no urinary retention, or any other unwanted side effects associated with opiates or sedation.

- They spend less time at the hospital for the procedure because postoperative recovery time is just minutes, since they receive no sedation and no opioid medications. They can just get up and go home, as they would do after a visit to the dentist.

- They have no need to have someone stay with them the evening after the surgery. Following outpatient procedures with general anesthesia in many facilities, patients are required to have a responsible adult stay with them for 12 to 24 hours. This is difficult for many patients, especially if they have children.

- Approximately 12% of apparently previously cognitively well patients undergoing anesthesia and noncardiac surgery will develop symptoms of cognitive dysfunction after their procedure.[2] There is no postanesthetic "brain fog" with WALANT because there is no sedation.

- Patients get to know and talk to their surgeon during the surgery for advice on how to care for the hand postoperatively, time off work, and other issues.

- There is no downtime from work or need for a babysitter to go for preoperative testing for sedation on a day before the surgery. Patients do not have to obtain an unnecessary electrocardiogram (ECG) or chest X-rays, attend an anesthesia consultation, or undergo preoperative blood tests.

- Hand surgery under pure local anesthesia is not expensive. Many patients in developing countries could afford hand surgery if they did not have to pay the large costs associated with sedation and general anesthesia in the main operating room.

- In the setting of scarce resources, reduced main operating room requirements often lead to increased operating room access for both surgeon and patient.

- When patients are afraid of needles, there is no unnecessary insertion with a 20-gauge intravenous cannula. All the patient will feel is a single brief prick with a 27- or 30-gauge needle in the hand when we inject the local anesthetic properly (see Chapter 5).

- Patients can see repaired structures working during the surgery after a loss of function such as tendon laceration, tenolysis, tendon transfer, hand fracture, or Dupuytren's contracture. This visual memory helps motivate them throughout postoperative therapy and recovery.

- Patients do not need to endure a tourniquet for even 5 minutes. We tell all our trainees that they need to put a tourniquet on their own arm or forearm for 5 minutes before they ever say, "Patients tolerate it well." The true meaning of this phrase might be, "Patients let me do it without complaining, even though it may hurt a lot."

- The fact that there is no need for a tourniquet is advantageous in patients who have lymphedema or arteriovenous shunts in the forearm.

- Patients do not need to fast or change medication schedules before the procedure, which is particularly helpful for diabetic patients.

- Patients with sore elbows, shoulders, or backs can position themselves comfortably for hand and elbow surgery because there is no tourniquet or anesthesiology equipment preventing them from shifting out of an uncomfortable position. They can easily turn on their side during the procedure.

- Patients do not need to get undressed for surgery when we use field sterility (see Chapter 10).

- WALANT is safer for patients than sedation, especially for individuals with medical comorbidities (▶ Video 2.2). All anesthesiologists agree that less sedation is safer sedation. The safest sedation is no sedation.

- Pressure sores and nerve palsies from incorrect positioning under general anesthesia are avoided.

- Surgeons are less likely to operate on the wrong hand or the wrong finger if the patient is wide awake with no sedation.

- Trauma patients can undergo surgery during the day in minor procedure rooms (see Chapter 10) instead of in the middle of the night in the main operating room. They do not need hospital admission to wait for or recover from sedation. Surgeons and nurses are more likely to be able to perform surgery well when rested during daytime hours than while tired at night.

- There is no need to discontinue anticoagulation medication in most cases because the epinephrine provides enough hemostasis to dry up the wound nicely.[3]

- It is possible to see a patient in consultation and operate on him or her the same day, because there is little to no preoperative workup required for pure local anesthesia. This is much less expensive and more convenient for patients who have to travel long distances to the surgeon's clinic or office.

- One study has shown that it may be safe for patients to drive home after WALANT hand surgery.[4]

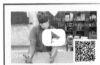

Video 2.4 Surgeon puts a tourniquet on his own arm to see what it feels like.

ADVANTAGES FOR SURGEONS

- We can make adjustments on repaired tendons and finger fractures after seeing active movement in comfortable, cooperative patients and make certain everything is working well before we close the skin. This decreases the rate of rupture and tenolysis after flexor tendon repair (see Chapter 19).

- Patients help to rupture adhesions in tenolysis and remember what they achieve in motion at surgery when they are unsedated.

- We have an easier time setting proper tension on tendon transfers before we close the skin by watching the patient move the transfer to test the tension.

- We see what is happening with active movement during the surgery in complex reconstructive cases to improve results.

- We do not have to look after patients who must be admitted to the hospital after hand surgery because of sedation complications such as nausea and vomiting.

- We can operate on patients with multiple medical problems safely and easily, because we give them no sedation. They walk in, have their hand surgery, and then get up and go home with their medical issues unchanged. The fact that they are morbidly obese, diabetic, or have severe lung disease has no bearing on the hand surgery itself, only on the sedation.

- We do not have to use cautery for most cases because epinephrine hemostasis is very good. We only open cautery as required, not as a routine. The epinephrine and natural clotting typically dry up the field by the time we get to skin closure. This can reduce operative time and the cost of cautery equipment, and possibly even prevent postoperative hematoma.

- There is no need to stop let-down bleeding from a tourniquet, because we do not use one.

- We do not need to stop anticoagulation therapy in many if not most cases, because epinephrine hemostasis is good. This is safer for the patient and decreases the liability for the surgeon.[3]

- We have an easier time in patients with lymphedema, dialysis access, or previous vascular surgery in which a tourniquet might cause problems.

- We get to educate the patient during the surgery for better outcomes and fewer complications. Time spent on intraoperative patient education can also decrease the time spent in the office on patient education (see Chapter 7 and Chapter 8).

- Patient compliance is improved. When you personally tell the patients to keep their hand elevated and immobile at the end of the surgery, they are more likely to comply than if a nurse tells this to them in the recovery room when they are still under the influence of sedation.

- We only need one nurse for most simple hand operations, such as carpal tunnel release. This increases efficiency and productivity and reduces costs (see Chapter 14). We can perform more cases in the same amount of time at less cost. It is never necessary to wait for the slowest member of a big team to finish his or her work so that we can proceed.[5]

- Simple operations such as carpal tunnel and trigger finger can be moved out of the main operating room. We can perform them in the clinic or office with field sterility for greatly improved turnover time and surgeon convenience (see Chapter 10).

- We can perform hand trauma procedures such as tendon repair and finger fracture with K-wiring during the day in minor procedure rooms instead of in the middle of the night in the main operating room.

- We can use lidocaine with epinephrine injection to flood the area, even in sedated or sleeping patients, to decrease bleeding and pain at the end of surgery. Many of us use lidocaine and epinephrine without a tourniquet, even when we have patients under general anesthesia.

- We can wash very dirty hand injuries in the emergency department with tap water after numbing the hand. There is level I evidence that this is as effective as sterile saline.[6]

- Simple wounds and fight bites can be managed in the emergency room (see Chapter 35).

Video 2.5 Washing a contaminated hand in a wide awake patient in the emergency department with tap water.

WHY NO SEDATION?

- There is no need for sedation for many if not most patients: the only two reasons patients needed sedation in the past for hand surgery were: (1) to tolerate the pain of the tourniquet and (2) to tolerate the pain of injection of the local anesthetic. These reasons are no longer valid because the use of epinephrine has removed the need for a tourniquet (see Chapter 3), and local anesthetic can be reliably injected in an almost pain-free manner (see Chapter 5).

- Sedated patients cannot remember intraoperative teaching from their surgeon and will miss this excellent communication opportunity because of the amnestic drugs.

- Some patients become uninhibited and harder to manage with even small amounts of sedation. They can end up requiring general anesthesia, with all its inconveniences.

- Pain-free, unsedated, cooperative patients can move their reconstructed fingers through a full range of motion during the surgery and remember how well the reconstructed hand functions. The surgeon can make changes during the procedure to improve the outcome, and patients are motivated to achieve the same movement they remember seeing on the operating table.

ADVANTAGES FOR ANESTHESIOLOGISTS

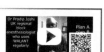

Video 2.6 An upper extremity block specialist anesthesiologist, who uses WALANT routinely, discusses where it fits in his practice.

- Anesthesiologists such as Dr Joshi in ▶ Video 2.6, who use WALANT all the time, clearly understand the advantage and really like the technique.
- WALANT is the safest form of sedation because there is no sedation.
- This is especially helpful in patients with many medical comorbidities to whom sedation adds unnecessary and unwanted risk.
- Avoiding endotracheal intubation also avoids droplet spread of diseases like COVID-19.
- There is no endotracheal intubation with WALANT. Intubation and general anesthesia should be avoided in all COVID-19 patients. Postoperative pulmonary complications associated with a high mortality of 20% occur in asymptomatic COVID-19 patients who undergo surgery with general anesthesia.[7,8]

References

1. Egemen Ayhan and Filiz Akaslan. Patients' perspective on carpal tunnel release with WALANT or intravenous regional anesthesia. Plast Reconstr Surg 2020;145(5):1197–1203
2. Needham MJ, Webb CE, Bryden DC. Postoperative cognitive dysfunction and dementia: what we need to know and do. Br J Anaesth 2017; 119(suppl_1):i115–i125
3. Becuwe L, Sleth JC, Favennec YE, Candelier G. Anestesia Local com o Paciente Totalmente Acordado e Sem Torniquete (WALANT) em fratura exposta de polegar sob terapia antitrombótica: superando um impasse. [Wide-Awake Local Anesthesia and No Tourniquet (WALANT) in open thumb fracture under antithrombotic therapy: overcoming an impasse] (Article in Portuguese). Rev Bras Anestesiol 2019;69(4):425–426
4. Thompson Orfield NJ, Badger AE, Tegge AN, Davoodi M, Perez MA, Apel PJ. Modeled wide-awake, local-anesthetic, no-tourniquet surgical procedures do not impair driving fitness: an experimental on-road noninferiority study. J Bone Joint Surg Am 2020;102(18):1616–1622
5. Warrender WJ, Lucasti CJ, Ilyas AM. Wide-awake hand surgery: principles and techniques. JBJS Rev 2018;6(5):e8
6. Moscati RM, Mayrose J, Reardon RF, Janicke DM, Jehle DV. A multicenter comparison of tap water versus sterile saline for wound irrigation. Acad Emerg Med 2007;14(5):404–409
7. COVIDSurg Collaborative. Mortality and pulmonary complications in patients undergoing surgery with perioperative SARS-CoV-2 infection: an international cohort study. Lancet 2020;396(10243):27–38
8. Lei S, Jiang F, Su W, et al. Clinical characteristics and outcomes of patients undergoing surgeries during the incubation period of COVID-19 infection. EClinicalMedicine 2020;21:100331

CHAPTER 3

SAFE EPINEPHRINE IN THE FINGER MEANS NO TOURNIQUET

Donald H. Lalonde, Robert E. Van Demark, Jr., and Chris Chun-Yu Chen

THE RISE AND FALL OF THE MYTH OF THE DANGER OF INJECTING EPINEPHRINE IN THE FINGER

- In the period before 1950, the belief developed among surgeons that epinephrine causes finger necrosis. This dogma became entrenched in medical school teachings, where we were told that we should not inject epinephrine into "fingers, nose, penis, and toes." Evidence-based medicine has now altered that misconception. This chapter tells the story of how it happened.

- Before we begin the chapter, times are changing. In a recent survey of the American Society for Surgery of the Hand (ASSH) members published in Journal of Hand Surgery Global Online open in June of 2020, only 2% of ASSH members are still worried about epinephrine in the finger[1].

Video 3.1 History of the rise and fall of the epinephrine danger myth (Lalonde, Canada).

THE LONG HISTORY OF SAFE USE OF EPINEPHRINE IN THE FINGER BY CANADIAN SURGEONS

- When the first author was a medical student at Queen's University in Kingston, Ontario, from 1975 to 1979, there was an excellent hand surgeon Dr Pat Shoemaker, who used epinephrine in the finger all the time. He did wide awake flexor tendon repair with field sterility in the emergency department and got good results. Some of his colleagues were skeptical and taught medical students the traditional view that epinephrine in the finger was dangerous and could cause finger necrosis as a result of vasoconstriction. Only Dr Shoemaker was "allowed" to do it because he was a hand surgeon who did not any have trouble "yet"! He never did get into trouble. He has long since retired and passed away.

Video 3.2 How ro reverse epinephrine vasoconstriction with phentolamine injection in the finger (Lalonde, Canada).

Video 3.3 How to reverse finger epinephrine vasoconstriction after accidental intrasheath injection if you got a white finger for trigger finger surgery (Lalonde, Canada).

- Dr Bob MacFarlane of London, Ontario, former president of the ASSH, became famous for his Dupuytren's research. He regularly performed wide awake Dupuytren's surgery with lidocaine and epinephrine hemostasis.

- Dr John Fielding, the first plastic surgeon in Ottawa, pioneered use of wide awake hand surgery with epinephrine hemostasis in that city. Many Ottawa surgeons followed his lead and used the technique routinely long before the first author did.

- Many other Canadian hand surgeons in other cities adopted the same technique.

SIX THINGS STIMULATED MY INTEREST FOR BEGINNING ROUTINE ELECTIVE EPINEPHRINE HEMOSTASIS USE IN THE FINGER FOR EVERY CASE IN 2001

- The first author knew of well over 100 surgeon-years of clinical safety in the practices of Drs Shoemaker, MacFarlane, Fielding, and others who routinely injected epinephrine in fingers. They were good surgeons. He trusted and respected their clinical judgment.

- He knew he could use phentolamine as an epinephrine vasoconstriction rescue agent if he needed it.

- He had been using epinephrine for carpal tunnel, flexor sheath ganglion, and trigger finger procedures for many years with no problems.

- He had used epinephrine in the finger many times before 2001, but not routinely, and he had not encountered any problems.

- We had great difficulty getting the main operating room for our hand trauma cases because of a chronic shortage of anesthesiologists at Saint John. Epinephrine hemostasis meant no tourniquet was required. It also meant we could operate on a patient with a traumatic hand injury outside the main operating room at our convenience, Monday through Friday, 9 AM to 5 PM, without having to admit patients or wait for an anesthesiologist.

- Dr Keith Denkler published his landmark paper in 2001.[1] Dr Denkler painstakingly reviewed 120 years of literature from 1880 to 2000, most of it by hand through *Index Medicus* volumes, and *did not find one case* of lidocaine with epinephrine finger necrosis in the world literature. This was my tipping point. After reading his paper, the first author decided to use epinephrine in every finger with good capillary refill on fingertip pulp palpation until he needed phentolamine rescue. He still has not needed it in 2020, but he has used it several times with accidental high-dose (1:1,000) epinephrine injections, and occasionally to shorten the time of ischemia.

FOUR MAIN CONCEPTS THAT SUPPORT THE FALL OF THE MYTH

- We can reliably reverse epinephrine vasoconstriction with phentolamine in the human finger.[2]

- There were no lost fingers and not one case required phentolamine rescue in a prospective study of 3,110 consecutive cases of elective epinephrine injection in the finger and hand by nine surgeons in six cities, called the *Dalhousie Project clinical phase*.[3] A similar study of over 1,111 fingers injected with epinephrine in 2010 by another group of surgeons yielded similar results.[4] A recent study of 400 infants,[5] and another study of over 12,000 patients in China, also showed no finger loss.[6]

- More than 100 cases of high-dose 1:1000 epinephrine[7,8] revealed that not one finger injected with a dosage 100 times the concentration of epinephrine that we use clinically actually died. If 1:1000 epinephrine does not cause finger loss, it is highly unlikely that 1:100,000 will ever cause a finger loss.

- The source of the epinephrine myth, created between 1920 and 1945, stemmed from the use of procaine (Novocaine).[8] It was the "new caine," invented in 1903 to add the existing cocaine. It was the only safely injectable local anesthetic until the introduction of lidocaine in 1948. More fingers died from procaine injection alone than from procaine plus epinephrine injection. Procaine starts with a pH of 3.6 and becomes more acidic as it sits on the shelf.[9] The U.S. Food and Drug Administration (FDA) instituted mandatory expiration dates on injectable medicines in 1979.[10] The "smoking gun" paper that established that procaine was the actual cause of finger deaths that had been blamed on epinephrine was a 1948 FDA warning published in the *Journal of the American Medical Association* that found batches of procaine with a pH of 1 destined for injection into humans![11]

WE PROVED THAT WE CAN RELIABLY REVERSE EPINEPHRINE VASOCONSTRICTION IN THE HUMAN FINGER; THE DALHOUSIE PROJECT

- We needed to prove that phentolamine did in fact reliably reverse epinephrine vasoconstriction in the human finger.[12]

- In 2002, in Halifax, we performed a prospective, randomized, double-blind controlled trial called the *Dalhousie Project*. In the *level I evidence experimental phase,* we injected both hands of 18 Dalhousie University alumnus hand surgeons (including me) who volunteered to have both their ring fingers injected in three sites with 1.8 mL of 2% lidocaine with epinephrine 1:100,000.[2] One hour later, we injected each of the three sites of one hand with 1 mg (1 mL) of phentolamine, and the three sites on the other hand were injected with 1 mL of saline solution. In the figure you can see the "phentolamine blush," where redness is returning around the three phentolamine injection sites one hour after we injected phentolamine in the left hand. The conclusion was that it took an average of 85 minutes for epinephrine-injected fingers to return to normal color after phentolamine injection, whereas it took an average of 320 minutes for epinephrine-injected fingers to return to normal color after injection of saline solution (no phentolamine).

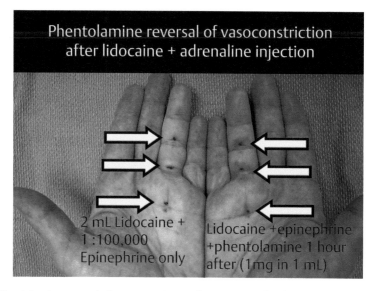

Fig. 3.1 Phentolamine reversal of vasoconstriction after injection of 2% lidocaine with epinephrine 1:100,000. In the left hand, the arrows indicate that 2 mL of lidocaine and epinephrine only were injected. In the right hand, the arrows indicate lidocaine and epinephrine were injected, and 1 hour later phentolamine was injected (1 mg in 1 mL).

MANAGING THE WHITE FINGERTIP WITH PHENTOLAMINE

- Most white fingertips will resolve without any treatment. However, to be on the safe side, you can reverse the white fingertip by injecting phentolamine wherever you have injected epinephrine before the patient leaves your facility.

- To reverse adrenaline vasoconstriction in the finger, inject 1 to 2 mg of phentolamine in 1 mL or more of saline solution into the subcutaneous fat wherever there is severe epinephrine pallor in the skin. This small extravascular dose will not affect blood pressure. The finger will pink up within an hour or two.

- When you inject lidocaine with 1:100,000 epinephrine in the proximal or middle phalanx subcutaneous fat, those areas will go white, but the fingertip or thumb tip will usually remain pink.

- If you inject the local anesthetic into the sheath instead of the subcutaneous fat, it diffuses to the distal phalanx, where it has a greater chance of making the fingertip white. Injection into the sheath for trigger finger causes a white fingertip; injection into the fat does not cause a white fingertip.

- Local anesthetic injected into the sheath hurts more than local anesthetic injected into the subcutaneous fat (see ▶ Video 17.4).

- There is a case of phentolamine reversal of duskiness in a finger the morning after lidocaine and epinephrine injection.[15] ▶ Video 3.4 shows another case by Robert E. Van Demark, Jr.

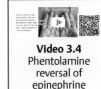

Video 3.4
Phentolamine reversal of epinephrine vasoconstriction the morning after epinephrine injection (Van Demark, Jr., USA).

- The first author has injected many thousands of fingers with epinephrine. He has not needed phentolamine rescue once. Many thousands of patients in China[6] and the rest of the world have also been safely injected with the same observation. Also, he has been treating patients with morphine for over 30 years and have not had to rescue one with naloxone. That does not mean he will not in the future, and he knows how to use it if he needs it.

- He has demonstrated phentolamine rescue to many visiting surgeons. He recommends that all hand surgeons try it at least once. This will help them and their nursing colleagues allay their epinephrine fear.

- What is phentolamine? Phentolamine is an alpha-adrenergic blocking agent introduced in 1957 as an antihypertensive agent in pheochromocytoma management. Phentolamine (Rogitine®) is the rescue agent for epinephrine vasoconstriction in the human finger.

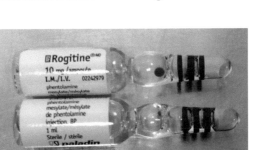

Fig. 3.2 Phentolamine (Rogitine) is the rescue agent for epinephrine vasoconstriction in the human finger.

- Phentolamine manufacturers recommend a dosage of phentolamine of 5 mg intravenously to lower blood pressure.[12]

- Phentolamine is also available in many countries as Trimix®, which is an injectable, three-drug, prescribed medication used to treat erectile dysfunction. The active ingredients in the mixture are usually alprostadil, papaverine, and phentolamine. We are aware of successful reversal of epinephrine vasoconstriction in the finger with Trimix.

- Phentolamine is also available in Europe and North America for dental use as Oraverse®. It is pure phentolamine 0.45 mg in a 1.8-mL dental cartridge. It reliably reversed phentolamine vasoconstriction in Dr Lalonde's fingers shown in ▶ Fig. 3.2.

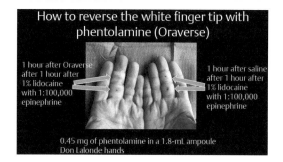

Fig. 3.3 Oraverse reversed epinephrine vasoconstriction in 1 hour in Dr Donald Lalonde's fingers.

- Terbutaline (selective b2-receptor agonist smooth muscle relaxant) was not effective in reversing epinephrine vasoconstriction in Don Lalonde's fingers. In 2017, he had a surgeon inject lidocaine with 1:100,000 epinephrine in both ring fingers. One hour later, 0.25 mg of terbutaline was injected in one of them and saline injected in the other finger at the same sites. He was unable to tell as to which finger got what, as was a third observing surgeon. Only the injecting surgeon knew which finger got the terbutaline. Not one of the three surgeons could see a difference between terbutaline and saline fingers (see ▶ Fig. 3.4). The return to pink time was the same in the terbutaline- and saline-injected fingers.

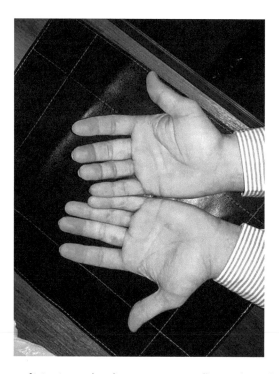

Fig. 3.4 After 1 to 4 hours of injection, terbutaline was not more effective than saline in Dr Lalonde's long fingers to reverse epinephrine vasoconstriction.

CONTRAINDICATIONS TO EPINEPHRINE IN THE FINGER

- In general, if there is good capillary refill when the fingertip is compressed and released before epinephrine injection into the finger, there will be good capillary refill after epinephrine injection unless the finger is devascularized with surgical dissection or manipulation.

- There were only five cases of finger loss implicating epinephrine in the literature[16,17,18,19,20] until the sixth unpublished one showed up in 2019 (shown in ▶ Video 3.5). In the first five cases, none of them convincingly proved that epinephrine was in fact at fault. Most importantly, none of them used phentolamine rescue. Three of the five cases were far from proving that epinephrine caused finger loss[16,18,19] and two other cases had blisters, which may have been from hot water burns.[17,20] Denkler reported 14 cases[1] of burned patients who attempted to "get their feeling back" by submersing their fingers in excessively hot water. This is the most common true cause of fingertip loss after local anesthesia.

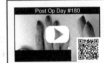

Video 3.5 Loss of hemi-fingertip in a Raynaud's patient in spite of phentolamine rescue (Lalonde, Canada).

- The sixth case shown in ▶ Video 3.5 shows that Raynaud's patients can run into problems. In spite of the fact that Dr Lalonde has injected in the fingers of more than five Raynaud's patients with no problems as shown in ▶ Fig. 3.5, ▶ Video 3.5 shows a patient who lost a hemi-fingertip after a trigger finger was injected in the fat in spite of phentolamine rescue 5 hours after surgery. This is the only case that we are aware of where phentolamine rescue has not been successful in the human finger.

- The case in ▶ Video 3.5 is extremely rare but demonstrates that patients who have hypoperfused digits may be at risk in spite of phentolamine rescue.

- Dr Lalonde's experience with Raynaud's patients is more like the one shown in ▶ Fig. 3.5.

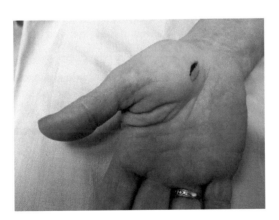

Fig. 3.5 Injection in the subcutaneous fat at the base of the thumb to remove a benign mass in this patient with Raynaud's phenomenon caused distal hyperemia with a full, red, hot thumb tip while the ulnar fingers remained colder and bluish. The epinephrine only causes vasoconstriction where it is located and functioning in the tissue. The distal nerve block lidocaine sympathectomy can temporarily improve flow in the distal finger beyond the location of the epinephrine.

- Venous compromise with WALANT distal radius fracture plate fixation has been reported as well.[21] The hand can turn blue after injection of tumescent local anesthesia, with venous compromise. However, it recovers as the tumescent local anesthesia liquid comes out and gets absorbed with the surgery.

TREATMENT OF ACCIDENTAL INJECTION OF HIGH-DOSE (1:1000) EPINEPHRINE IN THE FINGER

- Accidental injection of high-dose epinephrine occurs when people try to self-administer EpiPen or Ana-Kit injections to treat anaphylaxis in situations such as bee stings. Even though most of these individuals did not receive phentolamine rescue, in the hundreds of cases in the literature, there has been no reported finger loss.[22]

- You should treat these cases with phentolamine[1] to prevent ischemic axonotmesis and ischemic reperfusion pain, which can both occur when it takes 14 hours for a finger to pink up.[7] The dosage to reverse epinephrine vasoconstriction in the finger is to inject 1 to 2 mg of phentolamine in 1 mL or more of saline solution into the subcutaneous fat where the high-dose epinephrine was injected.

References

1. Grandizio Louis C, Graham Jove, Klena Joel C. Current trends in WALANT surgery: a surgery of American Society for Surgery of the Hand Members. Original Research 2020;2(4):186-190
2. Denkler K. A comprehensive review of epinephrine in the finger: to do or not to do. Plast Reconstr Surg 2001;108(1):114–124
3. Nodwell T, Lalonde D. How long does it take phentolamine to reverse adrenaline-induced vasoconstriction in the finger and hand? A prospective, randomized, blinded study: the Dalhousie Project experimental phase. Can J Plast Surg 2003;11(4):187–190
4. Lalonde D, Bell M, Benoit P, Sparkes G, Denkler K, Chang P. A multicenter prospective study of 3,110 consecutive cases of elective epinephrine use in the fingers and hand: the Dalhousie Project clinical phase. J Hand Surg Am 2005;30(5):1061–1067
5. Chowdhry S, Seidenstricker L, Cooney DS, Hazani R, Wilhelmi BJ. Do not use epinephrine in digital blocks: myth or truth? Part II. A retrospective review of 1111 cases. Plast Reconstr Surg 2010;126(6):2031–2034
6. Mantilla-Rivas E, Tan P, Zajac J, Tilt A, Rogers GF, Oh AK. Is epinephrine safe for infant digit excision? A retrospective review of 402 polydactyly excisions in patients younger than 6 months. Plast Reconstr Surg 2019;144(1):149–154
7. Tang JB, Gong KT, Xing SG, Yi L, Xu JH. Wide-awake hand surgery in two centers in China: experience in Nantong and Tianjin with 12,000 patients. Hand Clin 2019;35(1):7–12
8. Fitzcharles-Bowe C, Denkler K, Lalonde D. Finger injection with high-dose (1:1,000) epinephrine: does it cause finger necrosis and should it be treated? Hand (N Y) 2007;2(1):5–11

9. Thomson CJ, Lalonde DH, Denkler KA, Feicht AJ. A critical look at the evidence for and against elective epinephrine use in the finger. Plast Reconstr Surg 2007;119(1):260–266

10. Uri J, Adler P. The disintegration of procaine solutions. Curr Res Anest Anal 1950;29(4):229–234

11. Health Sciences Institute drug expiration dates. http://hsionline.com/2004/08/26/drug-expiration-dates-2/

12. Food and Drug Administration. Warning—procaine solution. JAMA 1948;138:599

13. Phentolamine description. https://www.drugs.com/pro/phentolamine.html

14. Ruiter T, Harter T, Miladore N, Neafus A, Kasdan M. Finger amputation after injection with lidocaine and epinephrine. Eplasty 2014;14:ic43

15. Muck AE, Bebarta VS, Borys DJ, Morgan DL. Six years of epinephrine digital injections: absence of significant local or systemic effects. Ann Emerg Med 2010;56(3):270–274

16. Zhu AF, Hood BR, Morris MS, Ozer K. Delayed-onset digital ischemia after local anesthetic with epinephrine injection requiring phentolamine reversal. J Hand Surg Am 2017;42(6):479.e1–479.e4

17. Ravindran V, Rajendran S. Digital gangrene in a patient with primary Raynaud's phenomenon. J R Coll Physicians Edinb 2012;42(1):24–26

18. Hutting K, van Rappard JR, Prins A, Knepper AB, Mouës-Vink C. [Digital necrosis after local anaesthesia with epinephrine]. Ned Tijdschr Geneeskd 2015;159:A9477

19. Ruiter T, Harter T, Miladore N, et al. Finger amputation after injection with lidocaine and epinephrine. Interesting Case, 3 November 2014, 3; 14: ic43. www.ePlasty.com

20. Sama CB. Post-traumatic digital gangrene associated with epinephrine use in primary Raynaud's phenomenon: lesson for the future. Ethiop J Health Sci 2016;26(4):401–404

21. Zhang JX, Gray J, Lalonde DH, Carr N. Digital necrosis after lidocaine and epinephrine injection in the flexor tendon sheath without phentolamine rescue. J Hand Surg Am 2017;42(2):e119–e123

22. Liu WC, Fu YC, Lu CK. Vascular compromise during wide-awake local anaesthesia no tourniquet technique for distal radial plating: a case report. J Hand Surg Eur Vol 2019;44(9):980–983

23. Lalonde D, Martin A. Epinephrine in local anesthesia in finger and hand surgery: the case for wide-awake anesthesia. J Am Acad Orthop Surg 2013;21(8):443–447

CHAPTER 4

ON USING TUMESCENT LOCAL ANESTHESIA

Donald H. Lalonde, Amir Adham Ahmad, and Alistair Phillips

WHAT IS TUMESCENT LOCAL ANESTHESIA?

- Wide awake hand surgery is all about injecting tumescent local anesthesia without a tourniquet and without sedation.

- Tumescing means injecting a large enough volume of lidocaine with epinephrine so that you can see it plump up the skin and feel it with your finger through the skin wherever you are going to cut, insert K-wires, or manipulate broken bones.

- Tumescent local anesthesia is like an extravascular Bier block, but the anesthetic is injected only where you need it. This technique avoids the risk associated with intravascular injection and the pain of a tourniquet.

WHY DO PATIENTS NOT NEED SEDATION FOR TUMESCENT LOCAL ANESTHESIA INJECTION?

- Because it does not hurt if injected properly (see Chapter 5).

- You can inject large areas such as the whole forearm and wrist with tumescent anesthetic in such a way that the patient barely feels the first sting of 27- or 30-gauge (0.3 or 0.4 mm) needles if you follow the simple guidelines presented in Chapter 5 on how to inject local anesthesia with minimal pain. Patients are amazed and delighted that the injection discomfort is minimal.

WHY IS TUMESCENT LOCAL ANESTHESIA SO EFFECTIVE?

- The smaller the nerve, the faster and more complete it gets numb when bathed with local anesthesia. Tumescent local anesthesia is extremely effective because it numbs all the small nerves completely by 30 minutes when epinephrine vasoconstriction has begun to plateau at peak efficiency in vasoconstriction.

- The larger the nerve, the longer it takes for anesthesia to peak. Median nerve numbness without ultrasound guidance continues to increase for 100 minutes after injection of tumescent local anesthetic around the nerve.[1] It is far more effective and faster to inject the median nerve at the common digital nerve trunk level just distal to the transverse carpal ligament (▶ Fig. 5.9 and ▶ Video 35.3).

- Although larger nerves can be blocked as part of tumescence, tumescent anesthesia is mainly small nerve block anesthesia. All of the nerves in the surgical area are bathed with local anesthesia, both large and small nerves. It is the small nerve effect from having local anesthesia everywhere that is faster and more effective than the large nerve blocks.

INJECT YOUR PATIENTS LYING DOWN IF POSSIBLE

- Fainting or vasovagal attacks are common when people see or get needles. It happens because there is not enough blood going to the brain. The brain reacts by bringing itself down to the lying position to improve brain blood flow. Fainting is less likely to happen if you inject patients lying down (see ▶ Video 6.1 on how to manage fainting).

- We often inject patients on a stretcher outside the procedure room if it is occupied.

- We often have the patients get up and sit with their partners after the injection if there are no fainting issues and the patient feels well. This gives the local anesthesia time to work.

IT IS BETTER TO INJECT LOCAL ANESTHESIA AT LEAST 30 MINUTES BEFORE SURGERY

- It is ideal to give the local anesthetic 30 minutes or more to work. It takes an average of 26 minutes for maximal cutaneous vasoconstriction to occur with 1:100,000 epinephrine.[2] It takes a similar amount of time for maximal numbness to occur with lidocaine. If you inject the patient in the recovery room or on a stretcher outside the operating room, the anesthetic will have time to work by the time you prep and drape the patient on the operating table.

- For short procedures, inject the first three patients and do the paperwork before you operate on the first patient. After you operate on the first one, inject the fourth patient while the nurse brings the second injected patient into the room (see Chapter 14 on how to schedule 15 or more cases in one day with one nurse).

- Decreased concentrations of epinephrine do not provide as intense a vasoconstriction, but they work very well. Dr Prasetyono has repeatedly shown that 1:1,000,000 epinephrine is very effective.[3]

- If your situation does not permit half an hour for the tumescent anesthetic to take effect, hemostasis is usually reasonable at 15 minutes after injection. The site will bleed a little more, but visibility will be acceptable.

NEVER ELICIT LARGE NERVE PARESTHESIAS WITH YOUR NEEDLE

- Causing paresthesia during injection of local anesthesia may mean that you may have lacerated nerve fascicles, and that is not a good thing. A 25-gauge needle is the width of a human fascicle. Try to get near the nerve and inject a large volume to make certain you surround the nerve with local anesthetic.
- Unless you are using ultrasound, it is better to keep the sharp needle tips 5 to 10 mm away from large nerves. If you inject tumescent local anesthetic near any nerve, it will numb if given enough time.

TUMESCENT LOCAL ANESTHESIA DOES NOT IMPAIR VISIBILITY

- Tumescent local anesthesia is as clear as water.
- In fact, tumescent local anesthetic hydrodissects the tissue planes for the surgeon and facilitates the dissection.
- A general rough guide for how much volume you will need is that each 20 mL of local anesthesia will cover an area of 10 × 10 cm (see atlas in Chapter 1).
- You can also inject large areas with tumescent local anesthetic much more quickly with less bruising and minimal pain by using blunt-tipped cannula needles (see more on cannula injection in ▶ Fig. 5.8 of Chapter 5).
- The use of tumescent local anesthetic injection with no tourniquet also helps you significantly in patients who are also having general anesthesia. Inject the tumescent solution as soon as the patient is asleep. It will decrease the bleeding, reduce the narcotic requirements administered by the anesthesiologist, and avoid having to deal with let-down bleeding that would occur when you release a tourniquet. You can then go scrub, prep, and drape the patient, and complete other tasks while the epinephrine takes effect.

SAFE DOSAGE OF LIDOCAINE WITH EPINEPHRINE

- The widely quoted maximal dose of lidocaine with epinephrine is 7 mg/kg. This is actually extremely safe. This number originated before 1950, at the dawn of lidocaine use. Since then, Vasconez and others have reported safe blood levels of lidocaine when they injected 35 mg/kg for liposuction.[4,5,6,7] We also know that 20 mg/kg produces safe blood levels of lidocaine when injected into the highly vascularized facial fat in facelift surgery.[8]

- Because we do not monitor most of our patients (see Chapter 6), we stay within the extremely safe dose of 7 mg/kg, which is all we need to perform most hand operations. In a 70 kg adult, this means the following:

$$7 \text{ mg/kg} \times 70 \text{ kg} = 490 \text{ mg or } 49 \text{ mL of 1\% lidocaine}$$

$$\text{with } 1{:}100{,}000 \text{ epinephrine}$$

- We, therefore, stick with 50 mL or 1% lidocaine with 1:100,000 epinephrine for all our surgeries and add saline when we need more volume.

Table 4.1 Safe dosage for an average adult	
Volume needed (mL) to stay with extremely safe dose of 7 mg/kg lidocaine	
<50	We use commercially available 1% lidocaine with 1:100,000 epinephrine (always buffered with 10 mL local anesthetic to 1 mL of 8.4% sodium bicarbonate to decrease the pain of injection).[4,9]
50–100	We dilute buffered 50 mL of commercially available 1% lidocaine with 1:100,000 epinephrine with 50 mL of saline solution to produce 100 mL of 0.5% lidocaine with 1:200,000 epinephrine.
100–200	We dilute buffered 50 mL of commercially available 1% lidocaine with 1:100,000 epinephrine with 150 mL of saline solution to produce 200 mL of 0.25% lidocaine with 1:400,000 epinephrine, which is clinically very effective both for local anesthesia and for vasoconstriction. The lower concentration just takes longer to work and does not last as long.

WHAT VOLUME AND CONCENTRATION OF LIDOCAINE/EPINEPHRINE SHOULD I INJECT?

- In the average adult:
  - **If we need less than 50 mL of volume**, we use 1% lidocaine with 1:100,000 epinephrine (always buffered with 10 mL local anesthetic added to 1 mL of 8.4% sodium bicarbonate to decrease the pain of injection).[9]
  - **If we need 50 to 100 mL of volume**, we dilute buffered 50 mL of 1% lidocaine with 1:100,000 epinephrine with 50 mL of saline solution to get 100 mL of 0.5% lidocaine with 1:200,000 epinephrine. *(Tip: 50 mL of local anesthetic will fit into a 50-mL bag of saline for a total of 100 mL.)*

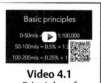

Video 4.1
Principles of tumescent local anesthesia.

  - **If we need 100 to 200 mL of volume**, we dilute buffered 50 mL of 1% lidocaine with 1:100,000 epinephrine with 150 mL of saline solution to get 200 mL of 0.25% lidocaine with 1:400,000 epinephrine, which is clinically very effective both for local anesthesia and for vasoconstriction. The lower concentration just takes longer to work and does not last as long. *(Tip: 100 mL of local anesthetic will fit into a 100-mL bag of saline for a total of 200 mL.)*

- You can mix lidocaine and epinephrine with saline solution in the small 50- or 100-mL bags that saline comes in. If you remove 10 mL of saline from a 50-mL bag and then add 40 mL of 1% lidocaine with 1:100,000 epinephrine, you now have 80 mL of 0.5% lidocaine with 1:200,000 epinephrine.

HOW LONG WILL TUMESCENT LOCAL ANESTHESIA LAST?

- You can finish most hand operations in the anesthesia time provided by lidocaine with epinephrine (5 hours in the wrist,[10] 10 hours in the finger[11]). We only use bupivacaine in operations that may last more than 3 hours. We add 10 mL of 0.5% bupivacaine with 1:200,000 epinephrine to the total injection mixture in these cases.

WHY NOT USE LONG-ACTING LOCAL ANESTHETICS LIKE BUPIVACAINE ALL THE TIME?

- Lidocaine with epinephrine lasts long enough to do most hand operations. As digital blocks, plain 1% lidocaine lasts 5 hours, 1% lidocaine with 1:100,000 epinephrine lasts 10 hours, the ***pain*** *relief part* of plain bupivacaine 0.5% lasts 15 hours, and adding 1:200,000 epinephrine to bupivacaine 0.5% only gives one extra hour of pain relief.[11,12]

- Lidocaine is like an on/off light switch where pain, touch, and pressure all come back at the same time. With bupivacaine, touch and pressure return at 30 hours whereas pain comes back at 15 hours![12] This is why patients come back to the emergency department the night after bupivacaine anesthesia to complain: "Doctor, my finger is still numb but it hurts!" They are not wrong, but the surgeon did not warn them about the annoying touch and pressure numbness that can last up to 2 days after bupivacaine injection.

- Bupivacaine and ropivacaine are cardiotoxic,[13] whereas lidocaine is injected as a 100-mg intravenous bolus to decrease pain in multiple trauma patients.[14,15]

- We did not spend 2 billion years evolving pain because it is bad for us. After an injury or an operation, it is our body's only way to tell us: "Hey would you quit that? I am trying to help you heal and you are screwing it up!!!" That is a little voice in the head that we should listen to after surgery. We can't hear the little voice with pain killers or local anesthetics silencing it. Patients who can feel a little pain 5 hours after surgery are more likely to keep their hand elevated and immobile to decrease bleeding that causes additional collagen deposition in the wound. We call it pain-guided healing.

THE GREATER THE CONCENTRATION OF EPINEPHRINE, THE LONGER AND MORE INTENSE THE VASOCONSTRICTION

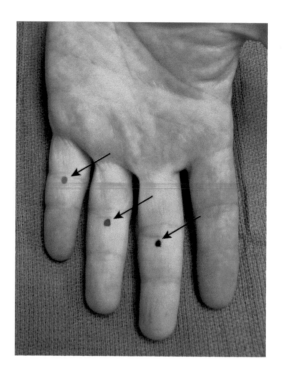

Fig. 4.1 Different concentrations of epinephrine last for different lengths of time. Dr Lalonde had three fingers simultaneously injected with 0.5 mL of different concentrations of epinephrine in three fingers.[1,16] The small finger (injected with epinephrine 1:100,000) pinked up completely after 6 hours. It took 10 hours for vasoconstriction to reverse in the ring finger after injection of 1:10,000 epinephrine. The long finger took 14 hours for the pink color to completely return after injection of 1:1000 epinephrine.

- Some surgeons use 1:1,000,000 epinephrine for WALANT[17] with good clinical results, but the epinephrine may not last as long as the 1:100,000 or 1:200,000, which most surgeons use.

- The designation 1:100,000 epinephrine means 1 g (1,000 mg or 1,000,000 µg) of epinephrine in 100,000 mL of saline solution, or 0.1 mg/10 mL, or 10 µg/mL.

- The designation 1:200,000 epinephrine means 1 g (1,000 mg or 1,000,000 µg) of epinephrine in 200,000 mL of saline solution, or 5 µg/mL.

DIFFERENT CONCENTRATIONS OF EPINEPHRINE PREMIXED WITH LIDOCAINE IN DIFFERENT COUNTRIES

- In Canada and the United States, the anesthetic comes premixed as 1% lidocaine with 1:100,000 epinephrine.

- At the time of writing, 1% lidocaine with 1:200,000 epinephrine is available as a premixed solution with lidocaine in many European countries, and this works very well for those surgeons. In Israel, premixed lidocaine with epinephrine is not available, and surgeons have to mix on their own. In Hong Kong and Brazil, premixed 2% lidocaine with 1:200,000 epinephrine is used. Egypt has premixed 2% lidocaine with 1:100,000 of epinephrine. Indonesia has 2% lidocaine with 1:80,000 epinephrine. Clearly, published evidence is not yet guiding the worldwide availability of a single optimal combination.

- You can mix lidocaine and epinephrine with saline solution in the small 50- or 100-mL bags that saline comes in. If you remove 10 mL of saline from a 50-mL bag and then add 40 mL of 1% lidocaine with 1:100,000 epinephrine, you now have 80 mL of 0.5% lidocaine with 1:200,000 epinephrine.

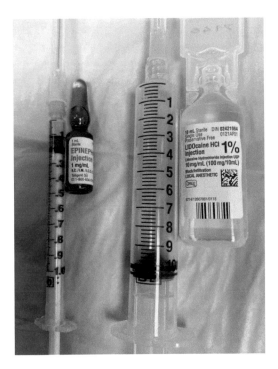

Fig. 4.2 You can take 0.1 mL (0.1 mg) of a 1 mL vial of 1:1,000 epinephrine (1 mg/mL) with an insulin syringe as seen in the figure and inject that into 10 mL of 1% lidocaine plain. You now have 10.1 mL of 1% lidocaine with 1:100,000 epinephrine.

- Another method (as recommended by Marco Felipe F.H. de Barros of Brazil) is to take one bottle of 20 mL of 2% plain lidocaine, add 0.4 mL of epinephrine 1:1,000 (1 mg/mL), which produces 2% lidocaine with 1:50,000 epinephrine. You can mix 20 mL of this 2% lidocaine with 1:50,000 epinephrine with an equal volume of 20 mL of saline solution to produce 40 mL of 1% lidocaine with 1:100,000 epinephrine.

- 50 mL of 1% lidocaine with 1:100,000 epinephrine contains 0.5 mL of 1:1,000 epinephrine seen in the bottle in ▶ Fig. 4.2.

SCARS, CREASES, AND PALMAR/DORSAL BORDERS: THREE NATURAL BARRIERS TO DIFFUSION OF TUMESCENT LOCAL ANESTHESIA

- Local anesthetic does not diffuse well across scars. You will most often need to inject local anesthetic on both sides of a linear scar, starting in unscarred healthy subcutaneous fat. For widely scarred areas, try to start proximal to distal injecting in healthy subcutaneous tissue all around the scarred area, and then finishing under the scar if necessary.

- All skin creases in the hand and wrist, such as the crease between the fingers and palm, have ligaments that bind the skin to deeper structures, such as the flexor sheath. These can slow the diffusion of tumescent local anesthetic to the other side of the crease. Local anesthetic will cross below a skin crease, but only slowly and if under pressure with large volumes. It is wisest to inject on both sides of creases, starting from proximal to distal, to decrease the pain of injection.

- Where palmar glabrous skin meets dorsal nonglabrous skin, there are cutaneous ligaments that act as a third barrier to diffusion of local anesthesia. This zone is also a natural embryologic "largely nerve-free territory" fusion line between the palm and dorsum of the hand, where the dorsal sensory system meets the palmar sensory system. Local anesthesia sometimes has difficulty diffusing across the fusion line because of the ligaments, and you might have to insert the needle both dorsally and volarly.

PERIOSTEAL INJECTION FOR PLATING LONG BONES SUCH AS THE RADIUS, ULNA, CLAVICLE, TIBIA, AND FIBULA

- See ▶ Fig. 44.4 and ▶ Fig. 44.5 for how to bathe the periosteum from proximal to distal when needing to plate long bone fractures.

- In the wrist and hand, the bones are so superficial that the periosteum gets bathed by subcutaneous tumescent fluid. In bigger long bones, tumescent bathing at the periosteal level is required to eliminate the pain and bleeding when plating fractures.

INFECTED HANDS

- In infected hands (see Chapter 35 for fight bite and flexor synovitis management), injecting directly into inflamed tissues does not work very well because: (1) it is painful, (2) the swollen tissues do not easily accept the extra local anesthetic volume, and (3) the hyperemia washes out lidocaine quickly, even with epinephrine.

- Instead of injecting into the infected area, inject tumescent local anesthetic first proximally and then around the affected site, and accept the fact that a little more bleeding will occur.

- In the clinic or emergency department in countries that regulate water cleanliness, you can wash a numbed infected draining hand in the sink, where a faucet delivers large volumes of clean water to wash out the pus from the wound (see ▶ Video 2.5). This also avoids contaminating clean main operating room theaters with pus.

References

1. Lovely LM, Chishti YZ, Woodland JL, Lalonde DH. How much volume of local anesthesia and how long should you wait after injection for an effective wrist median nerve block? Hand (N Y) 2018;13(3):281–284
2. McKee DE, Lalonde DH, Thoma A, Glennie DL, Hayward JE. Optimal time delay between epinephrine injection and incision to minimize bleeding. Plast Reconstr Surg 2013;131(4):811–814
3. Prasetyono TOH, Kusumastuti N. Optimal time delay of epinephrine in one-per-mil solution to visualize operation field. J Surg Res 2019;236:166–171
4. Burk RW III, Guzman-Stein G, Vasconez LO. Lidocaine and epinephrine levels in tumescent technique liposuction. Plast Reconstr Surg 1996;97(7):1379–1384
5. Nordström H, Stånge K. Plasma lidocaine levels and risks after liposuction with tumescent anaesthesia. Acta Anaesthesiol Scand 2005;49(10):1487–1490
6. Klein JA, Jeske DR. Estimated maximal safe dosages of tumescent lidocaine. Anesth Analg 2016;122(5):1350–1359
7. Klein JA. Tumescent technique for regional anesthesia permits lidocaine doses of 35 mg/kg for liposuction. J Dermatol Surg Oncol 1990;16(3):248–263
8. Ramon Y, Barak Y, Ullmann Y, Hoffer E, Yarhi D, Bentur Y. Pharmacokinetics of high-dose diluted lidocaine in local anesthesia for facelift procedures. Ther Drug Monit 2007;29(5):644–647
9. Frank SG, Lalonde DH. How acidic is the lidocaine we are injecting, and how much bicarbonate should we add? Can J Plast Surg 2012;20(2):71–73
10. Chandran GJ, Chung B, Lalonde J, Lalonde DH. The hyperthermic effect of a distal volar forearm nerve block: a possible treatment of acute digital frostbite injuries? Plast Reconstr Surg 2010;126(3):946–950
11. Thomson CJ, Lalonde DH. Randomized double-blind comparison of duration of anesthesia among three commonly used agents in digital nerve block. Plast Reconstr Surg 2006;118(2):429–432
12. Calder K, Chung B, O'Brien C, Lalonde DH. Bupivacaine digital blocks: how long is the pain relief and temperature elevation? Plast Reconstr Surg 2013;131(5):1098–1104
13. Balasanmugam C, Henriquez Felipe C, Rodriguez D, Kulbak G. Bradycardia, hypotension, and cardiac arrest: a complication of local anesthetics. Cureus 2019;11(2):e4033
14. Farahmand S, Hamrah H, Arbab M, Sedaghat M, Basir Ghafouri H, Bagheri-Hariri S. Pain management of acute limb trauma patients with intravenous lidocaine in emergency department. Am J Emerg Med 2018;36(7):1231–1235

15. Sin B, Gritsenko D, Tam G, Koop K, Mok E. The use of intravenous lidocaine for the management of acute pain secondary to traumatic ankle injury: a case report. J Pharm Pract 2018;31(1):126–129
16. Fitzcharles-Bowe C, Denkler K, Lalonde D. Finger injection with high-dose (1:1,000) epinephrine: does it cause finger necrosis and should it be treated? Hand (N Y) 2007;2(1):5–11
17. Prasetyono TO, Saputra DK, Astriana W. One-per-mil tumescent technique for bone and joint surgery in hand. Hand (N Y) 2015;10(1):123–127

CHAPTER 5

HOW TO INJECT LOCAL ANESTHETIC SO THAT IT DOES NOT HURT

Donald H. Lalonde

LOCAL ANESTHESIA DOES NOT HAVE TO HURT

- I spent the first 22 years of my practice hurting people with local anesthetic injection way more than I should have. I learned how not to hurt people with local injection in 2006. It is never too late to stop hurting people! If you want to hear the story of how and why that happened, look at ▶ Video 5.1.

- We now easily teach all of our medical students and residents[1] how to inject local anesthetic for carpal tunnel surgery so that all that the patient consistently barely feels is the little sting of a 27- or 30-gauge needle.

- Your patients will greatly appreciate that you have become almost magical by taking the time required to learn how to take the pain out of local anesthesia injection by following the simple rules listed below[2] (see ▶ Video 2.2 for patient's perspective on properly injected local anesthesia pain). Also see the link[3] for a longer 2020 lecture on this subject.

Video 5.1 The 2015 story of how Don Lalonde came to stop hurting people after 22 years of painful local anesthesia injections.

Video 5.2 How not to hurt people when you inject local anesthesia.

RULE 1: INJECT LOCAL ANESTHESIA WITH SMALL BORE, 27-GAUGE (0.4 MM) OR 30-GAUGE (0.3 MM) NEEDLES

- Stop using 25-gauge or larger needles. Bigger needles hurt more.

- Go find the person in your hospital who actually orders the needles. Ask him or her to see the form he or she fills out to make the orders. Point out to him or her where the 30-gauge, 0.5-inch needles are and ask him or her to click that box.

- Injecting large volumes quickly causes pressure pain. Using smaller needles will force you and remind you to slow down, which will decrease injection pain.

- Small needles need small syringes. In children, babies, digital blocks, and people who are very afraid of needles, I always start with a 30-gauge, 0.5-inch needle on a 3-mL syringe.

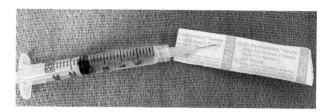

Fig. 5.1 Powerful weapon to decrease the pain of beginning the injection in children, sensitive patient and those afraid of needles—the 30-gauge, 0.5-inch needle on a 3-mL syringe.

RULE 2: CREATE SENSORY NOISE LIKE PINCHING THE SKIN INTO THE NEEDLE

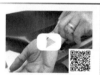

Video 5.3 Pinching the skin into the needle instead of pushing the needle into the skin.

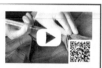

Video 5.4 Sensory noise when there is not enough skin to pinch.

- Pinch loose skin into the needle tip instead of moving the needle into the skin. The "sound" of the extrasensory input of the pinch drowns out the "sound" of the needle tip pain. This is like hearing a baby cry in a crowd versus hearing it cry in your room at 2 AM.

- Tell the patient you will **pinch the skin three times** while you count to 3. Ask them to **take a deep breath** when say the number 2. Ask them to try not to move if they feel a little poke when you get to 3. Pinch the skin firmly three times while you count. On the third pinch as you say the number 3, **pinch the skin into the needle** instead of pushing the needle into the skin. **Maintain the firm skin pinch to keep up sensory noise until the skin around the needle is completely numb.**

- If there is tight skin with nothing to pinch, as in the palm of the hand, press firmly on the tight skin just proximal to where you will insert the needle to create sensory "noise" to decrease pain felt by the patient.

- Ask the patient to look away. It may hurt the patient more if he or she watches the needle go in.[4]

- Icing the skin[5] and vibrating it[6] are other forms of sensory noise that can decrease the pain of needle entry.

- Ask the patient to take a deep breath just before you insert the needle. This is another good form of sensory noise (see ▶ Video 5.2).

RULE 3: NEVER LET THE NEEDLE GET AHEAD OF THE LOCAL ANESTHETIC AND "BLOW SLOW BEFORE YOU GO"

- Hitting live nerves with a sharp needle tip hurts! Never let your needle tip hit nerves that are not numb.

- Instead, blow slow before you go.

- Using longer needles will let you go further before having to reinsert the needle which may cause added pain. Our preferred "go-to" needle in most patients is the 27-gauge, 1.5-inches (3.8 cm) long.

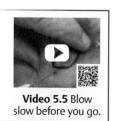

Video 5.5 Blow slow before you go.

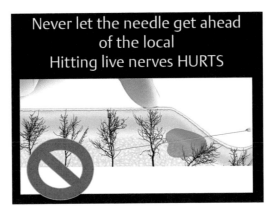

Fig. 5.2 Never let the needle get ahead of the local anesthetic. If this happens, the sharp needle tip will irritate nerve endings that are not numb. Inject the local anesthetic in an antegrade fashion so that the needle tip only enters numbed nerve territory. (Reproduced with permission from Strazar et al.[2])

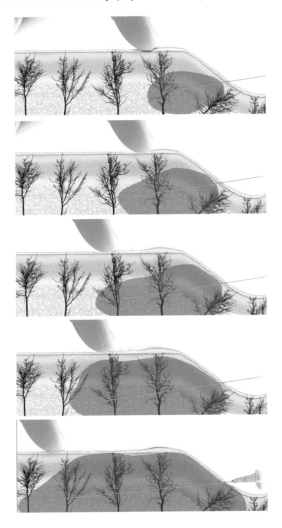

Fig. 5.3 Always repeat the phrase "blow slow before you go" in your head while you are injecting. It will help you to slow down and be patient. If you inject in an antegrade direction while advancing very slowly and steadily under the skin, the sharp needle tip will only enter numbed territory. There should always be at least 1 cm of visible or palpable local anesthetic ahead of the sharp needle tip. Feel it advance with the fingertip of your other hand. (Reproduced with permission from Strazar et al.[2])

RULE 4: LEARN FROM EACH PATIENT YOU INJECT BY ASKING HIM OR HER TO GIVE YOU A SCORE

- Ask each patient to score you every time you inject local anesthetic. I have my patients score me and all my medical students and residents every time we inject so we can see that our scores continue to improve.

- After the sting of the first needle entry is gone, ask the patient to tell you each time he or she feels pain during the injection process.

- If the patient does feel additional pain during the injection, stop moving the needle or back up a little and very, very slowly continue to inject in that one place until the pain is completely gone.

  - If the patient only feels the sting of the first needle stick, your pain score is 1 (hole-in-one).
  - If he or she feels pain a second time during the injection process, your medical student pain score drops to 2 (eagle).
  - If the patient feels pain three times, your resident scores a birdie, four times a bogie, and so on.
  - If you are a teacher, have all your trainees scored by all their patients every time they inject and ask them what their score was each time they inject. Your medical students and residents will want to get better and better. The patients will be more likely to be happy to have the learner participate in the surgery.

- Each patient you inject presents an opportunity for you to get better and better at injection. Each time we do not ask the patient to score us is a wasted opportunity to improve our technique.

- The most common reason that medical students and residents do not score a hole-in-one while injecting for carpal tunnel surgery is that they inject too quickly.[1] It takes about 4 to 5 minutes to consistently score a hole-in-one for carpal tunnel injection.

- The three most common causes of poor pain scores are:

  - Injecting too quickly.
  - Letting the sharp needle tip get ahead of the local anesthetic into unanesthetized areas.
  - Reinserting needles into "live," unanesthetized skin.

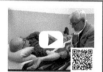

Video 5.6
Explaining pain scoring to patients so they can help you get better at hurting less every time you inject.

RULE 5: REINSERT NEEDLES WITHIN 1 CM OF THE BLANCHED (SWOLLEN)/UNBLANCHED (NOT SWOLLEN) BORDER

- Never reinsert the needle into unblanched skin. If there are not enough epinephrine molecules working there to cause vasoconstriction, chances are there is not enough lidocaine there for pain-free needle reinsertion.

- When you are injecting a large area (extensor indicis to extensor pollicis longus tendon transfer, for example), and you need to reinsert the injecting needle, reinsert the needle only into clearly blanched areas that are tumesced with visible or palpable local anesthetic (slightly firm to palpation). You should reinsert the needle 1 cm inside well-blanched skin beyond the border of the blanched/unblanched skin junction.

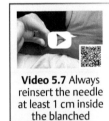

Video 5.7 Always reinsert the needle at least 1 cm inside the blanched (swollen)/ unblanched (not swollen) border so they never feel it.

RULE 6: TOO MUCH LOCAL ANESTHETIC IS BETTER THAN NOT ENOUGH LOCAL ANESTHETIC

- The more volume that you inject, the greater are the odds that the patient will feel no pain after you start to dissect. Try to avoid "top-ups" of local anesthetic that give patients unnecessary bad memories. Your patients do not want to feel pain during surgery any more than you want to wake up during a procedure in which you have been given a general anesthetic.

- Patients never complain about being too numb but frequently complain about not being numb enough. Stay within safe limits (50 mL of 1% lidocaine with 1:100,000 epinephrine as in Chapter 4) but always provide a little more volume than you need, except for the fingers, where you need only 2 mL per phalanx per side in the proximal and middle phalanges.

- Never run out of gas while flying an airplane, and never run out of local anesthesia if you need extra safe volume of solution (see Chapter 4) for a "top-up" because your patient is having pain during the surgery. Always plan to have extra local anesthetic in case you need it. You should aim to NEVER have to top-up because of the pain of local anesthesia during surgery, just like patients should never wake up during a general anesthesia.

- There should be at least 1 to 2 cm of tumesced (swollen, blanched) visible local anesthetic under the skin beyond wherever you plan to insert a sharp object or move a broken bone.

- The two most common causes of needing a "top-up" are:
  - Not injecting enough volume of tumescent local anesthetic.
  - Not giving the local anesthetic enough time to work (wait half an hour).

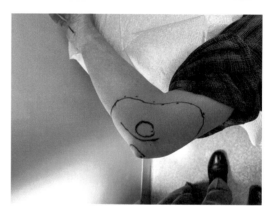

Fig. 5.4 Too much tumescent local anesthesia is better than not enough. Here you see 60 mL of 0.5% lidocaine with 1:200,000 epinephrine in the elbow for cubital tunnel decompression, 30 minutes after injection. The carpal tunnel got 20 mL of the same solution. These patients always feel *no* pain during the surgery.

RULE 7: STABILIZE THE SYRINGE WITH BOTH HANDS AND HAVE YOUR THUMB READY ON THE PLUNGER TO AVOID THE PAIN OF A MOVING NEEDLE

- It can take up to a minute for the needle site to numb after you place the needle under the skin, especially if you inject an insufficient bleb right under the dermis. This time, the patient will feel the sting with every little wobble of the needle moving in the skin.

- If you stabilize the syringe with two hands, and if your thumb is on the plunger ready to inject before the needle penetrates, you will minimize painful needle movement in unanesthetized skin.

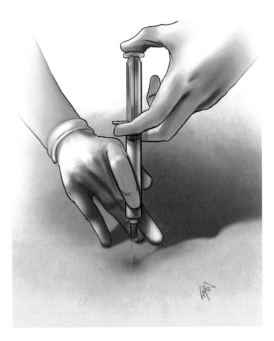

Fig. 5.5 Stabilize the needle so that it does not wobble until the skin is numb. Hold it with two hands and thumb ready on the plunger. If the syringe-holding hand is free and is not stabilized on the skin, the patient will feel every little needle movement until the local anesthetic has numbed the needle insertion site. (Reproduced with permission from Strazar et al.[2])

RULE 8: INJECT A VISIBLE BLEB (0.5 ML) WITH A PERPENDICULAR NEEDLE JUST UNDER THE DERMIS AND THEN PAUSE UNTIL THE PATIENT SAYS THE NEEDLE PAIN HAS GONE (ASK HIM OR HER TO TELL YOU WHEN THE PAIN HAS GONE)

• Nerves in the dermis are like trees with sensitive leaves, and in the fat are like branches and trunks. Injections in the dermis hurt more than in subcutaneous fat because you irritate more "leaves" with the pressure of intradermal injection.[7] Inject just under the dermis instead of in the dermis.

• Inserting the needle perpendicular (90 degrees) to the skin hurts less than if you come in parallel to it because you pierce fewer nerve endings with the sharp needle tip on the way to the subcutaneous fat.[8]

• Begin by injecting a visible bleb (0.5 mL) just under the dermis, then pause until the patient tells you the pain has all gone. You need to ask him or her to tell you when the pain has gone. You will then be able to start to count the number of subsequent times the patient feels pain, and score yourself as in rule 4.

• When the patient tells you the sting of the needle site has gone, inject an additional 1.5 mL very slowly without moving the needle.

• If you start to inject quickly or move the needle tip out of the numb zone, the patient will feel pain. After you have injected the initial 2 mL of anesthetic, you can change the angle from 90 degrees perpendicular to parallel to the skin without causing pain.

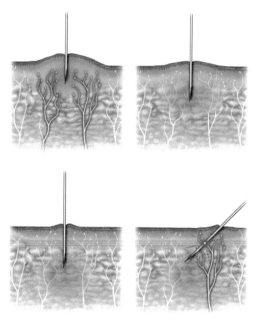

As soon as the needle is inserted, *blow in a visible bleb of 0.5 mL under the dermis, not in the dermis.* The needle should be inserted at 90 degrees so that fewer nerves are pierced. At a 90-degree angle, the patient will feel less pain than if the needle is inserted at a 45-degree angle. (From Strazar AR, Leynes PG, Lalonde DH. Minimizing the pain of local anesthesia injection. Plast Reconstr Surg 132:675, 2013.)

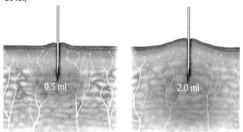

After you have injected 0.5 mL in the subcutaneous fat, hold still at least 15 seconds. Ask the patient to tell you when the sting of the needle is all gone. The first subcutaneous bleb or wheal must be visible or palpable under the skin in order for the needle insertion site to be properly numbed. After the patient tells you the sting of the needle is gone, inject an additional 1.5 mL very slowly without moving the needle. (From Strazar AR, Leynes PG, Lalonde DH. Minimizing the pain of local anesthesia injection. Plast Reconstr Surg 132:675, 2013.)

Fig. 5.6

RULE 9: BUFFER 1% LIDOCAINE AND 1:100,000 EPINEPHRINE WITH 10:1 8.4% SODIUM BICARBONATE AND DO NOT REFRIGERATE

- 1% lidocaine with 1:100,000 epinephrine has an average pH of 4.2, with a range of 3.3 to 5.5.[9] This can be 1,000 times more acidic than the normal body pH of 7.4. This is one reason it hurts when you inject it unbuffered.

- Alkalinizing the local anesthesia also makes it work faster and last longer.[10,11]

- A bottle of 50 mL of 8.4% sodium bicarbonate costs less than $10.

- Draw up 1 mL of bicarbonate and 10 mL of 1% lidocaine with 1:100,000 epinephrine in a 10-mL syringe. Conveniently, 10-mL Luer-lock syringes hold 11 mL of liquid, 20-mL syringes hold 22 mL of liquid, and 5-mL syringes hold 5.5 mL.

- Alternatively, inject 2 mL of bicarbonate into a 20-mL bottle of lidocaine with epinephrine.

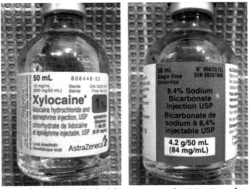

ᵃ 10 mL syringe actually holds 11 mL, and a 20 mL syringe holds 22 mL. Simply add 1 mL of 8.4% bicarbonate to 10 mL of 1% lidocaine and 1:100,000 epinephrine to make the pH body neutral.[1] Draw up 1 mL of sodium bicarbonate, then fill the rest of the 10 mL syringe to 11 mL with 1% lidocaine with 1:100,000 epinephrine. (From Strazar AR, Leynes PG, Lalonde DH. Minimizing the pain of local anesthesia injection. Plast Reconstr Surg 132:675, 2013.)

Fig. 5.7

- Refrigerated local anesthetic will result in a more uncomfortable injection for the patient than room-temperature local anesthetic.[12] We store our lidocaine with epinephrine at room temperature. Some centers keep their lidocaine and epinephrine refrigerated so that it lasts longer. This is not necessary if you simply adhere to the expiration dates on the bottle.

OTHER TIPS OF LESS PAINFUL SHARP NEEDLE INJECTION

- Always inject from proximal to distal to anesthetize nerves proximally. The tumescent local anesthetic will create nerve blocks proximally.

- If you are blocking a major nerve as part of tumescent local anesthesia, never elicit paresthesias! If you do, you may have lacerated the nerve with your needle. Remember that a 25-gauge needle is the width of a human fascicle. You want to get near the nerve and inject a large volume to make certain you surround the nerve with local anesthetic.

- You may want to stage your injections for more time efficiency. For example, start by injecting 10 mL in the palm. This blocks the digital nerves of the fingers of interest. See or inject other patients while this takes effect. Come back 30 minutes later to perform all your distal injections quickly in the distal palm and fingers now that the nerve blocks have worked.

- Do not inject directly into a scar or skin crease. Scarred skin is tender and does not distend easily with local anesthetic. Skin creases exist because structures such as the tendon sheath adhere to the skin at that point with cutaneous ligaments, which are accompanied by sensitive nerve branches that feel the sharp pain of needle insertion. See Chapter 4 for details of injecting creased and scarred skin.

RULE 10: USE BLUNT TIP CANNULA NEEDLES TO INJECT LARGE AREAS WITH LOCAL ANESTHETIC

- Blunt-tipped cannulas slide through fat without piercing nerves, unlike of sharp needle tips. They are more expensive (about $5 to $10), but definitely faster and less painful than sharp needle tips.[13]

Video 5.8 Cannula injection of tumescent local anesthetic for synovectomy and tendon transfer.

- You insert blunt-tipped cannulas into skin injection sites made with sharp needles with a bore of larger diameter than that of the cannula so the cannula enters the injection site opening easily. For example, you insert a 27-gauge (5.7 cm long) cannula into an injection site opening made with a 25-gauge needle in anesthetized skin.

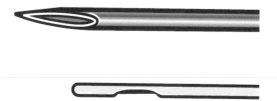

Fig. 5.8 The larger bore sharp needle tip (above) makes a hole for the smaller blunt tip cannula (below)

- See ▶ Video 26.4b for 37-mm, blunt-tipped, 27-gauge cannula injection for carpal tunnel surgery.
- See ▶ Video 38.5 for 40-mm-long, blunt-tipped, 25-gauge cannula in an injection site made with a 20-gauge needle for trapeziectomy.

OTHER HELPFUL HINTS FOR DECREASING THE PAIN OF LOCAL ANESTHESIA INJECTION

- Some local anesthesia manufacturers insist on refrigeration. Others allow storage at room temperature in a cupboard. Hospitals buy whichever is cheaper, even though it costs a lot more to store. When using refrigerated ones, you should warm it under a hot tap for a few seconds before taking the lid off to use it. Alternatively, you can remove it from the fridge the night before which saves time on the day. Cold local anesthesia hurts more than room temperature anesthesia.[12]

HOW TO TELL THAT YOUR LOCAL ANESTHESIA IS PROFOUND ENOUGH THAT YOUR PATIENT WILL NOT FEEL PAIN WHEN YOU CUT OR MOVE A FRACTURE

- Touch the numbed finger and ask the patient: "Does this finger still feel like it belongs to you, or does it feel like it belongs to someone else?" Most people who have had a finger anesthetized will understand this. Totally numb fingers feel like they belong to someone else.
- If the area is totally white with epinephrine, it will almost certainly be numb.
- The "pink rule": Never put a sharp object into pink (nonvasoconstricted) skin. If there is no functioning epinephrine there, there is no functioning lidocaine there.
- See ▶ Video 51.2 for painless manipulation of long bone fracture (tibia in this case) so you know it will not hurt when you plate it.

COMMON DIGITAL ROOT BLOCK WORKS MUCH FASTER AND IS MORE EFFECTIVE THAN A MEDIAN NERVE BLOCK AT THE WRIST

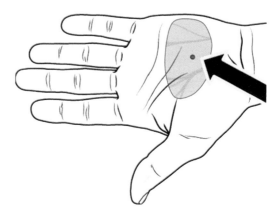

Fig. 5.9 Common digital trunk block.

- Inject at the root of the common digital nerve trunks in the palm of the hand just distal to the transverse carpal ligament where the nerve trunks divide in the fat pad you see all the time when you do carpal tunnel release.

- The smaller the nerve, the faster and more completely it numbs. This is much more effective and works much faster than a median nerve block proximal to the wrist crease, which can take 100 minutes to peak in effectiveness.[14]

- Inject 10 to 20 mL of 1% lidocaine with 1:100,000 epinephrine just deep to the palmar fascia and superficial to the fat pad without moving the needle. Watch and feel the tissues inflate if you don't have ultrasound vision. Draw back to make sure you are not in the palmar arch vessels. You should be injecting just proximal to the arch and just distal to the transverse carpal ligament.

- This will numb both median and ulnar nerve common digital roots.

References

1. Farhangkhoee H, Lalonde J, Lalonde DH. Teaching medical students and residents how to inject local anesthesia almost painlessly. Can J Plast Surg 2012;20(3):169–172
2. Strazar AR, Leynes PG, Lalonde DH. Minimizing the pain of local anesthesia injection. Plast Reconstr Surg 2013;132(3):675–684
3. Link to Lalonde lecture to ICTEC Indonesian Hand Society lecture July 2020. accessed July 26 2020. https://www.youtube.com/watch?v=lcSizvzD6LM
4. Höfle M, Hauck M, Engel AK, Senkowski D. Viewing a needle pricking a hand that you perceive as yours enhances unpleasantness of pain. Pain 2012;153(5):1074–1081

5. Aminabadi NA, Farahani RM. The effect of pre-cooling the injection site on pediatric pain perception during the administration of local anesthesia. J Contemp Dent Pract 2009;10(3):43–50

6. Nanitsos E, Vartuli R, Forte A, Dennison PJ, Peck CC. The effect of vibration on pain during local anaesthesia injections. Aust Dent J 2009;54(2):94–100

7. Arndt KA, Burton C, Noe JM. Minimizing the pain of local anesthesia. Plast Reconstr Surg 1983;72(5):676–679

8. Martires KJ, Malbasa CL, Bordeaux JS. A randomized controlled crossover trial: lidocaine injected at a 90-degree angle causes less pain than lidocaine injected at a 45-degree angle. J Am Acad Dermatol 2011;65(6):1231–1233

9. Frank SG, Lalonde DH. How acidic is the lidocaine we are injecting, and how much bicarbonate should we add? Can J Plast Surg 2012;20(2):71–73

10. Gupta S, Kumar A, Sharma AK, Purohit J, Narula JS. "Sodium bicarbonate": an adjunct to painless palatal anesthesia. Oral Maxillofac Surg 2018;22(4):451–455

11. Gupta S, Mandlik G, Padhye MN, Kini YK, Kakkar S, Hire AV. Combating inadequate anesthesia in periapical infections, with sodium bicarbonate: a clinical double blind study. Oral Maxillofac Surg 2014;18(3):325–329

12. Hogan ME, vanderVaart S, Perampaladas K, Machado M, Einarson TR, Taddio A. Systematic review and meta-analysis of the effect of warming local anesthetics on injection pain. Ann Emerg Med 2011;58(1):86–98.e1

13. Lalonde D, Wong A. Local anesthetics: what's new in minimal pain injection and best evidence in pain control. Plast Reconstr Surg 2014; 134(4, Suppl 2):40S–49S

14. Lovely LM, Chishti YZ, Woodland JL, Lalonde DH. How much volume of local anesthesia and how long should you wait after injection for an effective wrist median nerve block? Hand (N Y) 2018;13(3):281–284

CHAPTER 6

DEALING WITH SYSTEMIC ADVERSE REACTIONS TO LIDOCAINE AND EPINEPHRINE

Donald H. Lalonde

THE SAFETY OF SYSTEMIC LIDOCAINE AND EPINEPHRINE INJECTION

- The only drugs required for most hand surgery procedures are lidocaine (also called lignocaine) and epinephrine.

- Lidocaine was introduced in the late 1940s. For over 65 years, American dentists have injected lidocaine premixed with epinephrine in an average of many millions of patients per day with no monitoring, no intravenous insertion, and no preoperative testing and very few reported adverse reactions.[1,2] If there were common or serious problems with lidocaine and epinephrine injection, the American legal community would have been seeking financial compensation for their clients from dentists long ago.

- Adverse reactions to local anesthetics are usually a reaction to epinephrine, vasovagal syncope, or overdose toxicity. Patients may interpret adverse reactions as an allergy to local anesthetic. True allergy to amide local anesthetics is considered to be rare.[3,4,5]

7 MG/KG OF LIDOCAINE WITH EPINEPHRINE IS VERY SAFE

- The maximal dose of lidocaine with epinephrine, published before 1950, is 7 mg/kg. Since then, Vasconez and others have reported safe blood levels of lidocaine when they injected 35 mg/kg or more for liposuction.[6,7,8,9]

- In facelifting, where the blood flow is high, 21 mg/kg of lidocaine with epinephrine yielded 70% less than toxic blood levels at their highest.[10]

- Emergentologists inject 100 mg of lidocaine in slow intravenous boluses to treat various pain conditions.[11] Anesthesiologists inject 1 mg/kg of lidocaine intravenously for pain control in postoperative patients.[12] Others have used 5 mg/kg lidocaine intravenously over 6 hours to manage neurogenic pain.[13]

- Inadvertent intravenous small boluses of local anesthetic may occur with antegrade injection, as described in Chapter 4. However, toxicity from these tiny intravascular doses is very unlikely, given the above safety statistics.

SAFETY OF LIDOCAINE

- Lidocaine is much less cardiotoxic than other local anesthetics such as bupivacaine or ropivacaine (see the section on Longer-Lasting Local Anesthetics). In fact, internists commonly inject lidocaine to rescue ventricular arrhythmias.[14]

- Although there are many reports of lidocaine skin test "allergy" in patients,[15] many patients who test positive can be safely given lidocaine.[16] True anaphylaxis documentation is rare.

- A PubMed search for lidocaine anaphylaxis reveals 10 case reports in the past 10 years. Out of the 10 cases, 2 had incomplete details,[17,18] and the remaining 8 had other confounding variables, which made it hard to attribute the anaphylaxis solely to the lidocaine.[17,19,20,21,22,23,24,25] These reports are rare when you consider the many billions of lidocaine doses administered in dental offices in the world in the past six and a half decades. If life-threatening anaphylaxis to lidocaine actually does exist, it is likely to be extremely rare.[26]

- Lidocaine also appears to be safe to the fetus during pregnancy.[27]

TREATMENT OF SYSTEMIC ADVERSE REACTIONS TO LIDOCAINE AND EPINEPHRINE

- Lidocaine-induced seizures can occur with large intravenous doses administered too quickly, or with excessive doses injected subcutaneously. With the doses and slow injection technique outlined in Chapter 4 and Chapter 5, this complication is likely to be rare or nonexistent. The treatment of lidocaine-induced seizures is airway control and benzodiazepines. The treatment of lidocaine toxicity is lipid emulsion Intralipid (1.5 mg/kg).[5] Lipid rescue protocol recommends an initial Intralipid 20% bolus of 1.5 mL/kg over 1 minute. This should be followed immediately with a continuous infusion at 0.25 mL/kg/minute. A single bolus is typical, but should be repeated or the infusion increased if spontaneous circulation fails to return or blood pressure declines.

- The antidote of epinephrine vasoconstriction is phentolamine. The myth that epinephrine vasoconstriction is dangerous in fingers is addressed in Chapter 3. This chapter only deals with systemic effects.

- The medical literature is almost devoid of reports of serious systemic adverse reactions to the epinephrine that accompanies the lidocaine, even in patients with cardiac disease.[28] However, if there is a concern about giving a patient with cardiac disease epinephrine-containing local anesthetic, we can monitor these patients and/or give them lower dosages of epinephrine.

- Epinephrine still provides good hemostasis in doses as low as 1:400,000[29] or 1:1,000,000.[30] We routinely use 1:400,000 epinephrine when we need 100 to 200 mL of volume for larger cases and find the hemostasis perfectly acceptable, as long as we give the epinephrine half an hour to work (see Chapter 4).

- Epinephrine in a local anesthetic can cause transient elevation of the heart rate and blood pressure, but the clinical importance of this effect remains unclear.[31] Adverse outcomes among hypertensive patients are infrequent, and hemodynamic outcomes, which are possible risk indicators, reflect only minimal change.[32]

MONITORING IS NOT NECESSARY DURING WIDE AWAKE HAND SURGERY

- Canadian hand surgeons have well over 40 years of extensive experience in wide awake hand surgery without monitoring and without significant adverse events.

- Moh's surgeons in the United States use exactly the same drugs that we do in the highly vascular face without monitoring and with an excellent safety record.[33]

- Almost all of those who read this text have been to the dentist and received lidocaine with epinephrine with zero blood pressure or electrocardiogram (EKG) monitoring and have not suffered ill effects given the same drugs we give for WALANT—lidocaine with epinephrine.

LONGER-LASTING LOCAL ANESTHETICS

- Ropivacaine and bupivacaine both last longer than lidocaine, but they have a lower safety profile.[5] In large doses, bupivacaine[34,35] and ropivacaine[36,37,38] can be cardiotoxic and fatal. Lipid emulsion therapy has been used for both bupivacaine[39] and lidocaine[40] rescue.

- For digital blocks, bupivacaine-induced useful numbness to pain lasts only half as long (15 hours) as the annoying pressure and touch numbness (30 hours).[41] That is why patients with bupivacaine digital blocks complain that their injured finger is still numb, but it hurts.

- Lidocaine's pain and numbness to touch and pressure all come back at the same time, like an on/off light switch.

- You can finish most hand operations in the anesthesia time provided by lidocaine with epinephrine (5 hours in the wrist,[42] 10 hours in the finger[43]). We use bupivacaine only in operations that may last more than 2.5 to 3 hours or in procedures such as a trapeziectomy, where postoperative pain may be severe.

THE EPINEPHRINE "RUSH" AND THE VASOVAGAL ATTACK (FAINTING)

- Although lidocaine and epinephrine are probably two of the safest drugs in use, injecting them can have two relatively common adverse events. These are the epinephrine "rush" and the vasovagal attack in response to receiving a needle injection.

THE EPINEPHRINE RUSH

- About one-third of patients can feel an epinephrine "rush," "jitter," "shakiness," "nervousness," or a feeling "like you have had too much coffee" for up to 20 to 30 minutes after an injection of local anesthetic.

- Forewarned is forearmed. We warn all of our patients that they may get this rushy feeling after we inject them. We tell them that this is not an allergy; it is a normal reaction to the epinephrine we have injected with the lidocaine, and the sensation will go away in 20 to 30 minutes.

- Catechol-o-methyl transferase and monoamine oxidase are two enzymes that rapidly break down epinephrine in plasma[44] so that its half-life inside blood vessels is only 1.7 minutes.[45] However, extravascular epinephrine degradation is slower. The molecules must first get into blood vessels either by diffusion or through the lymphatics. You can frequently see white lymphatic vasoconstriction tracks in the forearm when you inject epinephrine into the hand.

AVOIDING THE FAINT

- Loss of consciousness that occurs with a faint or vasovagal attack occurs because there is not enough blood going to the brain. Nature's solution is to bring the head down by fainting to allow more blood to get to the brain with gravity.

- Have the patient lie down if he or she is sitting. (We do not recommend anesthetic injection in the sitting position because there is less blood going to the brain than when someone is lying down.)

- A bandage change or cast removal can trigger fainting. Needles with or without local anesthetic are another common trigger.

MANAGING FAINTING

- Patients can faint even if you inject them lying down.

Recognizing that Someone Is Going to Faint

- The following are signs that a patient is about to faint. The patient may say, "I'm not feeling well," or "I think I'm going to be sick (vomit)." If you look at the patient, he or she may be pale in the central upper face (glabella, between the eyes, upper nose, or perioral skin).

PATIENTS CAN FAINT EVEN IF YOU INJECT THEM LYING DOWN

If your patient is showing signs that he or she is about to faint, get more blood to the brain with the following gravity-changing maneuvers:

- Lie the patient down if he or she is sitting up.

- If the patient is lying down, put your hand beneath the knees and raise the knees up to flex the hips and knees so the thigh blood can run down toward the brain.
- Remove the pillow from under the head and place it under the feet.
- Lower the head of the stretcher to the Trendelenburg position (head down, feet up).

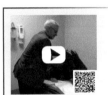

Video 6.1
Managing the patient who is going to faint.

THE ANXIOUS PATIENT

- Most anxious patients can be reassured with a quiet, soothing voice and manner. Most will tolerate wide awake hand surgery if they can tolerate a dental procedure.
- Music can be helpful to decrease anxiety.
- Some anxious patients do better with sedation. You can give them small oral doses of medication or provide full main operating room sedation with an anesthesiologist. The downside is that the patient will not be able to receive and remember intraoperative teaching and may not be able to help you by cooperatively moving the hand to assess its function during surgery.

References

1. Gaffen AS, Haas DA. Survey of local anesthetic use by Ontario dentists. J Can Dent Assoc 2009;75(9):649
2. Jeske AH. Xylocaine: 50 years of clinical service to dentistry. Tex Dent J 1998;115(5):9–13
3. Bina B, Hersh EV, Hilario M, Alvarez K, McLaughlin B. True allergy to amide local anesthetics: a review and case presentation. Anesth Prog 2018;65(2):119–123
4. Rood JP. Adverse reaction to dental local anaesthetic injection—"allergy" is not the cause. Br Dent J 2000;189(7):380–384
5. Gitman M, Fettiplace MR, Weinberg GL, Neal JM, Barrington MJ. Local anesthetic systemic toxicity: a narrative literature review and clinical update on prevention, diagnosis, and management. Plast Reconstr Surg 2019;144(3):783–795
6. Burk RW III, Guzman-Stein G, Vasconez LO. Lidocaine and epinephrine levels in tumescent technique liposuction. Plast Reconstr Surg 1996;97(7):1379–1384
7. Klein JA. Tumescent technique for regional anesthesia permits lidocaine doses of 35 mg/kg for liposuction. J Dermatol Surg Oncol 1990;16(3):248–263

8. Nordström H, Stånge K. Plasma lidocaine levels and risks after liposuction with tumescent anaesthesia. Acta Anaesthesiol Scand 2005;49(10):1487–1490

9. Klein JA, Jeske DR. Estimated maximal safe dosages of tumescent lidocaine. Anesth Analg 2016;122(5):1350–1359

10. Ramon Y, Barak Y, Ullmann Y, Hoffer E, Yarhi D, Bentur Y. Pharmacokinetics of high-dose diluted lidocaine in local anesthesia for facelift procedures. Ther Drug Monit 2007;29(5):644–647

11. Tanen DA, Shimada M, Danish DC, Dos Santos F, Makela M, Riffenburgh RH. Intravenous lidocaine for the emergency department treatment of acute radicular low back pain, a randomized controlled trial. J Emerg Med 2014;47(1):119–124

12. Barreveld A, Witte J, Chahal H, Durieux ME, Strichartz G. Preventive analgesia by local anesthetics: the reduction of postoperative pain by peripheral nerve blocks and intravenous drugs. Anesth Analg 2013;116(5):1141–1161

13. Tremont-Lukats IW, Hutson PR, Backonja MM. A randomized, double-masked, placebo-controlled pilot trial of extended IV lidocaine infusion for relief of ongoing neuropathic pain. Clin J Pain 2006;22(3):266–271

14. Dogru K, Duygulu F, Yildiz K, Kotanoglu MS, Madenoglu H, Boyaci A. Hemodynamic and blockade effects of high/low epinephrine doses during axillary brachial plexus blockade with lidocaine 1.5%: a randomized, double-blinded study. Reg Anesth Pain Med 2003;28(5):401–405

15. Janas-Naze A, Osica P. The incidence of lidocaine allergy in dentists: an evaluation of 100 general dental practitioners. Int J Occup Med Environ Health 2019;32(3):333–339

16. Corbo MD, Weber E, DeKoven J. Lidocaine allergy: do positive patch results restrict future use? Dermatitis 2016;27(2):68–71

17. Al-Dosary K, Al-Qahtani A, Alangari A. Anaphylaxis to lidocaine with tolerance to articaine in a 12 year old girl. Saudi Pharm J 2014;22(3):280–282

18. Khokhlov VD, Krut' MI, Sashko SIu. [Anaphylactic shock following administration of lidocaine after negative skin test]. Klin Med (Mosk) 2012;90(7):62–64

19. Lee MY, Park KA, Yeo SJ, et al. Bronchospasm and anaphylactic shock following lidocaine aerosol inhalation in a patient with butane inhalation lung injury. Allergy Asthma Immunol Res 2011;3(4):280–282

20. Soong WJ, Lee YS, Soong YH, et al. Life-threatening anaphylactic reaction after the administration of airway topical lidocaine. Pediatr Pulmonol 2011;46(5):505–508

21. Sinha M, Sinha R. Anaphylactic shock following intraurethral lidocaine administration during transurethral resection of the prostate. Indian J Urol 2008;24(1):114–115

22. Culp JA, Palis RI, Castells MC, Lucas SR, Borish L. Perioperative anaphylaxis in a 44-year-old man. Allergy Asthma Proc 2007;28(5):602–605

23. Kim H, Lee JM, Seo KS, Kwon SM, Row HS. Anaphylactic reaction after local lidocaine infiltration for retraction of retained teeth. J Dent Anesth Pain Med 2019;19(3):175–180

24. Osman BM, Maga JM, Baquero SM. Case report: management of differential diagnosis and treatment of severe anaphylaxis in the setting of spinal anesthesia. J Clin Anesth 2016;35:145–149

25. Chan TYK. Fatal anaphylactic reactions to lignocaine. Forensic Sci Int 2016;266:449–452

26. Specjalski K, Kita-Milczarska K, Jassem E. The negative predictive value of typing safe local anesthetics. Int Arch Allergy Immunol 2013;162(1):86–88
27. Moore PA. An increased rate for major birth anomalies was not found following dental treatment requiring local anesthesia during pregnancy. J Evid Based Dent Pract 2016;16(1):75–76
28. Sanatkar M, Sadeghi M, Esmaeili N, et al. The evaluation of perioperative safety of local anesthesia with lidocaine containing epinephrine in patients with ischemic heart disease. Acta Med Iran 2013;51(8):537–542
29. Kämmerer PW, Krämer N, Esch J, et al. Epinephrine-reduced articaine solution (1:400,000) in paediatric dentistry: a multicentre non-interventional clinical trial. Eur Arch Paediatr Dent 2013;14(2):89–95
30. Prasetyono TO, Biben JA. One-per-mil tumescent technique for upper extremity surgeries: broadening the indication. J Hand Surg Am 2014;39(1):3–12.e7
31. Abu-Mostafa N, Aldawssary A, Assari A, Alnujaidy S, Almutlaq A. A prospective randomized clinical trial compared the effect of various types of local anesthetics cartridges on hypertensive patients during dental extraction. J Clin Exp Dent 2015;7(1):e84–e88
32. Bader JD, Bonito AJ, Shugars DA. Cardiovascular effects of epinephrine in hypertensive dental patients. Summary. Agency for Healthcare Research and Quality evidence report/technology assessment: Number 48. AHRQ Publication Number 02–E005. Rockville, MD: The Agency, Mar 2002. https://www.ncbi.nlm.nih.gov/books/NBK11858/
33. Larson MJ, Taylor RS. Monitoring vital signs during outpatient Mohs and post-Mohs reconstructive surgery performed under local anesthesia. Dermatol Surg 2004;30(5):777–783
34. Dudley MH, Fleming SW, Garg U, Edwards JM. Fatality involving complications of bupivacaine toxicity and hypersensitivity reaction. J Forensic Sci 2011;56(5):1376–1379
35. Cordell CL, Schubkegel T, Light TR, Ahmad F. Lipid infusion rescue for bupivacaine-induced cardiac arrest after axillary block. J Hand Surg Am 2010;35(1):144–146
36. Jiang X, Huang W, Lin X. Ropivacaine-induced cardiac arrest and paraplegia after epidural anesthesia. Minerva Anestesiol 2012;78(11):1309–1310
37. Gnaho A, Eyrieux S, Gentili M. Cardiac arrest during an ultrasound-guided sciatic nerve block combined with nerve stimulation. Reg Anesth Pain Med 2009;34(3):278
38. Hübler M, Gäbler R, Ehm B, Oertel R, Gama de Abreu M, Koch T. Successful resuscitation following ropivacaine-induced systemic toxicity in a neonate. Anaesthesia 2010;65(11):1137–1140
39. Harvey M, Cave G, Chanwai G, Nicholson T. Successful resuscitation from bupivacaine-induced cardiovascular collapse with intravenous lipid emulsion following femoral nerve block in an emergency department. Emerg Med Australas 2011;23(2):209–214
40. Dix SK, Rosner GF, Nayar M, et al. Intractable cardiac arrest due to lidocaine toxicity successfully resuscitated with lipid emulsion. Crit Care Med 2011;39(4):872–874
41. Calder K, Chung B, O'Brien C, Lalonde DH. Bupivacaine digital blocks: how long is the pain relief and temperature elevation? Plast Reconstr Surg 2013;131(5):1098–1104

42. Chandran GJ, Chung B, Lalonde J, Lalonde DH. The hyperthermic effect of a distal volar forearm nerve block: a possible treatment of acute digital frostbite injuries? Plast Reconstr Surg 2010;126(3):946–950

43. Thomson CJ, Lalonde DH. Randomized double-blind comparison of duration of anesthesia among three commonly used agents in digital nerve block. Plast Reconstr Surg 2006;118(2):429–432

44. Kopin IJ. Monoamine oxidase and catecholamine metabolism. J Neural Transm Suppl 1994;41:57–67

45. Rosen SG, Linares OA, Sanfield JA, Zech LA, Lizzio VP, Halter JB. Epinephrine kinetics in humans: radiotracer methodology. J Clin Endocrinol Metab 1989;69(4):753–761

CHAPTER 7

TIPS ON EXPLAINING WALANT TO PATIENTS BEFORE SURGERY

Nikolas Alan Jagodzinski, Alistair Phillips, and Donald H. Lalonde

MANAGING PATIENT FEARS BEFORE SURGERY

- For patients, fear of the unknown and anxiety about pain are the two biggest concerns about being awake during hand surgery.

- If we explain the process to patients calmly, clearly, and with confidence, we can easily quell the fear of the unknown for most patients.

- If we inject local anesthetic almost painlessly, as described in Chapter 5, it really does make the local anesthetic injection and most upper and lower limb surgery almost pain-free, except for the initial pinch with a 27- or 30-gauge needle. The patient will be amazed at how brief and minor the discomfort is.

THINGS TO TELL PATIENTS DURING THE CONSULTATION SO THAT THEY UNDERSTAND THE PROCEDURE BETTER

- A good opening line of a consultation is: "The great thing about this operation is that it is done under local anesthesia which is much safer, quicker, and easier for you than general or regional anesthesia." This usually reassures patients that this is the norm for this procedure and not something out of the ordinary.

- "Wide awake surgery is as simple as when you go to the dentist for a filling, but usually hurts less. We put in the freezing/numbing medicine, we perform the surgery, and then you get up and go home."

- "Most patients will tell you that it is a more pleasant experience than going to the dentist"[1] (see ▶ Video 2.3 for patient impressions).

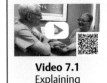

Video 7.1 Explaining WALANT to a patient.

Video 7.2 More things to tell patients to remove fear of the unknown.

THINGS TO TELL PATIENTS ABOUT PREPARING FOR THE DAY OF SURGERY (QUOTES OF THE EXACT WORDS WE SAY TO PATIENTS)

- You will not need to undergo any tests before surgery. That means you do not need to leave work or pay a babysitter to go for tests on the day before your surgery. You just need to arrive on the day of surgery.

- You do not have to stop taking any medication before surgery.

- You do not have to fast before surgery or change any diabetic treatment routine.

- The usual amount of time you will be in the hospital is the time of surgery plus 30 to 40 minutes to inject the local anesthesia and give it time to work.

- Bring a book to read or your phone to pass the 30 minutes minimum it takes for ideal local anesthesia to work.

- After the surgery, there is no need to wait around in the hospital to recover. You just get up and go home.

- You do not need to get undressed (for patients for whom field sterility will be used, see Chapter 10). You will simply roll up your sleeve and have the surgery. You may want to wear short sleeves or a loose long-sleeve shirt so the bandage fits in easily. If you had an operation under regional or general anesthesia you would need to undress and change into a hospital gown.

- You can bring in earphones/music, a movie, or a virtual reality device to use during the surgery if you want.

- Technically, you could drive a car home after your surgery because you did not get sedation. However, you are "impaired," since you will only have one normally functioning hand. Because you are not used to this situation, driving may not be safe. If you were in an accident and it was your fault, it would be hard for you to justify in court that you were driving with one hand impaired, even if you were sedation-free and pain-free while the local anesthetic was still working.

- You will not need to have someone stay with you the evening of surgery, because you will not have had sedation. It will be safe for you to be alone with your children or elderly parents the evening of surgery. If you were to have sedation, the hospital would tell you that you need to have someone stay with you at home the evening of surgery.

FOR PATIENTS WHO ARE AFRAID OF NEEDLES (QUOTES OF THE EXACT WORDS WE SAY TO PATIENTS)

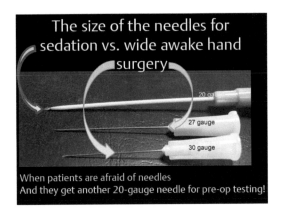

Fig. 7.1 Comparison of the relative size of needles for sedation and wide awake hand surgery. The 20-gauge cannula is used for sedation; a 20-gauge needle is used for preoperative testing. The 27-gauge or 30-gauge needles are used for WALANT.

- We will not put in an intravenous needle in your hand so you will avoid that unnecessary pain in your unoperated hand.

- You will be amazed at how little the freezing/numbing medicine hurts when we put it in slowly with a tiny needle. Most people just feel one little needle prick in the hand, and then they feel no pain at all (see Chapter 5).

- The needle prick you will feel will be smaller than the sting of an intravenous insertion if we were using a general anesthetic because we use a much smaller needle.

- *For those who are especially afraid of needles and therefore request sedation:* If you have sedation, you will have two needle sticks with bigger needles than the single prick you will feel if we numb you with a local anesthetic. You get two bigger needles if you want to be asleep: the first larger one is for blood tests, then you get another one with an intravenous line inserted to put you to sleep.

- In ▶ Video 7.3, a patient describes the impression of pain of a local anesthetic needle for trapeziectomy versus the pain of intravenous needle insertion. This patient just had 40 mL of local anesthetic to numb up the radial hand, as described in Chapter 5 and Chapter 27.

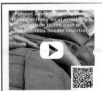

Video 7.3 Patient compares the pain of trapeziectomy local anesthesia injection to the pain of intravenous line insertion.

THINGS TO TELL PATIENTS ABOUT THE DAY OF SURGERY (QUOTES OF THE EXACT WORDS WE SAY TO PATIENTS)

- You will be amazed at how little the freezing/numbing medicine hurts when we put it in slowly with a tiny needle. Most people just feel one little needle prick in the hand, and then they feel no pain at all (see Chapter 5).

- You will have time to talk to me before and while we inject the local anesthetic. We inject it slowly so it will not hurt while I am injecting and we can talk comfortably.

- Occasionally, people become faint when they get a needle. Has this ever happened to you? We inject local anesthesia while you are lying down to avoid this. If you tend to faint, we will tilt the stretcher so your head is lower than your feet, and this will help to prevent your fainting.

- After we finish the injection, you may feel a bit jittery, as if you have had too much coffee, or like you are a little nervous. It is not your nerves. It is because there is a little adrenaline in the numbing medicine, and these feelings are completely normal and not dangerous. If it does happen, the shaky feeling goes away all by itself in 5 to 30 minutes. This is a normal reaction to adrenaline, and you are not allergic to it.

- You will then go back to the waiting room to give the numbing medicine time to work for at least half an hour. You can read, play on your phone, or listen to music.

- You do not have to worry about what will happen to you because you are awake. You can just ask us anything at any time during or after surgery and we will gladly explain things to you or solve any problems you might have.

- It is very uncommon for anyone to feel pain during the surgery, but if you did, you would just tell me and I would add more local anesthetic.

- All you will feel is the cold and wet of us washing your hand and maybe a little pulling and tugging during the surgery.

- If you have a sore shoulder or back, let us know and we will help you adjust to a more comfortable position, such as on your side, during the surgery. We can't do that when you are sedated because we cannot know if your body is in a painful position.

- We will not be putting any uncomfortable tourniquet on your arm (for those who have had experience with a tourniquet or have heard about it).

- You can watch the surgery if you wish. Many patients do enjoy watching parts of the surgery. Some tell their friends that watching the surgery should be on their "bucket list." However, you do not have to watch anything if you do not want to.

- While operating, we can also discuss details about how you should care for your hand after the surgery. You will remember our discussions because you are not sedated.

- After the surgery, you will just get up and go home with your hand held higher than your heart. Your hand will be "on strike" for 2 or 3 days. We don't want you to move your fingers during that time so you do not bleed inside the wound. This will also allow the swelling to go away and will decrease your pain.

- You will not have nausea and you will not vomit because you are not sedated.

- You will not have trouble urinating after surgery because you are not sedated.

- *For tendon or bone reconstruction patients:* You will be able to help me get a better result. After I fix your tendon/bone, you can move it to make sure it is working properly. Sometimes I need to adjust what I have done because your repaired tendon does not want to fit in the tunnel it lives in after I fix it. If you move your broken finger after I fix it, I can be sure that I have it straight. We are more likely to get a good result if you are awake to help me get it right. You cannot move it if you are asleep or sedated during the procedure.

REGIONAL ANESTHESIA VERSUS WALANT PATIENT EDUCATION (QUOTES OF THE EXACT WORDS WE SAY TO PATIENTS)

- Staying awake is safer than sedation because the safest sedation is no sedation. This is especially important for you because of your other medical problems (such as your lung problem …).

- Sometimes, regional anesthesia blocks do not work. Because of this, you will still need all of the preoperative anesthetic appointments, blood tests, fasting, getting undressed, etc. in case you need sedation or general anesthesia as a backup to a failed regional block.

- We don't use a tourniquet in WALANT. Under regional anesthesia with a tourniquet, it can be sometimes painful in spite of the block. Even with the best regional block, tourniquet pain can be significant after 90 minutes. Any tourniquet pain can cause the patient to squirm about to try and get comfortable. Uncomfortable patients make it harder for the surgeons to do their job well and easier for surgical mistakes to occur.

- In one study, patients who had bilateral carpal tunnel surgery with intravenous regional anesthesia (Bier block) on one side and WALANT on the other side preferred the WALANT side.[1]

Reference

1. Ayhan E, Akaslan F. Patients' perspective on carpal tunnel release with WALANT or intravenous regional anesthesia. Plast Reconstr Surg 2020;145(5):1197–1203

CHAPTER 8

TEACHING PATIENTS AND RESIDENTS DURING SURGERY DECREASES COMPLICATIONS

Donald H. Lalonde and Duncan McGrouther

TALKING TO PATIENTS DURING SURGERY CAN BE A GAME CHANGER

- Talking to patients during surgery not only gives them something to think about and puts their minds at ease, but also provides them with information about all aspects of their problem, the likely course of recovery and rehabilitation, and gives you the opportunity to address any questions they may have.

- During the years when we performed hand surgery with sedation, there was no point in educating patients during the surgery. They would not remember what we told them because of mind-altering drugs. With each passing year of wide awake hand surgery, it is becoming more and more apparent *that patient education during surgery is very helpful in many ways.* You can educate your patients about postoperative care and how to avoid complications while you are operating, and this is a better use of your time than talking with the nurses about the weather.

- The time you spend talking to patients during the surgery is time you do not need to spend with them in the office before or after the surgery.

Video 8.1 Advice to patient during skin cancer excision in the hand.

- Investing time to educate the patient during the surgery will save the time that would be lost on complications that may occur because the patient did not know how to look after his or her hand postoperatively. When the surgeon stresses the importance of keeping the hand elevated for a couple of days after surgery, patients are much less likely to walk around with their hand dangling down. This decreases internal bleeding, swelling, and pain. It enables patients to get off all pain medicine sooner.

- Educated patients understand the importance of their rehabilitation protocols, are more likely to be compliant with postoperative instructions, and may require fewer follow-up appointments.

- You often find out important details about the patient's life and activities that you did not learn about in the initial consultation, especially in trauma patients.

- Patients love personal education in a nonrushed fashion from their surgeon. They are able to develop a one-on-one bond with you that was not possible in the days when sedation meant they had no memory of the procedure, and they did not feel that they were an active participant in the process.

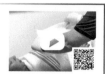

Video 8.2 Advice to patient during prepping for a hand fracture pinning.

- Also see ▶ Video 14.1 and ▶ Video 14.2 for patient education during local anesthesia injection during carpal tunnel surgery.

INTRAOPERATIVE EDUCATION ABOUT HOW TO TAKE PAIN MEDICINE FOR MOST HAND OPERATIONS

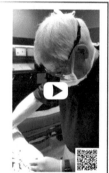

- Intraoperative education is a useful strategy to simply educate patients on the fact that all they will need for most operations is ibuprofen or acetaminophen.[1,2]

- Dr Lalonde and most European, Asian, and South American surgeons never prescribe narcotics after carpal tunnel surgery and patients do very well without them. See how he explains this to patients during surgery in ▶ Video 8.3a. This is also applicable to most other minor hand operations.

- In ▶ Video 8.3b, a patient is given intraoperative advice during Dupuytren's contracture release. See the intraoperative advice and the postoperative patient result of good intraoperative education on how to take pain medicine properly.

Video 8.3a Explaining how to take pain medicine after carpal tunnel surgery to avoid the need for narcotics.

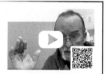

Video 8.3b Explaining how to take post-op pain medication during Dupuytren's surgery.

DIRECT QUOTES TO PATIENTS ON PAIN MANAGEMENT

- What do you normally take for pain for a headache? Advil? Tylenol?
  If they say Advil or Tylenol, I tell them that is all they are going to need when the local anesthesia comes out in 4 to 5 hours.[2,3] You can take up

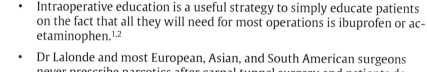

to 800 mg of Advil or Motrin (ibuprofen) and up to 1 g of Tylenol (acetaminophen) when the numbing medicine wears off. You can take ibuprofen and acetaminophen at the same time, because the two medications work in different ways.

- There are two kinds of pain with any operation: (1) the pain of the cut, and (2) the pain of "Gee, doctor, now it only hurts when I put my hand down or when I move." The pain of the cut lasts a day or two, and you can take Advil or Tylenol for that pain. Stop taking pain medicine as soon as you get into the pain of "Gee, doctor, now it only hurts when I put my hand down or when I move" and listen to your body. That pain is your friend. It is your body telling you, "Hey there, I am not ready for that. I am trying to heal in here and you are screwing it up! Stop that!" That little voice inside your head is one that you should listen to. You can't hear that little voice in your head if you have ibuprofen in your ears!

- This is called pain-guided healing. It is alco called common sense or instinct. Just don't do what hurts!

- We did not spend 2 billion years evolving pain because it is bad for us; it is our body's only way of telling us how to behave so we can heal faster.

- Don't baby your hand, but don't do anything that hurts. If you try to do something and it does hurt, don't try it again that afternoon. Do not try it again for 2 or 3 days. Healing takes days and weeks, not minutes and hours. You will get better faster if you listen to your body. It is very wise. It will tell you what you can and cannot do, but the only language it speaks is pain.

- Don't put your hand down and do things with it until you are off ALL pain medicine so you KNOW what hurts, and until it does not hurt to put it down and do things.

- See ▶ Video 36.6 for patient education on pain management in distal interphalangeal (DIP) joint fusion surgery.

DIRECT QUOTES TO PATIENTS ON HAND ELEVATION AND IMMOBILIZATION

- Keep your hand higher than your heart for the next day or two. Consider that it is "on strike."

- Don't move your fingers or put your hand down until all of the numbing medicine is gone and until you are off all pain medications and you KNOW what hurts.

- If you keep your hand up and quiet, it will swell less, hurt less, and bleed less inside. Treat it like a sleeping baby. Don't disturb it! If you walk around with your hand dangling down, it will swell more, bleed more inside, hurt more, and take you longer to get better. Internal bleeding makes a clot and it takes weeks for your body to dissolve it. This slows recovery.

- The look of your hand will be like a report card. If you come in here in 3 days with a swollen sore hand, it is because you have not been keeping it higher than your heart, and you have been walking around with your hand dangling down. If you come in here with both hands looking the same, it is because you listened to the rules and kept your hand higher than your heart. You will get better much faster.

INTRAOPERATIVE ADVICE QUOTES TO PATIENTS ON SHOWERING, BANDAGING, AND INFECTION FOR MOST SOFT TISSUE HAND OPERATIONS (CARPAL TUNNEL, DUPUYTREN'S, ETC.)

- You can remove your "Hollywood" bandage (a 3-inch gauze roll so named because it is mostly applied for its visual effect) before you take a shower tomorrow with a naked hand. There is no problem with getting your wound wet in the shower. It is a myth that you can't water fresh wounds; fresh wounds love running water. You don't need to rub soap in it, but it is OK to let soap or shampoo run over it. After the shower, you can gently pat the wound site dry with a towel. Put on a clean, dry bandage and reuse or recycle the Hollywood bandage over the Band-Aid. The bandage does not need to be sterile, just clean.

- The Hollywood bandage is only there for visual effects to remind you and those around you that you can't do the things you normally do because you have had an operation. They will not shake your hand or ask you to do something that may hurt your hand. Stop using the outer bandage in 3 to 7 days.

- When the liquid stops oozing out, the germs cannot swim into your wound, and no bandage is required. You may want to keep the bandage on for the Hollywood effect for sympathy or to protect yourself from small children and eager hand-shakers.

Video 8.4
Intraoperative advice on showering and bandaging after carpal tunnel, trigger finger.

- Also see ▶ Video 9.5 for good advice on elevation, pain medicine, pain-guided healing, activity, and showering for an 8-year-old during the surgery.

- Redness on or around the incision is normal; redness less than the width of your thumb is healthy inflammation. The redness means that your body is bringing more blood to the wound edges to help with healing. Bruising in your forearm can also be normal. Infection is uncommon after a carpal tunnel procedure. Signs of infection include redness that goes all over your palm and up your forearm, with more and more pain in the incision instead of less and less pain, fever, chills, and real pus coming out of the wound (as opposed to a little clear liquid or blood in the first 2 or 3 days, which is normal).

EXAMPLES OF WAYS INTRAOPERATIVE PATIENT EDUCATION DECREASES THEIR RISK OF POSTOPERATIVE COMPLICATIONS AND REOPERATION

- With complicated procedures such as a flexor tendon repairs or K-wired finger fractures, patients leave the operating room with a full understanding of how to take good care of their hand after surgery to get a better result. They understand that if they move the hand too much, the repair will fall apart. If they do not move it at all, everything will become stuck and they may need a second operation to improve stiffness.

- Talking with patients during flexor tendon repair about how to look after their hand after surgery can decrease your rupture and tenolysis rates (see ▶ Video 19.7a and ▶ Video 19.7c).

- A 10-year-old is given advice in ▶ Video 8.5 during flexor tendon repair about how to look after the finger in the days after surgery. ▶ Video 9.3 shows this patient's whole care.

- See ▶ Video 15.2 to see a surgeon and therapist explaining the Saint John postoperative flexor tendon repair protocol to a patient during surgery.

- Talking with patients during finger fracture repair about how to look after their hand after surgery can decrease your stiff finger rate.

- ▶ Video 41.1 shows how patient education starts during injection of local anesthesia for a finger fracture K-wiring. ▶ Video 41.8 shows more intraoperative education in the same patient at the end of the case. His result at 4 weeks is shown in ▶ Video 41.TT6.

- Patients know when their fingers look crooked; they have been looking at their own fingers for years. They can tell you if you have properly reduced their crooked finger before you leave the operating room as in ▶ Video 41.6. If it is still crooked, you can fix it right there and then so you don't need to come back.

- In ▶ Video 41.9, advice is given to another K-wired finger fracture patient.

Video 8.5
Intraoperative advice to a 10-year-old on how to look after her hand after surgery (for more on this patient, see ▶ Video 9.3).

Video 8.6
Intraoperative education to patient having distal interphalangeal (DIP) joint fusion.

THINGS NOT TO SAY AND NOT TO DO TO A PATIENT DURING SURGERY

- Never say something like "Oops." Create an atmosphere of calm, efficiency, and competence.

- A totally silent frowning surgeon may seem scary to patients, while one who speaks too much without listening can also fail to reassure. The good doctor version of the "bedside manner" is the "operating table side manner." Treat patients with kindness and useful information that you would like to have if you were the patient.

- Do not ask the scrub nurse for things with scary words like knife, blade, scalpel. Use terms like "a number 15."

- Do not pass bloody swabs or instruments in front of the patient if you can avoid it.

THINGS TO SAY TO PATIENTS WHEN YOU BEGIN THE INJECTION OF LOCAL ANESTHETIC

- It is good to begin with a calm, comfortable conversation about weather, family, or football before you inject the local anesthetic. Wait to focus on talking about the hand until the patient is more relaxed.

- Your instructions to the patient should be polite and simply worded:
  - "Can you please lie down comfortably on your side? Would you kindly place your hand flat on the stretcher?"
  - "Try not to move when I put the needle in. If you pull away (which is normal when you get a little sting), the needle will come out before the medicine goes in, and I will need to put the needle in a second time. If you hold still, you will only feel one little stick instead of two. I will help you by holding your hand and counting to three. OK? At the count of two, take a nice deep breath. When I get to three, try not to move...." (see Chapter 5 for minimal pain injection tips).

- After you have started putting in the lidocaine and epinephrine, and the pain is completely gone, tell the patient it will take a little while for you to finish putting in the numbing medicine. "If I do it slowly, it will not hurt at all."

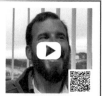

Video 8.7 Patient's impression of intraoperative education after initial fear of being awake.

- As you inject the local anesthetic and have confirmed that the patient will no longer be feeling pain during the injection process, ask whether he or she has any questions about the surgery or about the care of the hand, when to go back to work, and other postsurgery issues. Take this 5-minute opportunity to answer questions and to tell the patient how to look after the hand after surgery.

EDUCATING TRAINEES TO PERFORM WALANT SURGERY

- If you are teaching residents or medical students during the surgery, say positive things like "Well done! That was a perfect stitch," and so on. You may not normally be this complimentary to trainees, but patients are reassured when you like what the trainee is doing. This attitude goes a long way toward increasing patient's confidence in the surgical teaching event.

- If you don't like what the resident is doing, nonverbal communication such as covering the wound with your hand is very effective.

- Say things such as "I know that some surgeons like to use the scissors this way when they do this part of the operation, but I like to use them this way, because ..." as you take over the surgery.

- Softly saying, "Pause ...here is another way I use to get to the same goal" is also a good way to stop the action as you put your hand over the wound and take over the instruments.

- This is clearly not the time or the place to reprimand a resident.

- Teachers and trainees both like the "no-rush" environment of the no tourniquet time clock. It is more conducive to comfortable learning because the hurried approach of limiting tourniquet time creates unnecessary anxiety.[3]

References

1. Alter TH, Ilyas AM. A prospective randomized study analyzing preoperative opioid counseling in pain management after carpal tunnel release surgery. J Hand Surg Am 2017;42(10):810–815
2. Ilyas AM, Miller AJ, Graham JG, Matzon JLA. A prospective, randomized, double-blinded trial comparing acetaminophen, ibuprofen, and oxycodone for pain management after hand surgery. Orthopedics 2019;42(2):110–115
3. Tang JB, Xing SG, Ayhan E, Hediger S, Huang S. Impact of wide-awake local anesthesia no tourniquet on departmental settings, cost, patient and surgeon satisfaction, and beyond. Hand Clin 2019;35(1):29–34

CHAPTER 9

TIPS ON GOOD LOCAL ANESTHESIA IN INFANTS AND CHILDREN

Donald H. Lalonde, Geoffrey Cook, Steven Koehler, and Chao Chen

HOW TO EXPLAIN WALANT TO CHILDREN BEFORE YOU INJECT THE LOCAL ANESTHETIC

- Most reasonable children do very well with WALANT hand surgery.[1] The key is to provide good local anesthesia (see Chapter 5) with a skillful injection so that all they feel is a minor single sting of a 30-gauge or smaller gauge needle. The other necessary skill is the ability to make them feel comfortable with your attitude and words.

- The most important factor in gaining the patient's trust and cooperation is how you talk to the child before you inject the local anesthetic. Using a calm, soft-spoken voice with a gentle manner and engaging conversation is very helpful. If you are not comfortable having a nice prolonged conversation with the child, perhaps you should plan on performing the surgery with the patient under general anesthesia.

- The child must be old enough to understand your explanation and to hold still while you insert the first needle.

- If you can get the child to hold still to tolerate the stick of a 30-gauge needle in the finger or hand, you can perform the surgery with WALANT.

Video 9.1 Local injection in the thumb of a 4-year-old girl (Lalonde, Canada).

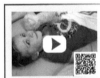

Video 9.2 Flexor tendon repair in a 6-year-old girl with patient impressions at 13 years of age (Lalonde, Canada).

THE FOLLOWING CONVERSATION WORKS WELL WITH CHILDREN

"Do you believe in magic?"

Most children will say "No." If they say "yes," the same conversation can happen.

Video 9.3
Explaining "magic medicine" injection of local anesthesia to an 8-year-old for redo trigger thumb (Lalonde, Canada).

Video 9.4 Talking to the 8-year-old in Video 9.3 during the surgery so that she is comfortable (Lalonde, Canada).

Video 9.5
Postoperative advice given to the mother and 8-year-old in Video 9.3 during the surgery (Lalonde, Canada).

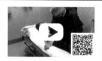

Video 9.6 Flexor tendon injection in a 10-year-old (Lalonde, Canada).

"Neither do I (or I don't), but today I am going to show you some real magic. I am going to put some magic medicine underneath your skin. After I put it there, I will be able to fix your finger and it WILL NOT HURT AT ALL. I PROMISE YOU.

The only problem with putting in the magic medicine is that you have to feel one tiny needle to get the medicine in there. All you need to do is hold still and not move.

I will help you by holding your hand.

If you pull your hand away before the medicine goes in, the needle will come out and I will have to stick it back in.

If you hold still, you will only feel one little short sting. If you move, you will feel two stings.

Do you think you can hold still?"

- If the child gets a totally panicked look in the eyes that indicates he or she cannot hold still for the injection, general anesthesia is advisable.

- You need to keep your promise by making certain that all the child feels is the first sting, as shown in Chapter 5. Be sure that you have more than enough volume of anesthetic rather than not enough. Children should NEVER have to have "top-ups."

- I usually have my body between the patient's eyes and his or her hands. Note that in ▶ Video 9.3, my body is in an awkward position on the wrong side of the table for this video so that you can see the patient and the injection.

- After you inject the local anesthetic, this is what you can tell the patient:

  "I told you all you would feel was one little stick and then no pain.

  I was not lying, was I?"

  They say, "No."

  "I am not lying now. The surgery will not hurt you one little bit now that the magic medicine is in there."

- You can establish a wonderful relationship with most children during WALANT surgery.

- You can avoid all the risks and inconveniences of pediatric sedation and general anesthesia for many, if not most, cases.

- The same benefits of the patient's seeing active movement in an operation such as flexor tendon repair or a finger fracture hold true for children as for adults.

WALANT HAND SURGERY FOR BABIES

- For accessory finger nubbins in a newborn, have the mothers start to feed the infants for a minute or two until they are in that "feeding zone trance."

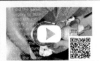

- Gently massage and pinch the skin for 30 seconds before inserting the needle so the feeding child is used to someone touching his or her hand.

- Pinch while pushing the skin up into the needle (see Chapter 5) and keep pinching until you see the skin blanch and you know the needle site is numb.

Video 9.7 Details of local anesthesia to remove extra digits in newborn (both hands and feet in this case) (Lalonde, Canada).

- Pinch the skin into the tip of a half inch 30-gauge needle to the depth of just below the dermis at a point just proximal to the extra digit base. Inject enough 1% lidocaine with 1:100,000 epinephrine with 10% by volume of 8.4% bicarbonate so that you can see the tissue swell up under the nubbin. The needle pain momentarily distracts the baby from drinking milk, but he or she usually just carries on feeding quickly because the discomfort is brief and minor. Do hold the hand gently but firmly in case the child does move.

- Do the surgery in the mother's arms with the baby sleeping as they often do when they finish eating.

- The younger they are, the better it is, because they fall asleep after they eat as a newborn. Dr Lalonde likes 2 weeks of age to give the parents a little time to adapt to the baby first.

Video 9.8 Excision of a fifth finger nubbin in a 4-week-old baby (Lalonde, Canada).

- Parents really appreciate avoiding general anesthesia in their babies and infants.

TIPS AND TRICKS FOR PEDIATRIC WALANT HAND SURGERY

- Start with a 30-gauge needle and a 3-mL syringe instead of a 27-gauge needle.

- Have the local anesthetic in your pocket, out of sight and ready to inject, without the child seeing the syringe. Have the child look away before you take the syringe out of your pocket and while you insert the needle.

Video 9.9 Extensor tendon repair in 7-year-old and patient's impressions 10 years later (Cook, Canada).

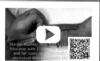

Video 9.10 Plating mid radius and ulna fractures in a 12-year old (Koehler, USA).

Video 9.11 Tenolysis in a 4-year-old distracted by a video on a phone (Chen, China).

- Simply pressing firmly on the skin proximal to where you will insert the needle can create sensory input "noise" that decreases the pain felt by the patient. (See Chapter 5 for a list of rules on how to inject local anesthetic with minimal pain.)

NO TOURNIQUET FOR CASES IN WHICH A GENERAL ANESTHETIC IS ADMINISTERED

- The benefits of epinephrine vasoconstriction and painless awakening from the lidocaine also apply when patients are asleep.

- For pediatric repair of a trigger thumb performed under general anesthesia, inject under the skin at the center of the incision until you see the tissues are a little swollen and firm. Usually no more than 1 mL is required in these tiny thumbs.

- For operations like syndactyly in which children will be having general anesthesia, you can still avoid the tourniquet and let-down bleeding. As soon as the anesthesiologist has the child asleep and lets you proceed, inject the lidocaine with epinephrine wherever you will dissect. Then you can go scrub and prep the patient. By the time you make the first incision, the epinephrine will have started to work.

COMMUNICATION AND INJECTION SKILLS

With a little practice in communication and injection techniques, most hand surgeons can easily provide almost pain-free local anesthesia to children to make their hand surgery experience and that of their parents a safe, pleasurable, and educational one.

Reference

1. Wang HC, Lin GT. Percutaneous release for trigger thumb in children under general and local anesthesia. Kaohsiung J Med Sci 2004;20(11):546–551

CHAPTER 10

MOVING SURGERY OUT OF THE MAIN OPERATING ROOM WITH EVIDENCE-BASED FIELD STERILITY

Donald H. Lalonde, Nikolas Alan Jagodzinski, and Robert E. Van Demark, Jr.

FIELD STERILITY VERSUS FULL STERILITY

- In this book, *field sterility*, as shown below, means creating a localized sterile field with four towels or a small 40 × 40 cm drape with a hole in it. We only expose and sterilize the part we are operating on or need to see move during the surgery. The surgeon has a mask and sterile gloves, but no sterile gown. Laminar airflow is not required.

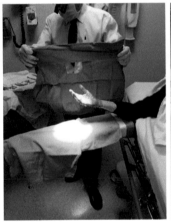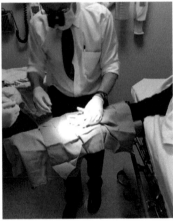

Fig. 10.1 Most carpal tunnel procedures in Canada are performed with field sterility in a minor procedure room outside of the main operating room.[1]

- In this book, *full sterility* means standard operating room (OR) full draping with the entire patient covered in sterile drapes, with surgeons and nurses in sterile operating gowns, caps, masks, and gloves.

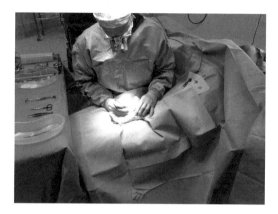

Fig. 10.2 Full sterility for carpal tunnel procedures in the main operating room is still commonly used in many cities of the world outside of Canada.

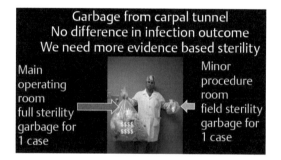

Fig. 10.3 Main operating room sterility for carpal tunnel procedures produces 10 times as much trash, is four times more expensive, and is not different in infection outcome when compared with field sterility in procedure rooms.

CUSTOM-BASED STERILITY VERSUS EVIDENCE-BASED STERILITY

- Custom-based sterility is based on concept like: "If some sterility is good, more must be better," and "We have always done it this way." This has led to evidence-free standards of care in the way much sterility is practiced today. Example: Blue OR hats have more bacteria than pink OR hats.

- Evidence-based sterility is based in science with studies looking at true infection rates with different levels of sterility, and an examination of the cost–benefit ratio of outcomes as they affect patients.

- Infection after a total knee prosthesis can result in loss of the implant and osteomyelitis with great morbidity and cost to patients. The cost of full OR sterility is clearly justified in this case.

- Infection after carpal tunnel surgery with field sterility is rare and usually responds to suture removal and oral antibiotics with very little morbidity and cost to the patient. Space suit sterility is not justifiable in view of patient cost or morbidity.

- How much sterility is required for different operations needs to be looked at in this type of evidence-based context. For an in-depth look at the evidence behind main OR sterility, Google "Lalonde's evidence-based sterility" and you will get the following open access review article.[2]

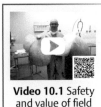

Video 10.1 Safety and value of field sterility for minor hand surgery.

FULL STERILITY VERSUS FIELD STERILITY FOR MINOR HAND SURGERY PROCEDURES: WHAT IS THE INFECTION EVIDENCE?

- What is the evidence for field sterility infection in hand surgery? In a prospective consecutive series of 1,504 field sterility carpal tunnel procedures in 5 North American cities by 6 surgeons,[3] only 6 patients developed superficial infections, none of which required incision and drainage; no intravenous antibiotics were given, no reoperation was necessary, and none of the patients required hospital admission. Two infections resolved with suture removal and no antibiotics, and only four patients required oral antibiotics. None of these patients had been given preoperative antibiotics. The infection rate in the 1,504 case series was 0.39%, almost identical to the Mohs 20,821 case series described below.[4]

- A second prospective series of 1,035 minor hand surgery cases with field sterility[5,6] produced an infection rate of 1.1% with very little morbidity in the few infected patients. All responded to oral antibiotic therapy. Out of the 11 infected patients, 8 were insulin-dependent diabetics.

- A retrospective series comparing main OR versus procedure room carpal tunnel surgery revealed no difference in infection rates, but a 10 times greater expense in the main OR.[7]

- Closed reduction and field sterility K-wiring of hand fractures in two comparative studies in USA showed the same infection rates as full main OR sterility.[16,17] Both studies showed increased efficiency and cost saving of the field sterility groups. A third study of K-wiring fractures in a New York emergency room also showed safe infection levels.[18]

- Plastic surgeons and dermatologists all over the world have excised small skin cancers and benign lesions with field sterility outside the main OR for well over 80 years, with no significant infection issues. The standard of care of Mohs surgery skin cancer excision in the United States and around the world is field sterility outside the main OR. A recent prospective American cohort study of 20,871 cases of Mohs surgery with field sterility revealed an infection rate of 0.37% with only 78 infections.[1] This infection rate is almost identical to the 1,504 case series field sterility carpal tunnel infection rate discussed above.

- The blood supply to the hand is excellent, which is why most hand lacerations sutured in the emergency department do not develop infection, even though many of those lacerations occurred in severely contaminated hands. Before such lacerations occur, injured patients get no prepping and draping and yet infection is still uncommon.

- When antibiotics such as cephalosporins are required, they can be given orally with 90% of the bioavailability of the intravenous route in 30 minutes.[13,14,15,23]

MAIN OPERATING ROOM STERILITY VERSUS FIELD STERILITY FOR MINOR HAND SURGERY PROCEDURES: WHAT IS THE FINANCIAL AND PATIENT MORBIDITY COST?

- Cost savings to the patients are enormous in minor hand surgery procedures such as carpal tunnel, trigger finger, and K-wiring fractures[4,5,6,11,12,19,20,21,22] (see Chapter 2 and Chapter 11).

- One study revealed that minor procedure room WALANT carpal tunnel surgery was twice as efficient and cost one quarter the cost of main OR WALANT surgery, even without the anesthesiology costs.[24]

- Canadian surgeons perform simple hand trauma operations in Calgary, Saskatoon, Ottawa, Saint John, and many other cities with field sterility. These Canadian hand surgeons are repairing tendons and K-wiring most fractures outside the main OR in clinical procedure rooms, Monday through Friday, 8 AM to 5 PM. Calgary has dedicated field sterility clinic trauma rooms on weekend daytime hours as well. Patients get a better tendon repair at 2 PM than at 2 AM when surgeons and nurses are sleepy.

- The patient morbidity in field sterility, WALANT carpal tunnel and trigger finger operations in minor procedure rooms is minimal. The patient doesn't need to suffer the embarrassment of getting undressed and being transported on a stretcher. There is no unnecessary monitoring. There is no uncomfortable intravenous insertion. He or she simply rolls up a sleeve and has the surgery in a minor procedure room like at the dentist. He or she then gets up and goes home.

- We can wash very dirty hand injuries in the emergency department with tap water after numbing the hand. There is level I evidence that this is as effective as sterile saline.[25]

- See US patient's and surgeon's impressions of instituting minor procedure room sterility in their practice in ▶ Video 12.1.

WHEN DO WE USE THE MAIN OPERATING ROOM WITH FULL STERILITY FOR HAND SURGERY?

- We perform most of our hand surgeries in the clinic or office because using the main OR is much slower and much more expensive; the only added benefit is absolute sterility.

- The only time we perform WALANT procedures in the main OR is when we need full sterility because infection would be very detrimental to patients. Examples of cases that we take to the main OR are permanent implant cases such as plates, screws, and joint replacements.

References

1. Peters B, Giuffre JL. Canadian trends in carpal tunnel surgery. J Hand Surg Am 2018;43(11):1035.e1–1035.e8
2. Yu J, Ji TA, Craig M, McKee D, Lalonde DH. Evidence-based sterility: the evolving role of field sterility in skin and minor hand surgery. Plast Reconstr Surg Glob Open 2019;7(11):e2481
3. Leblanc MR, Lalonde DH, Thoma A, et al. Is main operating room sterility really necessary in carpal tunnel surgery? A multicenter prospective study of minor procedure room field sterility surgery. Hand (N Y) 2011;6(1):60–63
4. Alam M, Ibrahim O, Nodzenski M, et al. Adverse events associated with Mohs micrographic surgery: multicenter prospective cohort study of 20,821 cases at 23 centers. JAMA Dermatol 2013;149(12):1378–1385
5. Hashemi K, Blakeley CJ. Wound infections in day-case hand surgery: a prospective study. Ann R Coll Surg Engl 2004;86(6):449–450
6. Jagodzinski NA, Ibish S, Furniss D. Surgical site infection after hand surgery outside the operating theatre: a systematic review. J Hand Surg Eur Vol 2017;42(3):289–294
7. Halvorson AJ, Sechriest VF II, Gravely A, DeVries AS. Risk of surgical site infection after carpal tunnel release performed in an operating room versus a clinic-based procedure room within a Veterans Affairs medical center. Am J Infect Control 2020;48(2):173–177
8. Sieber D, Lacey A, Fletcher J, Kalliainen L. Cost savings using minimal draping for routine hand procedures. Minn Med 2014;97(9):49
9. Bismil M, Bismil Q, Harding D, Harris P, Lamyman E, Sansby L. Transition to total one-stop wide-awake hand surgery service-audit: a retrospective review. JRSM Short Rep 2012;3(4):23
10. Chatterjee A, McCarthy JE, Montagne SA, Leong K, Kerrigan CL. A cost, profit, and efficiency analysis of performing carpal tunnel surgery in the operating room versus the clinic setting in the United States. Ann Plast Surg 2011;66(3):245–248
11. Gillis JA, Williams JG. Cost analysis of percutaneous fixation of hand fractures in the main operating room versus the ambulatory setting. J Plast Reconstr Aesthet Surg 2017;70(8):1044–1050
12. Steve AK, Schrag CH, Kuo A, Harrop AR. Metacarpal fracture fixation in a minor surgery setting versus main operating room: a cost-minimization analysis. Plast Reconstr Surg Glob Open 2019;7(7):e2298
13. Verhaegen J, Verbist L. Oral cephalosporins. Acta Clin Belg 1992;47(6):377–386
14. Apocephalex monograph used for the Saint John Regional Hospital Pharmacy Department accessed April 14, 2020 https://pdf.hres.ca/dpd_pm/00046862.PDF
15. Keflex product monograph used by the Saint John Regional Hospital Pharmacy Department accessed April 14, 2020 https://pdf.hres.ca/dpd_pm/00045523.PDF
16. Dua K, Blevins CJ, O'Hara NN, Abzug JM. The safety and benefits of the semi-sterile technique for closed reduction and percutaneous pinning of pediatric upper extremity fractures. Hand (N Y) 2019;14(6):808–813

17. Garon MT, Massey P, Chen A, Carroll T, Nelson BG, Hollister AM. Cost and complications of percutaneous fixation of hand fractures in a procedure room versus the operating room. Hand (N Y) 2018;13(4):428–434

18. Starker I, Eaton RG. Kirschner wire placement in the emergency room. Is there a risk? J Hand Surg [Br] 1995;20(4):535–538

19. Kazmers NH, Stephens AR, Presson AP, Yu Z, Tyser AR. Cost implications of varying the surgical setting and anesthesia type for trigger finger release surgery. Plast Reconstr Surg Glob Open 2019;7(5):e2231

20. Thiel CL, Fiorin Carvalho R, Hess L, et al. Minimal custom pack design and wide-awake hand surgery: reducing waste and spending in the orthopedic operating room. Hand (N Y) 2019;14(2):271–276

21. Albert MG, Rothkopf DM. Operating room waste reduction in plastic and hand surgery. Plast Surg (Oakv) 2015;23(4):235–238

22. Van Demark RE Jr, Becker HA, Anderson MC, Smith VJS. Wide-awake anesthesia in the in-office procedure room: lessons learned. Hand (N Y) 2018;13(4):481–485

23. Béïque L, Zvonar R. Addressing concerns about changing the route of antimicrobial administration from intravenous to oral in adult inpatients. Can J Hosp Pharm 2015;68(4):318–326

24. Leblanc MR, Lalonde J, Lalonde DH. A detailed cost and efficiency analysis of performing carpal tunnel surgery in the main operating room versus the ambulatory setting in Canada. Hand (N Y) 2007;2(4):173–178

25. Moscati RM, Mayrose J, Reardon RF, Janicke DM, Jehle DV. A multicenter comparison of tap water versus sterile saline for wound irrigation. Acad Emerg Med 2007;14(5):404–409

CHAPTER 11

WALANT AND VALUE IN HEALTH CARE: IMPROVING OUTCOMES AND LOWERING COST

Peter J. L. Jebson, Kevin T. K. Chan, Levi L. Hinkelman, Daniel Hess, Robert E. Van Demark, Jr., Mark Baratz, Leigh-Anne Tu, and Donald H. Lalonde

KEY POINTS

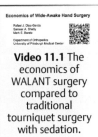

Video 11.1 The economics of WALANT surgery compared to traditional tourniquet surgery with sedation.

- The cost associated with hand surgery procedures is dependent on the surgical setting and anesthetic type.

- Wide awake local anesthesia without a tourniquet (WALANT) is an established, popular, safe, and cost-effective technique for performing hand surgery.

- Simple hand procedures (carpal tunnel, trigger finger/thumb, de Quervain's, mass excision) can be safely performed using WALANT in the ambulatory or clinic procedure suite with field sterility.

- WALANT is particularly beneficial in the United States where rising health care costs are not sustainable and demonstrating value (outcome/cost) is increasingly demanded and financially rewarded.

- Although WALANT clearly demonstrates value, hand surgeons are not being reimbursed commensurately (no difference in professional fee). There is increasing interest on the part of payers to reimburse a site of service payment differential or develop alternative payment models such as bundled payments.

- In the United States, there is also a purposeful shifting of financial risk to patients. Increasing health insurance premium payments and higher co-pays and deductibles are part of an effort for patients to have "skin in the game." As a direct result, patients are becoming consumers particularly for elective "shoppable" services.

- There is a trend toward increasing transparency in health care. Payers are sharing the cost of care with the public and creating "narrow networks" of preferred providers who deliver value.

- Employers are facing unsustainable rising employee health care costs and are developing preferred provider networks to ensure they are paying for value.

- Incorporating WALANT into your practice including performing simple hand procedures in the ambulatory or clinic procedure suite delivers value for patients and payers and will give you a competitive edge in the evolving value-based care paradigm. Consider direct-to-employer offerings and negotiating site of service differential reimbursement with commercial payers. However, to do this requires a thorough understanding of your direct and indirect costs.

- Performing hand surgery using WALANT with the associated lowering of cost is particularly advantageous in risk-based reimbursement and population health management arrangements. This is particularly appealing to our primary care colleagues who are a major referral source to hand surgeons.

DECREASED PATIENT COSTS

- Patients ultimately pay for the whole cost of their health care, either directly with cash or indirectly through public taxes or private insurance plan payments. Hand surgery using WALANT is associated with lower overall cost regardless of where the surgery is performed (operating room [OR], outpatient surgery center [OSC], ambulatory, or clinic procedure suite, or office).[1]

- WALANT is associated with lower opioid consumption and lower odds of developing medical or surgical complications postoperatively compared with standard anesthesia patients.[2]

- Simple hand procedures using WALANT can be safely performed with field sterility or disposable packs and instrument trays designed to reduce the amount of opened and unused material.[3,4]

- Avoiding the OR (main OR) or OSC means less time away from work, lower child care costs, fewer parking fees, and other incidental expenses associated with an overnight or prolonged hospital stay.

- Avoiding the use of sedation permits the surgery to be performed without an anesthetist and mitigates against the development of nausea and vomiting and associated postanesthesia care unit costs.

- Many facilities (OSC or OR) require patients to have someone stay with them the evening and/or night of sedation. There are no "babysitter" requirements for patients who have wide awake surgery. Patients can go home, look after their children, and resume their normal activities without having someone accompany and monitor them as they recover from sedation.

- WALANT utilizes local anesthetic only, which is less expensive than regional or general anesthesia.

- Performing hand surgery with WALANT in the ambulatory or clinic procedural suite eliminates the need for routine intravenous antibiotics, which is not supported in the literature for clean procedures of short duration. Antibiotics for such cases would unnecessarily subject patients to increased risk (and cost) of side effects including *Clostridium difficile* colitis, urinary tract infection, and anaphylaxis. If required, oral cephalosporins have 90% of the bioavailability of their intravenous counterpart (see Chapter 10).

- Hand surgery with WALANT in the ambulatory or clinic procedural suite can be safely performed without the need for preoperative testing. Patients therefore do not incur the cost of an evaluation and testing, which often includes travel, time away from work, and/or arranging for a babysitter.[5]

- Hand surgery with WALANT in the ambulatory or clinic procedural suite can be safely performed in diabetic patients, those on anticoagulants, and those with a pacemaker with no adjustment of their medications or normal daily routines.

- A detailed direct and indirect cost analysis study determined that performing carpal tunnel, trigger finger/thumb, or de Quervain's surgery with WALANT in a clinic procedural suite using field sterility without a preoperative evaluation or intravenous antibiotics resulted in an average savings of $3,603 for trigger finger/thumb release, $3,490 for carpal tunnel release, and $3,282 for de Quervain's release compared to surgery at a traditional location (OR or OSC). This resulted in less out-of-pocket expense for patients with high co-pay and/or deductible health insurance coverage plans.[5]

- It is possible to see a patient in consultation and operate on him or her the same day as there is little or no preoperative workup required for local anesthesia. This is a significant cost saving for patients who travel long distances to the surgeon's facility.

- Intraoperative testing for tendon gapping with active movement after repair has decreased the need for and costs of reoperation for postoperative complications such as tendon rupture and tenolysis.[6,7]

- There is less risk of a wrong-site surgery with awake, nonsedated patients.

DECREASED PAYER COSTS

- WALANT is associated with lower opioid consumption.[2]

- WALANT utilizes local anesthetic only, which is less expensive than regional or general anesthesia.

- Performing simple hand surgery with WALANT in the ambulatory of clinical minor procedure room is less expensive than an OSC or hospital OR.[8,9,10,11,12,13,14,15]

- Using WALANT for hand surgery obviates the need for an anesthetist for regional or general anesthesia.

- Avoiding the use of sedation or general anesthesia mitigates against the development of nausea and vomiting and associated postanesthesia care unit costs.

- Performing hand surgery with WALANT and field sterility requires less supplies.

- Performing hand surgery with WALANT in the ambulatory or clinical procedural suite eliminates the need for intravenous antibiotics and the costs associated with such side effects as *C. difficile* colitis, urinary tract infection, and anaphylaxis (patient safety).

- Hand surgery with WALANT in the ambulatory or clinical procedural suite can be safely performed without preoperative consultation and/or testing.

- The bond that develops between the surgeon and patient with clear intraoperative communication and education decreases the risk of patient's discontent and litigation.

- Government and commercial payers are becoming increasingly aware of evidence-based medicine supporting the use of WALANT, surgery in the ambulatory or clinical procedural suite, and less expensive field sterility. Because of this, it may be financially impractical to continue utilizing other anesthesia techniques or perform surgery in an OSC or OR (e.g., bundled payment).[8,9,12,13,14,15]

INCREASED REVENUE FOR THE SURGEON

- Incorporating WALANT into your practice and performing simple hand procedures in the ambulatory or clinical procedural suite delivers value for patients and payers and will give you a competitive edge. This is particularly relevant when you consider the trend of greater transparency in health care and "more skin in the game" for patients with respect to out-of-pocket expenses. As a result, you will experience higher demand as patients seek you out.

- Delivering value in hand surgery will enable you to offer direct-to-employer arrangements and negotiate site of service differential reimbursement with commercial payers.

- Utilizing WALANT to perform simple hand surgeries in the ambulatory or clinical procedure suite is more efficient than at an OSC or OR. One study demonstrated that the surgeon could perform twice as many WALANT carpal tunnel releases in the same amount of time by moving the cases from the main OR to a minor procedure room with field sterility.[8]

- Using WALANT to provide value will enable you to be a part of a narrow or preferred provider network with more referrals.

- WALANT results in high patient satisfaction. Satisfied patients are more apt to refer family and friends for care and improve your brand via social media postings.

- Performing minor hand surgeries using WALANT in the ambulatory or clinical procedural suite between cases at an OSC or OR results in efficient use of time and an overall higher number of surgeries performed during your block time.[22]

DECREASED COSTS FOR PRACTICES AND HEALTH SYSTEMS

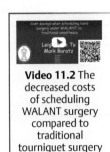

Video 11.2 The decreased costs of scheduling WALANT surgery compared to traditional tourniquet surgery with sedation.

- Hand surgery with WALANT can be performed safely with field sterility using less supplies with a reduction of medical waste.[10,17,18] Less expensive draping and gowning is required for field sterility.[8] Our office minor procedure suite standard setup consists of one surgical prep, two disposable large paper drapes, three disposable linen towels, one suture, one scalpel blade, one small soft dressing, and reusable instruments. We wear a disposable hat, gloves, and mask. We do not wear a gown.

- There are no anesthesia costs other than the cost of the local anesthetic agent. There are no anesthesiologist fees or their allied personnel salaries and benefits including health care premiums!

- Performing hand surgery with WALANT in an office procedure suite requires less staff. We work with a medical assistant or athletic trainer with OR certification. In the OSC or OR, salaries and benefits for extra nurses required for sedation are avoided.

- Performing surgery at an OSC or OR is associated with higher instrument sterilization costs.

- Health systems that offer their own health insurance plan gain additional margin contribution from the savings generated by those "covered lives" who undergo hand surgery using WALANT.

- Office minor procedure rooms can obtain accreditation from the American Association for Accreditation of Ambulatory Surgery Facilities (AAAASF) in the United States and the Canadian Association for Accreditation of Ambulatory Surgical Facilities (CAAASF) in Canada for procedures using pure local anesthesia (no sedation). Accreditation for a procedure suite that does not use sedation is much easier and less expensive to obtain than accreditation for a facility that uses sedation or general anesthesia.

- If you do not use sedation or regional anesthesia, there are no associated medication or equipment costs.

- Using WALANT in an OSC or OR means there is no need for recovery room nurses and their salaries and benefits because patients simply get up and go home after surgery.

- There is less risk of wrong-sided surgery with awake, nonsedated patients with no associated medicolegal expenses or cost of second victim's (e.g., OR staff, nursing, anesthetist, surgeon) lost productivity and counseling.

- There is no need for patient gowns, paper footwear, and surgical caps, because patients do not undress for field sterility surgery (see Chapter 10).

SOCIETAL BENEFITS

- Prescription opioid abuse is highly prevalent in the United States. Between 2002 and 2017, there was a fourfold increase in the total number of deaths related to opioids. WALANT patients are less likely to fill an initial opioid prescription in the postoperative period compared to those who underwent a standard anesthetic technique.[2] Lowering the number of opioid pills in society has an unquantifiable benefit on the cost of drug-related crime, legal costs, rehabilitation treatment, and lost productivity.

- Lowering the cost of care and delivering value contribute to a lower percentage of our gross domestic product (GDP) spent on health care.[19,20,22]

- There is less risk of wrong-sided surgery with awake, nonsedated patients and therefore less potential disability and litigation associated costs.

- Medical waste is a significant societal burden. The health care industry is the second-largest contributor to waste in the United States with more than 4 billion tons of medical waste produced per year. The US health care industry accounts for 10% of the total greenhouse gas emissions, 9% of criteria air pollutants, and 5 to 7 kg/bed/day of care related solid waste. ORs generate 25 to 35% of a hospital's total waste volume and consume on average 56% of total hospital supply expenses.[4] Transitioning simple hand procedures to WALANT, especially if done in the office, allows the surgeon to directly control the amount of waste generated by each procedure by minimizing medical equipment, unnecessary draping, and unused surgical supplies.[16]

LEAN AND GREEN HAND SURGERY: THE SIOUX FALLS, SOUTH DAKOTA STORY AND CHALLENGE

- Health care in the United States is expensive and wasteful. With the cost of US health care approaching nearly 18% of the GDP and over $10,000 per person, the United States spends more on health care than any other country.[23] In a recent review article, the estimated cost of waste in the US health care system ranges from $760 billion to $935 billion, representing 25% of total health care costs.[24] The potential savings range from $191 billion to $282 billion.

- A recent article by Bravo and colleagues discusses environmentally responsible hand surgery. While reviewing the current "Lean and Green" surgery literature, several strategies are mentioned to decrease our waste production.[16] The options include: The reprocessing of single-use devices, sterilization options, and the role of recycling in surgical waste disposal.

- In 2014, Dr Mark Baratz spoke at the American Association for Hand Surgery meeting on the Greening of Hand Surgery (see ▶ Video 11.1). He discussed the idea of a "minimal custom pack design." His group analyzed the contents of their surgical packs and removed all unnecessary items. When Dr Donald Lalonde was visited by Dr Robert E. Van Demark, Jr. in New Brunswick, Canada, he saw "field sterility" for WALANT cases. When he compared Don's back table for a carpal tunnel release (▶ Fig. 11.1) to his own carpal tunnel setup in South Dakota (▶ Fig. 11.2), Robert thought there was room for improvement as he pondered Dr Baratz's philosophy.

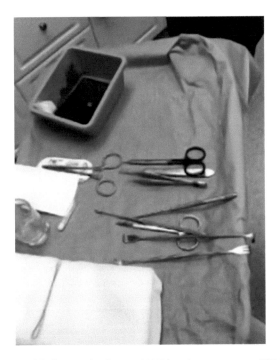

Fig. 11.1 Basic instrument table for Dr Lalonde's WALANT hand surgery cases, 2014.

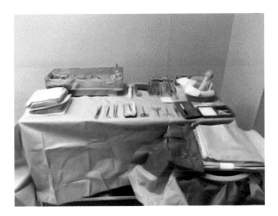

Fig. 11.2 Previous basic instrument table for Dr Van Demark's hand surgery cases, 2014.

• As Dr Van Demark started using WALANT in his practice, it seemed like a perfect time to transition to the "minimal custom pack design" for his cases. His personal tipping point came when he studied the amount of waste generated by just one carpal tunnel procedure (▶ Fig. 11.3). He began a series of meetings with administration and staff to create new custom packs for minor surgery. Their new "Lean and Green" surgical packs have led to a dramatic change in the waste generated for the majority of their minor hand cases (▶ Fig. 11.4). The amount of supplies on the surgical back table has also decreased (▶ Fig. 11.5). Using the new surgical packs, they have seen cost savings of $10.64 and a decrease in surgical waste of 5.06 lbs for each surgical procedure. Since starting their "Lean and Green" project in 2014, his hospital system in Sioux Falls, South Dakota has saved $34,452.32 and decreased surgical waste production by 16,384 lbs or 8.2 tons. Patient satisfaction has remained high: 99% of patients felt that their procedure was the same or better than a dental visit.[26]

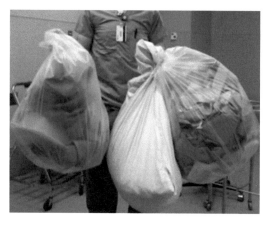

Fig. 11.3 The amount of waste generated from one carpal tunnel case in the main operating room in Sioux Falls, South Dakota before instituting the "Lean and Green" surgical packs, 2014.

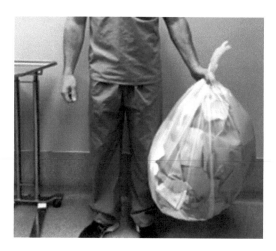

Fig. 11.4 The amount of waste generated from one carpal tunnel case in Sioux Falls, South Dakota after instituting the "Lean and Green" surgical packs, 2019.

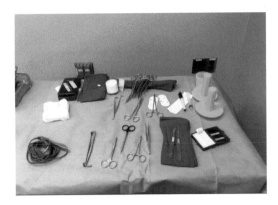

Fig. 11.5 The new basic instrument table for Dr Van Demark's hand surgery cases, 2019.

- At the 2019 American Society for Surgery of the Hand (ASSH) Annual Meeting, Jebson reported on 320 patients treated by one surgeon. Using only 1% lidocaine with epinephrine, surgery was performed in a dedicated office procedure room. The estimated cost savings for this patient population ranged from $2,200 to $2,800 per patient. The authors estimated the total yearly savings for one surgeon to be from $704,000 to $896,000. In addition, patient satisfaction was high; 99% of the patients would have surgery again in the office procedure room.[27]

- The Lean and Green Hand Surgery Initiative has been adopted by the American Association for Hand Surgery (AAHS), ASSH, American Society for Reconstructive Microsurgery (ASRM), and American Society for Peripheral Nerve (ASPN). The goals are to reduce costs, reduce waste, improve safety, and increase patient satisfaction. It is estimated that there are approximately 2,000 hand surgeons practicing in the United States. If every surgeon would do 100 cases in a year (a total of 200,000 cases/year) dramatic savings could be realized. Using our practice, savings of $10.64 per case and 5.06 lbs of saved waste, there would be a cost savings of $2.13 million and a decrease of 1,012,000 lbs (506 tons) of waste.

- The additional savings seen with WALANT are huge. Using Jebson's estimated savings of $2,200 to $2,800 per patient with wide awake anesthesia and no preoperative testing, the savings for 200,000 cases would range from $440 to $560 million.[27]

- We would challenge everyone to critically look at their own practice and see if you have an opportunity to join the "Lean and Green" initiative.

References

1. Bismil M, Bismil Q, Harding D, Harris P, Lamyman E, Sansby L. Transition to total one-stop wide-awake hand surgery service-audit: a retrospective review. JRSM Short Rep 2012;3(4):23
2. Lalchandani G, Halvorson R, Rahgozar P, Immerman I. Wide-awake local anesthesia for minor hand surgery associated with lower opioid prescriptions, morbidity, and costs: a nationwide database study. J Hand Surg Am Global 2020;2:7–12

3. Albert MG, Rothkopf DM. Operating room waste reduction in plastic and hand surgery. Plast Surg (Oakv) 2015;23(4):235–238

4. Thiel CL, Fiorin Carvalho R, Hess L, et al. Minimal custom pack design and wide-awake hand surgery: reducing waste and spending in the orthopedic operating room. Hand (N Y) 2019;14(2):271–276

5. Chan K, Edlund A, Jebson PJL. Office based hand surgery using wide awake local anesthesia no tourniquet (WALANT) delivers true value. Manuscript in submission.

6. Lalonde DH, Martin AL. Wide-awake flexor tendon repair and early tendon mobilization in zones 1 and 2. Hand Clin 2013;29(2):207–213

7. Higgins A, Lalonde DH, Bell M, McKee D, Lalonde JF. Avoiding flexor tendon repair rupture with intraoperative total active movement examination. Plast Reconstr Surg 2010;126(3):941–945

8. Leblanc MR, Lalonde J, Lalonde DH. A detailed cost and efficiency analysis of performing carpal tunnel surgery in the main operating room versus the ambulatory setting in Canada. Hand (N Y) 2007;2(4):173–178

9. Chatterjee A, McCarthy JE, Montagne SA, Leong K, Kerrigan CL. A cost, profit, and efficiency analysis of performing carpal tunnel surgery in the operating room versus the clinic setting in the United States. Ann Plast Surg 2011;66(3):245–248

10. Alter TH, Warrender WJ, Liss FE, Ilyas AM. A cost analysis of carpal tunnel release surgery performed wide awake versus under sedation. Plast Reconstr Surg 2018;142(6):1532–1538

11. Codding JL, Bhat SB, Ilyas AM. An economic analysis of MAC versus WALANT: a trigger finger release surgery case study. Hand (N Y) 2017;12(4):348–351

12. Rhee PC, Fischer MM, Rhee LS, McMillan H, Johnson AE. Cost savings and patient experiences of a clinic-based, wide-awake hand surgery program at a military medical center: a critical analysis of the first 100 procedures. J Hand Surg Am 2017;42(3):e139–e147

13. Kazmers NH, Presson AP, Xu Y, Howenstein A, Tyser AR. Cost implications of varying the surgical technique, surgical setting, and anesthesia type for carpal tunnel release surgery. J Hand Surg Am 2018;43(11):971–977.e1

14. Foster BD, Sivasundaram L, Heckmann N, et al. Surgical approach and anesthetic modality for carpal tunnel release: a nationwide database study with health care cost implications. Hand (N Y) 2017;12(2):162–167

15. Kazmers NH, Stephens AR, Presson AP, Yu Z, Tyser AR. Cost implications of varying the surgical setting and anesthesia type for trigger finger release surgery. Plast Reconstr Surg Glob Open 2019;7(5):e2231

16. Bravo D, Gaston RG, Melamed E. Environmentally responsible hand surgery: past, present, and future. J Hand Surg Am 2020;45(5):444–448

17. Holoyda KA, Farhat B, Lalonde DH, et al. Creating an outpatient, local anesthetic hand operating room in a resource-constrained Ghanaian hospital builds surgical capacity and financial stability. Ann Plast Surg 2020;84(4):385–389

18. Gil JA, Goodman AD, Harris AP, Li NY, Weiss AC. Cost-effectiveness of initial revision digit amputation performed in the emergency department versus the operating room. Hand (N Y) 2020;15(2):208–214

19. Gabrielli AS, Lesiak AC, Fowler JR. The direct and indirect costs to society of carpal tunnel release. Hand (N Y) 2020;15(2):NP1–NP5

20. Far-Riera AM, Pérez-Uribarri C, Sánchez Jiménez M, Esteras Serrano MJ, Rapariz González JM, Ruiz Hernández IM. Estudio prospectivo sobre la aplicación de un circuito WALANT para la cirugía del síndrome del túnel carpiano y dedo en resorte [Prospective study on the application of a WALANT circuit for surgery of tunnel carpal syndrome and trigger finger]. Rev Esp Cir Ortop Traumatol 2019;63(6):400–407

22. Caggiano NM, Avery DM III, Matullo KS. The effect of anesthesia type on nonsurgical operating room time. J Hand Surg Am 2015;40(6):1202–9.e1
23. Papanicolas I, Woskie LR, Jha AK. Health care spending in the United States and other high-income countries. [published correction appears in JAMA. 2018 May 1;319(17):1824] JAMA 2018;319(10):1024–1039
24. Shrank WH, Rogstad TL, Parekh N. Waste in the US health care system: estimated costs and potential for savings. JAMA 2019;322(15):1501–1509
26. Van Demark RE Jr, Smith VJS, Fiegen A. Lean and Green hand surgery. J Hand Surg Am 2018;43(2):179–181
27. Jebson PJ. (2019 September) SYMPOSIUM 09: Practical Tips to Improve Patient Outcomes and Prepare for Value Based Healthcare. Symposium conducted at American Society for Surgery of the Hand Annual Meeting, Las Vegas, NV.

CHAPTER 12

WALANT AND "THE WHY": ADMINISTRATION, ANESTHESIOLOGY, NURSING, AND PAYERS

Peter J. L. Jebson, Kevin T. K. Chan, Levi L. Hinkelman, Daniel Hess, Julie E. Adams, Michael W. Neumeister, Robert E. Van Demark, Jr., Peter C. Amadio, and Donald H. Lalonde

STRATEGY FOR IMPLEMENTING A WALANT HAND SURGERY PROGRAM IN YOUR INSTITUTION OR PRACTICE

- The well-known author Simon Sinek has stated "bad decisions are made on false assumptions" and "It all starts with why." Make sure you understand and can articulate "the why" to all key stakeholders.[1]

- Before attempting to implement a WALANT program, contact surgeons who have been successful. Visit them and observe their facilities, workflow, and resources. Speak with their manager, staff, and administrators. Consider taking your administrators with you to get institutional buy-in.

- Review the literature and all the advantages of WALANT in Chapter 2 and prepare thoughtful, succinct, well-organized, evidence-based presentations and handouts for all key stakeholders. Emphasize the *value* of WALANT (refer Chapter 11 with respect to outcome, cost savings, and patient safety). Present in a respectful way being certain to listen carefully to objections and concerns.

- Schedule one-on-one meetings with key influential stakeholders but understand they are not always aligned and often have different motivations (i.e., their "margin"—better reimbursement at an outpatient surgery center [OSC] or operating room [OR] versus office or clinic procedure suite). You will be more successful if you understand the perspectives of others and anticipate objections and questions.

- Start with simple hand procedures in the OSC or OR. Monitor outcomes and obtain patient satisfaction surveys particularly if you want to transition some case types to an ambulatory or clinical procedure suite (i.e., carpal tunnel, trigger finger/thumb).

- As you become more comfortable and competent begin performing more complex cases in the OSC or OR.

- The key is to start small, demonstrate success including patient satisfaction, low complication rate, and quantification of the cost savings for patients and payers.

- Before proceeding with a WALANT hand surgery program in an ambulatory clinic space, you need to make sure you adhere to all state and federal laws and regulations including accreditation.

- Make sure that BEFORE you start performing procedures in the office or clinical procedure suite you and/or your payer relations team negotiate a site of service reimbursement differential (or bundle payment) with commercial payers or employers. It is imperative that you determine your direct and indirect costs for each episode of care as part of the process.

- After COVID began in 2020, the British Society for Surgery of the Hand, the British Orthopedic Association, and the British Orthopedic Foot and Ankle Society, the British Association of Plastic, Reconstructive and Aesthetic Surgeons, the British Association of Hand Therapists, and the British Society for Orthopedic Children's Surgery all worked together to recommend that surgeons should "aim to perform all hand and wrist surgery under local anesthetic block or 'wide-awake local anesthetic no tourniquet' (WALANT) (https://www.boa.ac.uk/uploads/assets/ee39d8a8-9457-4533-9774e973c835246d/4e3170c2-d85f-4162-a32500f54b1e3b1f/COVID-19-BOASTs-Combined-FINAL.pdf; https://www.boa.ac.uk/uploads/assets/ae07ade5-6483-4fdd-bfe40f04350a7074/BOA-BSSH-BOFAS-LA-Pathway-guidelines-FINAL.pdf)"[2] to decrease the risk of COVID droplet spread for health care workers and patients alike. Under general anesthesia or sedation, one 2020 American study counted eight OR staff or personnel per case.[3] ▶ Fig. 12.1 is taken from https://www.boa.ac.uk/uploads/assets/ae07ade5-6483-4fdd-bfe40f04350a7074/BOA-BSSH-BOFAS-LA-Pathway-guidelines-FINAL.pdf which can be accessed through https://www.boa.ac.uk/resources/boa-pathway-guidelines-for-resumption-of-local-anaesthetic-musculoskeletal-procedures-in-adults.html which can be accessed through https://www.boa.ac.uk/.

 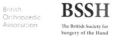

Recommended LA Pathway

The recommended pathway is suitable for both elective and trauma procedures. However treatment of trauma cases should not be inappropriately delayed by using this pathway for their care; local guidelines should be followed if they facilitate urgent trauma surgery through a different, C19-status unknown pathway.

The aims of the LA pathway are:

- To avoid transmission C19 from patients to staff and vice versa
- To avoid the logistic, personal and economic effect of unwarranted self-isolation
- To treat patients expeditiously
- To avoid lengthening waiting lists
- To encourage development and use of minor procedures facilities to treat appropriate cases.

Fig. 12.1 Statement of preferred local anesthetic pathway for hand and foot surgery published in England on August 3, 2020 at https://www.boa.ac.uk/uploads/assets/ae07ade5-6483-4fdd-bfe40f04350a7074/BOA-BSSH-BOFAS-LA-Pathway-guidelines-FINAL.pdf

THE ADMINISTRATION

- *All health care providers and systems are being challenged to lower the cost of care and demonstrate value. Hand surgery using WALANT delivers value (Chapter 11). Leverage this during your presentations, discussions, and negotiations.*

Video 12.1 First impressions of a new WALANT procedure room in Sioux Falls, South Dakota, USA.

- Health care is highly complex and matrixed. There is often misalignment, regulatory hurdles, and barriers. Patience is required as the process can be very frustrating. You will be successful if you understand the administrator's perspective and avoid an adversarial "us against them" relationship.

- Some compelling arguments are: you can improve patient satisfaction ratings, bring more work to the facility, increase the number of patients and cases done in a day, decrease the staff count for many procedures, open up ORs for "bigger" cases, and decrease the amount of wasted materials.

- WALANT surgery is more efficient. In one Canadian study, they performed twice as many carpal tunnel releases at one-quarter the cost by doing surgery in a minor procedure room instead of the main hospital OR.[4] An American study showed similar findings.[5]

- If resistance is encountered, suggest the implementation of a "pilot study," "quality improvement project," or "new patient-centered care initiative" to support your request.

- If there are minor procedure rooms already in existence, offer to use them to improve room utilization. Consider offering evening office surgery hours which has been extremely well received by patients in our practice.

- Administrators care about "market share." Hand surgery using WALANT is a programmatic differentiator that can help increase market share. Alternatively, market share may be lost if the competition can implement and promote sooner than you.

- The administrative and operations teams are responsible for the completion of all regulatory, compliance, and certification requirements.

- Before implementing a WALANT program in the office or clinical procedural suite the administrative team should determine the direct and indirect cost of the episode of care and negotiate favorable reimbursement including a site of service differential and contractual arrangement that rewards value!

- Remind them that building an office-based procedure suite is a fraction of the cost of a new OR in the hospital or OSC.

- It is important to understand that under the current reimbursement model, some hospitals have little interest in adopting wide awake anesthesia. This is changing. With the passage of the Accountable Care Act (ACA) in 2010, there has been a paradigm shift in reimbursement. There has been a shift from volume to value to control unsustainable health care costs and to improve the quality (outcomes) of care.[6,7] One of the goals of the ACA is to "control costs by regulating health care delivery and reimbursement." As part of the ACA, Accountable Care Organizations (ACOs) will play a major role in this transition. An ACO is a network of health care providers that provides care to a defined group of patients. To achieve ACO designation, the following guidelines need to be met[6]:

- "Express willingness to be accountable for quality, cost, and overall care of Medicare beneficiaries for minimum of 3 years."
- "Minimum of 5,000 Medicare beneficiaries with a strong core of primary care physicians."
- "Legal structure to receive and allocate payments."
- "Report on quality, cost, care-coordination measures, and meet patient-centeredness criteria."

- ACOs will be financially responsible for this group of patients. ACOs may be at risk for losing money if costs are higher than expected. In addition, Medicare and insurers will offer financial rewards for saving money and meeting quality guidelines.[6] Payment to ACOs will be an amount equal to a percentage of money saved through cost efficiency.[6]

- When faced with this new economic reality of ACOs and bundled payments, hospitals and health care systems will be interested in adopting new delivery systems that can be cost-effective while providing quality care with high patient satisfaction.

NURSING

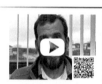

Video 12.2 Initially skeptical patient's impression of WALANT tendon repair.

- Introduce the WALANT concept to nursing leaders and key decision-makers in the perioperative areas with one-on-one meetings, Power-point presentations, and supporting documents.

- Engage them as a key stakeholder and appeal to their innate compassion and commitment to patient safety and quality care.

- Give in-service presentations to the OR and OSC nursing staff explaining "the why" behind hand surgery with WALANT. Share key information regarding outcomes, benefits, and improved safety with the lack of sedation.

- Show how WALANT is safer and better tolerated particularly with respect to postoperative confusion, nausea, and vomiting.

- Discuss the additional benefits including improved efficiency (less turnover time and increased number of patients receiving care/time, lowering of costs for the health system, high patient and family satisfaction).

- Have the nurses who seem more receptive to the WALANT concept be the first to participate. Find an early adopter and you will gradually win over their peers when they see how easy and uncomplicated it is for patients compared to what they have had to do before.

- Share with them how WALANT is cost effective for patients and payers including the government![8–14]

- Have patience and be persistent. Ask them to try it for the patients'.

ANESTHESIOLOGY

- Changing the culture of the anesthesia team: most of their concerns are because they are unfamiliar and have never tried the wide-awake approach. Most of the perceived issues go away quickly after even a short exposure to the technique.

- Show ▶ Video 12.3 to your anesthesia colleagues.

- Validate the concerns of your anesthesiology colleagues regarding their loss of revenue and impact on their compensation. Let them know you are implementing the program as part of your commitment to lower the cost of care and deliver value for patients and payers.

- Explain to them that WALANT can free them up to provide care for more complex surgeries that require regional and/or general anesthesia.

- Point out that they themselves are not subject to monitoring when they undergo dental treatment. WALANT utilizes the same drug they receive at the dentist—lidocaine and epinephrine.

- Share your presentations and the literature with them regarding outcomes and cost when using WALANT. They are likely not familiar with the technique and proven benefits.

- Try working with your anesthesiologist to inject only propofol for the local anesthetic injection part of the case. The patient can then wake up and participate in movement of reconstructed/repaired parts without the effects of tourniquet ischemia. You can still educate patients and they will remember important information if they are not given amnestic agents, which would void their ability and opportunity to receive intraoperative education. In addition, patients would not need nausea-producing medications.

- Choose tenolysis, flexor tendon repairs, and extensor indicis proprius (EIP) to extensor pollicis longus (EPL) tendon transfers for your initial cases as they historically have required general or regional anesthesia. Operative personnel will thereafter easily understand the advantages of patients remaining awake, cooperative, and pain-free without the tourniquet and sedation. Team members will understand how better outcomes can improve patient care in these operations.

- Choose the first few patients wisely for their good disposition and cooperative demeanor.

- Other good cases to start without sedation are patients with severe medical comorbidities in whom sedation or general anesthesia would be extremely risky.

Video 12.3 An anesthesiologist who uses WALANT routinely discusses where it fits in his practice.

NEXT STEPS

- After meeting one-on-one with key leaders, arrange a meeting of the "convinced" to create an action plan to institute the wide-awake alternative for at least some of the patients as a starting point. Doing it in small steps may be wiser.

- After you meet with key decision-makers one-on-one, consider creating a WALANT implementation group or committee with all the rest of the stakeholders so they can express their concerns and address them as a group.

PAYERS

- Physicians typically lack an understanding of the actual cost of care and experience in negotiating with payers. In addition, many health care organizations do not share costs and reimbursement contractual arrangements. However, this does not mean that you should not be engaged or an advocate for change.

- Make sure you understand the true cost of an episode of care (direct and indirect) including differences based on location of surgery known as site of service (i.e., OSC, OR, procedural suite).

- Make sure you understand your current fee schedule and the site of service reimbursement differential for all hand surgeries where WALANT may be safely used including in a procedural suite or office setting.

- Collaborate with your organization's payer relations/contracting team. Educate them on WALANT, the associated lowering in cost of care (see next section), and the potential to safely perform common hand procedures in a procedural suite or office setting in lieu of the OSC or OR.

- Provide your payer relations/contracting team and payers presentations and handouts espousing the value of hand surgery with WALANT. Quantify the actual savings using your modeling and the existing literature.

- Partner with your payer relations/contracting team to identify opportunities to negotiate better reimbursement for an episode of care using WALANT particularly when performed in a procedural suite or the office. Find out who the key decision-makers are. Attend meetings where reimbursement negotiations are discussed. Explain this new approach, which will increase patient satisfaction and safety while decreasing costs.

- Make sure you are being adequately reimbursed ("paying for value").

- Consider risk-based agreements for certain highly predictable surgeries (i.e., bundle payment).

- Consider direct-to-employer agreements where you can deliver high-quality care at a lower cost (utilizing WALANT for common hand surgeries in the office or procedural suite).

- Have the payer relations/contracting team identify alternative payment models that they are participating in thereby lowering the cost of care and improving the overall margin by utilizing WALANT (i.e., bundle payments, population health management, etc.). This is particularly advantageous in a health system with its own health insurance plan.

- Make sure that BEFORE you start performing procedures in the office or clinical procedure suite you or your payer relations team have negotiated and formalized an acceptable site of service reimbursement differential with commercial payers or employers.

- Eventually, insurance companies and governments will understand that sedation and the main OR are not essential for operations such as carpal tunnel surgery. They will be happy to save the money and increase the safety and satisfaction of their insured customers. It is to their great advantage to negotiate a lower facility fee with you than what they pay the hospital.

DECREASED PAYER COSTS

- WALANT utilizes local anesthetic only which is less expensive than regional or general anesthesia.

- Performing simple hand surgery with WALANT in the ambulatory or clinical procedural suite is less expensive than an OSC or hospital OR.[4,5,9,11,13,14]

- Using WALANT for hand surgery obviates the need for an anesthetist for regional or general anesthesia.

- Avoiding the use of sedation or general anesthesia mitigates against the development of nausea and vomiting and associated postanesthesia care unit costs.

- Performing hand surgery with WALANT and field sterility requires less supplies.

- Performing hand surgery with WALANT in the ambulatory or clinical procedural suite eliminates the need for intravenous antibiotics and the costs associated with such side effects as *Clostridium difficile* colitis, urinary tract infection, and anaphylaxis (patient safety).[13,14]

- Hand surgery with WALANT in the ambulatory or clinical procedural suite can be safely performed without preoperative consultation and/or testing.[13,14]

- The bond that develops between the surgeon and patient with clear intraoperative communication and education decreases the risk of patient discontent and litigation.

- WALANT is associated with lower opioid consumption and lower odds of developing medical or surgical complications postoperatively compared with standard anesthesia patients.[15]

- Hand surgery with WALANT in the ambulatory or clinical procedural suite can be safely performed in diabetic patients, those on anticoagulants, and those with a pacemaker with no adjustment of their medications or normal daily routines.[14]

- A detailed direct and indirect cost analysis study determined that performing carpal tunnel, trigger finger/thumb, and de Quervain's surgery with WALANT in a clinical procedural suite using field sterility without a preoperative evaluation or intravenous antibiotics resulted in an average savings of $3,603 for trigger finger/thumb release, $3,490 for carpal tunnel release, and $3,282 for de Quervain's release compared to surgery at a traditional location (OR or OSC). This resulted in less out-of-pocket expense for patients with high co-pay and/or deductible health insurance coverage plans.[14]

- There is less risk of a wrong-site surgery with awake, nonsedated patients.[9]

COMMONLY ENCOUNTERED CONCERNS AND QUESTIONS

- **"My friend had an anesthetic for the same surgery so why are you recommending this technique?"**

Acknowledge that some surgeons still use regional or general anesthesia or sedation with local anesthesia. Confirm that the surgery could be performed with sedation, but that would require the use of an OSC or hospital. Inform the patient that sedation is associated with risks and complications including aspiration, nausea, and vomiting.[13,16,17] Let them know that avoiding sedation is in their best interest. If sedation is preferred the patient is reminded of the loss of control, need for fasting, intravenous access, accompanying driver requirement, stopping or adjustment of certain medications, and the undressing and wearing of the stylish surgical gown!

Inform them that WALANT is a new technique that has been proven to be safe with high patient satisfaction, less morbidity than with other anesthesia techniques, and less overall cost including out-of-pocket expenses (deductibles and co-pays).[4,5,9–14,17,18]

Share with the patient that multiple studies have demonstrated high patient satisfaction with WALANT. Another study compared the patient's perspective of wide awake anesthesia and local anesthesia with sedation. Sedated patients spent more time in the hospital, required more preoperative testing, and reported greater nausea and vomiting postoperatively.[19] A British study of 100 consecutive patients assessed the patient's experience with wide awake hand surgery. A vast majority (91%) felt that the procedure was less painful or comparable to what they would experience from a dental visit; 86% would prefer to have wide awake anesthesia if they needed hand surgery again; and 90% would recommend WALANT to a friend.[18]

Remind the patient that dental offices have safely used only lidocaine with epinephrine without monitoring for over 60 years. Let them know that preventable harm such as wrong-sided surgery is much less likely to occur in nonsedated patients than in those who are asleep or heavily sedated.

Some patients do experience anxiety and prescribing a mild anxiolytic prior to the procedure can be helpful.

- **"I am very nervous about having surgery while I am awake."**

Validate the patients' concerns and let them know that it is very normal to be nervous. Reassure them that the technique is very safe with high patient satisfaction. Calmly explain the process to them. Encourage them to bring a friend or family member with them on the day of surgery. Consider playing low level relaxing music in the OR/procedure suite.

Inform the patient about how many such surgeries you have performed and what to expect. In a calm, confident soft-spoken manner, share the advantages of the technique versus using sedation including cost, convenience, easier recovery, and side effects.

Have them speak to patients who have already successfully undergone the same surgery and technique. Consider developing an educational video with patient testimony to help alleviate patients' fears and anxiety.

On rare occasion, consider prescribing an oral anxiolytic to be taken preoperatively. The patients will need to be reminded to have someone chaperone them postoperatively.

- **"What happens if I feel pain during the surgery?"**

Reassure the patient that it is extremely rare to feel any pain during the procedure. Remind them that they may feel you touching their hand. Let them know that on the rare chance that they feel any pain, you will inject more local anesthetic and the pain will go away.

If the surgeon follows the simple guidelines of tumescent local anesthetic administration and minimal pain injection of local anesthetic, this should be as infrequent as patients waking up during general anesthesia (see Chapter 4 and Chapter 5). Surgeons or anesthesiologists giving the local anesthetic should always be prepared to inject more local anesthetic volume while staying within the safe dosage limit.

- **"I get claustrophobic and don't want drapes covering me."**

Reassure the patient that you understand their fear.

Consider not using large surgical drapes at all. We have found that when performing simple hand procedures in the procedural suite or office setting, drapes that cover the patient's face and obscure vision of the surgical field and team are not necessary.

Let them know the purpose of the drapes—to protect them and to decrease the potential of infection. Draping that leaves the head free can easily accommodate such patients and maintain an adequate sterile field.

- **"I have a high pain threshold, but I hate needles."**

This is a remarkably common statement by patients. Reassure them that you understand their concerns and anxiety. Validate and have empathy.

Explain to the patient that advances in local anesthesia make it possible to use much smaller needles (27 or 30 gauge) that hurt less. Compare the insertion of the needle to that of a mild bee sting. Have a calm demeanor and use distraction techniques at the time of injection including conversation or desensitization like a dentist gently squeezing and shaking a gum at the time of needle insertion.

- **"I don't want to know or hear what is going on during the surgery."**

Explain to patients that they can choose to know or not know what the surgeon is doing. If they would like to be totally "out of the know," they can bring in music with headphones or watch a video on their tablet and ignore the whole event. If they change their mind and would like a "play-by-play" of the surgery, this can easily be accommodated by experienced wide awake procedure surgeons. Surprisingly, many patients become curious and want to see parts of their surgery.

- **"It is not safe to inject epinephrine in the finger or hand."**

Many health care workers are still not aware that the old dogma that epinephrine should not be used in the fingers is no longer valid. Share the literature with them.[20-23] Demonstrate the reversal of epinephrine vasoconstriction in the finger with phentolamine in your next simple hand operation, such as trigger finger release.

- **"What about the ill effects of epinephrine on cardiac function without monitoring?"**

Acknowledge that occasionally patients may feel a temporary increase in their heart rate or slight anxiety. However, point out that monitors have not been used for the millions of lidocaine and epinephrine injections that occur every day without problems in dental offices. Ask the objecting person if he or she ever had a monitor when he or she personally had lidocaine with epinephrine at a dental treatment.

Consider monitoring patients with portable monitors for the first few months of your implementation process. It will eventually become apparent that patients do not need monitoring for lidocaine and epinephrine injection any more than they would at a dentist's office.

Point out that there are areas in your hospital and/or community where doctors inject lidocaine with epinephrine daily without monitors (Mohs surgery clinic, plastic surgery skin cancer and nevus excision, line insertion, and other instances).

When patients do have a preoperative cardiac concern, decrease the concentration of epinephrine to between 1:400,000 and 1:1,000,000 and perform the procedure wide awake in the main OR with monitoring.

- **"My facility is not set up so that I can inject patients before they come into the operating room."**

Ideally, you should inject the local anesthetic at least 25 to 30 minutes before incision to allow optimal epinephrine vasoconstriction. In some facilities, this may be challenging in that there is no perceived space available for preoperative blocking. Although 25 to 30 minutes is ideal, you can begin a procedure sooner than that if necessary. You will need to tolerate initial temporary bleeding, which is only mildly annoying.

Consider setting up a workflow where you can inject patients on their stretcher in the preoperative holding area or in the recovery room.

You could also inject patients as soon as they arrive in the OR before you scrub and prepare and drape the patients.

- **"My facility requires a witnessed preinjection time out or pause: This may be difficult if I inject local anesthetic outside the operating room."**

Always adhere to patient safety measures including sign your site and surgical time outs to avoid wrong site surgery/injury and preventable harm.

Start by performing the injections in the holding area or recovery room with a nurse present as a witness. Discuss with the patient safety committee that having a witness is not necessary in the cooperative nonsedated patient.

- **"Should I still use a patient safety checklist since the patient is awake?"**

Patient safety is imperative. The hand is the most common area for a wrong site surgery. A safety checklist in the awake patient should still be utilized. In fact, the patient becomes part of the checklist process. Patient safety checks were developed because of preventable patient harm such as wrong-sided surgery and giving medications that they were allergic to. Some of these issues arose because sedated patients cannot speak for and protect themselves. If the patient and all members of the care team participate in the process and the use of sedation is avoided, these OR errors don't occur.

- **"If the surgery is more difficult than I anticipated, how do I keep the patient calm?**

For the most part, this situation can be avoided with appropriate procedure and patient selection.

Surgeons and nurses who cannot remain calm and confident should not embark on surgery with a wide-awake patient.

The staff and surgeon are both responsible for creating a calm, relaxed environment for the patient. The patient is easily calmed if the surgeon and the nurse are relaxed with a matter-of-fact attitude. It is critical that the staff and surgeon remain calm if the procedure is not going as planned. Having good body language and the correct speech cadence and tone is vital.

If the case cannot be safely completed, inform the patient and let him or her know that you are going to close the incision(s) and reschedule the procedure(s) with a general or regional anesthetic. Assure them that you are doing so in their best interest.

- **"I cannot work at my facility unless I have an anesthesiologist in the room."**

Seek to understand the reason for this policy. Reassure those involved that WALANT is a proven, evidence-based, safe technique. Using sedation is not necessary and places the patient at risk for complications.

If the facility is inflexible, have the anesthesia provider limit the injection of propofol for the 2 minutes required for you to inject the lidocaine and epinephrine. As soon as you have injected the local anesthetic, the anesthesiologist can wake the patient. Avoiding all amnestic medication and opiates will allow you to teach patients during the injection and the procedure and have them remember your advice. They will not have nausea. They will also be able to cooperate and show you movement of reconstructed structures without the motor block. Alternatively, your anesthesiologist may change his or her role to that of a consultant who is not necessarily present for your whole case.

Many hospital ORs have dedicated "local anesthesia" rooms where surgeons operate safely without any anesthesia personnel. Other hospitals have still not done it this way. Point out that dentists work under pure local anesthesia without an anesthesiologist. Local anesthesia without monitoring is safely performed in many other aspects of health care including the emergency department and clinic where skin cancer excision, minor procedures, and bone marrow aspiration are performed.

Anesthesia providers who are interested in developing skills in the injection of tumescent local anesthetic without sedation are more than welcome to start using the technique. This would free up surgeon's time. Anesthesiologists could be injecting local anesthetic in the preoperative area or room while the surgeon is operating on patients in the procedure room.

- **"What about the patients hearing me speak with my staff during the procedure?"**

Use this to your advantage to educate the patient during surgery to decrease complications (see Chapter 8).

At the beginning of the procedure let the patient know that he or she may hear you speak with your team during the surgery and that this a normal part of the procedure. Introduce the staff to the patients and clarify what role they play in their care. Always be careful about what you say and act in a professional manner at all times. Some patients find it beneficial to update them as you proceed. Informing them about what percentage of the procedure has been completed can be reassuring. Help make the patients feel at ease with simple conversation enquiring about their family, interests, and hobbies. Do NOT ignore the patient by conversing only with your staff.

You can keep conversation to a minimum, but it is true that the wide-awake approach does pressure surgeons to talk to patients during surgery. If you are the type of surgeon who does not like this type of interaction, perhaps WALANT is not for you. However, this can be an excellent intraoperative opportunity for patient education to decrease the risk of unnecessary postoperative complications.

- **"What if a medical student, resident, or advanced practice provider (PA or NP) is participating in the surgery?"**

Inform the patient prior to the procedure that you work with and educate medical students, residents in training, and advanced practice providers. Remind them that they are an integral part of the care team and that you were a learner once! Let them know that the learner may participate in the procedure but under your supervision and tutelage. Many patients have a great respect for their good fortune in having a master responsible for their surgery when they see a surgeon teaching a learner (Chapter 8). Be careful about what you say and how you act. If the surgeon has a calm, reassuring manner, this can be a very positive experience for the patient. On the other hand, if a surgeon is rough and aggressive in his or her teaching technique, the patient may be better off asleep!

It is true that the patient will be much more aware of who did what parts of the surgery, especially if the surgeon is not there for part of the operation. This increased transparency and truth-revealing to patients may be too much for the surgeon to bear, in which case the surgeon may prefer the patient asleep.

- **"If I use wide awake surgery, the patient becomes aware of frustrations and inefficiencies such as delays, dropped instruments, and lack of needed equipment."**

Make the patient aware that such unanticipated (and frustrating) events seem to occur routinely. Reassure them that such events will not distract the team from rendering the best care possible. Inform them that personnel entering and leaving the OR or procedure suite is just part of the normal workaday life of a surgical team. When things go slightly awry, convey a sense of matter-of-fact calm that will reassure the patient with our attitude and our reaction to adversity. In this way patients will witness us at our best behavior, not at our worst behavior.

THE SIOUX FALLS, USA EXPERIENCE BY DR *ROBERT E. VAN DEMARK, JR.*

I am an orthopedic hand surgeon employed by a large Midwestern health care system. In my practice there are 15 orthopedic surgeons, 3 podiatrists, 2 primary care sports medicine physicians, and 33 midlevel providers. Our hospital has 20 ORs with an additional 6 ORs devoted to orthopedics.

Because of the rapid growth of our group, we began to have OR access problems in 2013. At that same time, we started using wide awake or WALANT for some of our hand cases. We felt that with the use of wide awake surgery, we could move some local cases out of the hospital and into an office-based procedure room.

The challenge was to convince our administration that an in-office procedure room would be a win-win situation for everyone. When we approached our administration, they were reluctant to proceed with a minor procedure room outside of the hospital. We needed to educate them and address four concerns:

- What is WALANT or wide awake anesthesia?
- Is WALANT surgery safe for patients?
- Will patients be satisfied with WALANT surgery?
- Does this make financial sense for the system?

WHAT IS WALANT SURGERY?

Initially there was some confusion concerning wide awake anesthesia. Administration thought we were planning to have a complete OR suite built in the office. We really needed to explain what is involved during WALANT surgery. The concept of "minor procedure room field sterility" is new to many outside the spheres of Mohs surgery and plastic surgery in the United States. Our hand surgery colleagues in Canada have used wide awake surgery and minor field sterility extensively for a long time.[21] Minor field sterility includes the following components:

- Extremity preparation with iodine or chlorohexidine.
- A single drape.
- Minor instrument tray.
- Masks and sterile gloves with no gowns.
- No prophylactic antibiotics.
- Local anesthesia only.

IS WALANT SURGERY SAFE FOR PATIENTS?

Multiple studies have looked at the safety record of wide awake hand surgery done in the outpatient setting with minor field sterility (Chapter 10). In a large Canadian multicenter study of 1,504 carpal tunnel procedures, the superficial infection rate was 0.4% and the deep infection rate was 0%.[24] Similar results have been reported in other series.[9,18,19,25-29]

Our group recently reviewed our in-office procedure room experience. In a group of 566 patients, there were no deep infections and a 0.4% superficial infection rate.

WILL PATIENTS BE SATISFIED WITH WALANT SURGERY?

Multiple studies have demonstrated high patient satisfaction with wide awake anesthesia. A multicenter study from Canada and the United States compared the patient's perspective of wide awake anesthesia to local anesthesia with sedation. In comparing the two groups, sedated patients spent more time in the hospital, required more preoperative testing, and reported greater nausea and vomiting postoperatively. The majority of patients (93%) in both groups liked the anesthesia they had received and would choose it again.[19]

A British study reviewed the experience of 100 consecutive patients undergoing wide awake hand surgery. The study found that 91% of the patients felt that the procedure was less painful or comparable to what they would experience from a dental visit, 85% of patients would choose wide awake anesthesia if they needed hand surgery again, and 90% would recommend to a friend.[10]

The majority of our in-office patients (99%) rated the procedure room experience the same as or better than a dental visit.

DOES THIS MAKE SENSE FOR THE SYSTEM?

Data has been published on the significant cost savings of using a procedure room instead of a hospital OR. Costs associated with an anesthesiologist, preoperative testing, intravenous sedation, intraoperative monitoring, and recovery room go away with the use of local anesthesia with no sedation.[4,5,9–14,17,18,29–31]

The Bismil study of 1,000 consecutive wide awake procedure patients from the UK showed a savings of £750,000 ($1,160,000) for the National Health Service. Over a 10-year period, there was a total savings of £2 million.[29]

After several long months of meetings and talks, our practice developed a procedure room in the office at a fraction of the cost of a new OR in the hospital ($15,000 versus $5 million). We remodeled a cast room in our clinic and began doing wide awake cases in 2015 (▶ Fig. 12.2). After a few months, it larger to accommodate additional equipment.

In 2017, our hand clinic was remodeled, and we moved into a new and larger (215 sq.ft.) procedure room (▶ Fig. 12.3). This allowed more room for a mini C-arm and cautery. The new larger procedure room has been well received by patients and our staff.

In early 2019, access to ORs became an issue. Much to my surprise, the hospital administration approached our group and suggested the development of a wide awake procedure room located in the hospital Pain Clinic. This project was fast-tracked and in two months (March, 2019) we began doing our first wide-awake local cases using local field sterility in the hospital-based procedure room (▶ Fig. 12.4). This room has decompressed the ORs in the Orthopedic Center suites and has improved scheduling access for our partners.

The new hospital procedure room is approximately 375 sq.ft. and has been a great addition. Patients don't have to change into a gown and can watch TV during the procedure (▶ Fig. 12.5). One pleasant surprise is the decrease in turnover time. In our main hospital ORs, the turnover time between cases can range from 30 to 60 minutes. In the new procedure room, 10 minutes is the average time between cases.

We are currently looking at the cost and patient outcomes of the wide-awake cases done in our in-office procedure room, the new hospital procedure room, and in the main ORs.

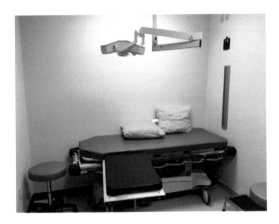

Fig. 12.2   Early in-office procedure room, 2015.

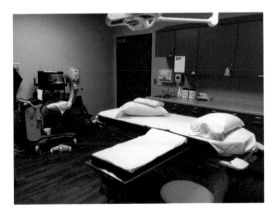

Fig. 12.3   Second-generation in-office procedure room, 2017.

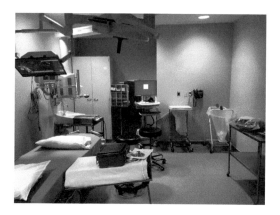

Fig. 12.4   Third-generation hospital-based wide-awake procedure room, 2019.

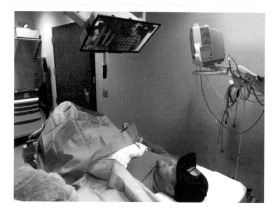

Fig. 12.5   Hospital-based wide-awake procedure room, 2019.

For a 2020 lecture by Dr Van Demark on **"Getting started with WALANT in your hospital"** go to http://mediafire.com/file/b3m7kyg8yps7e40/van+demark+getting+started+with+WALANT+in+your+hospital.mp4/file.[38]

References

1. Sinek S. Start with Why: How Great Leaders Inspire Everyone to Take Action. Penguin Group (USA) Publishing; 2009
2. British BOA, BSSH, BOFAS pathway guidelines recommending local anaesthetic musculoskeletal procedures in adults. Published August 3, 2020. https://www.boa.ac.uk/uploads/assets/ee39d8a8-9457-4533-9774e973c835246d/4e3170c2-d85f-4162-a32500f54b1e3b1f/COVID-19-BOASTs-Combined-FINAL.pdf Accessed August 16, 2020
3. Diamond S, Lundy JB, Weber EL, et al. A call to arms: emergency hand and upper-extremity operations during the COVID-19 pandemic. J Hand Surg Glob Online 2020;2(4):175–181
4. Leblanc MR, Lalonde J, Lalonde DH. A detailed cost and efficiency analysis of performing carpal tunnel surgery in the main operating room versus the ambulatory setting in Canada. Hand (N Y) 2007;2(4):173–178

5. Chatterjee A, McCarthy JE, Montagne SA, Leong K, Kerrigan CL. A cost, profit, and efficiency analysis of performing carpal tunnel surgery in the operating room versus the clinic setting in the United States. Ann Plast Surg 2011;66(3):245–248

6. Adkinson JM, Chung KC. The patient protection and Affordable Care Act: a primer for hand surgeons. Hand Clin 2014;30(3):345–352, vi–vii

7. Mathews AW. Can accountable-care organizations improve health care while reducing costs? Wall Street Journal. January 23, 2012 https://www.wsj.com/articles/SB10001424052970204720204577128901714576054

8. Codding JL, Bhat SB, Ilyas AM. An economic analysis of MAC versus WALANT: a trigger finger release surgery case study. Hand (N Y) 2017;12(4):348–351

9. Rhee PC, Fischer MM, Rhee LS, McMillan H, Johnson AE. Cost savings and patient experiences of a clinic-based, wide-awake hand surgery program at a military medical center: a critical analysis of the first 100 procedures. J Hand Surg Am 2017;42(3):e139–e147

10. Kamal RN, Behal R. Clinical care redesign to improve value in carpal tunnel syndrome: a before-and-after implementation study. J Hand Surg Am 2019;44(1):1–8

11. Kazmers NH, Presson AP, Xu Y, Howenstein A, Tyser AR. Cost implications of varying the surgical technique, surgical setting, and anesthesia type for carpal tunnel release surgery. J Hand Surg Am 2018;43(11):971–977.e1

12. Alter TH, Warrender WJ, Liss FE, Ilyas AM. A cost analysis of carpal tunnel release surgery performed wide awake versus under sedation. Plast Reconstr Surg 2018;142(6):1532–1538

13. Van Demark RE Jr, Becker HA, Anderson MC, Smith VJS. Wide-awake anesthesia in the in-office procedure room: lessons learned. Hand (N Y) 2018;13(4):481–485

14. Chan K, Edlund A, Jebson PJL. Office-based hand surgery using WALANT results in significant cost savings and value. Manuscript in preparation

15. Miller A, Kim N, Ilyas AM. Prospective evaluation of opioid consumption following hand surgery performed wide awake versus with sedation. Hand (N Y) 2017;12(6):606–609

16. Ayhan E, Akaslan F. Patients' perspective on carpal tunnel release with WALANT or intravenous regional anesthesia. Plast Reconstr Surg 2020;145(5):1197–1203

17. Lalonde D, Martin A. Tumescent local anesthesia for hand surgery: improved results, cost effectiveness, and wide-awake patient satisfaction. Arch Plast Surg 2014;41(4):312–316

18. Teo I, Lam W, Muthayya P, Steele K, Alexander S, Miller G. Patients' perspective of wide-awake hand surgery—100 consecutive cases. J Hand Surg Eur Vol 2013;38(9):992–999

19. Davison PG, Cobb T, Lalonde DH. The patient's perspective on carpal tunnel surgery related to the type of anesthesia: a prospective cohort study. Hand (N Y) 2013;8(1):47–53

20. Thomson CJ, Lalonde DH, Denkler KA, Feicht AJ. A critical look at the evidence for and against elective epinephrine use in the finger. Plast Reconstr Surg 2007;119(1):260–266

21. Lalonde D, Bell M, Benoit P, Sparkes G, Denkler K, Chang P. A multicenter prospective study of 3,110 consecutive cases of elective epinephrine use in the fingers and hand: the Dalhousie Project clinical phase. J Hand Surg Am 2005;30(5):1061–1067

22. Fitzcharles-Bowe C, Denkler K, Lalonde D. Finger injection with high-dose (1:1,000) epinephrine: does it cause finger necrosis and should it be treated? Hand (N Y) 2007;2(1):5–11

23. Chowdhry S, Seidenstricker L, Cooney DS, Hazani R, Wilhelmi BJ. Do not use epinephrine in digital blocks: myth or truth? Part II. A retrospective review of 1111 cases. Plast Reconstr Surg 2010;126(6):2031–2034

24. Leblanc MR, Lalonde DH, Thoma A, et al. Is main operating room sterility really necessary in carpal tunnel surgery? A multicenter prospective study of minor procedure room field sterility surgery. Hand (N Y) 2011;6(1):60–63

25. Hanssen AD, Amadio PC, DeSilva SP, Ilstrup DM. Deep postoperative wound infection after carpal tunnel release. J Hand Surg Am 1989;14(5):869–873

26. Rhee PC. The current and possible future role of wide-awake local anesthesia no tourniquet hand surgery in military health care delivery. Hand Clin 2019;35(1):13–19

27. Koegst WH, Wölfle O, Thoele K, Sauerbier M. Der "Wide Awake Approach" in der Handchirurgie - ein komfortables Anästhesieverfahren ohne Blutleere. [The "wide awake approach" in hand surgery: a comfortable anaesthesia method without a tourniquet]. Handchir Mikrochir Plast Chir 2011;43(3):175–180

28. Jagodzinski NA, Ibish S, Furniss D. Surgical site infection after hand surgery outside the operating theatre: a systematic review. J Hand Surg Eur Vol 2017;42(3):289–294

29. Bismil M, Bismil Q, Harding D, Harris P, Lamyman E, Sansby L. Transition to total one-stop wide-awake hand surgery service-audit: a retrospective review. JRSM Short Rep 2012;3(4):23

30. Via GG, Esterle AR, Awan HM, Jain SA, Goyal KS. Comparison of local-only anesthesia versus sedation in patients undergoing staged bilateral carpal tunnel release: a randomized trial. Hand (N Y) 2020;15(6):785–792

31. Kamnerdnakta S, Huetteman HE, Chung KC. Use and associated spending for anesthesiologist-administered services in minor hand surgery. Plast Reconstr Surg 2018;141(4):960–969

32. Zuckerman JD, Jahangir AA. What's important: rational health-care reform: an American Orthopaedic Association (AOA) 2016 OrthoTalk. J Bone Joint Surg Am 2017;99(7):613–615

33. Leslie BM, Blau ML. Survival strategies in a changing practice environment. J Hand Surg Am 2014;39(5):1012–1016

34. Yuan F, Chung KC. Defining quality in health care and measuring quality in surgery. Plast Reconstr Surg 2016;137(5):1635–1644

35. Squitieri L, Chung KC. Measuring provider performance for physicians participating in the merit-based incentive payment system. Plast Reconstr Surg 2017;140(1):217e–226e

36. Squitieri L, Chung KC. Value-based payment reform and the Medicare Access and Children's Health Insurance Program Reauthorization Act of 2015: a primer for plastic surgeons. Plast Reconstr Surg 2017;140(1):205–214

37. Sterbenz JM, Chung KC. The Affordable Care Act and its effects on physician leadership: a qualitative systematic review. Qual Manag Health Care 2017;26(4):177–183

38. 2020 lecture by Dr Van Demark on "Getting started with WALANT in your hospital" http://mediafire.com/file/b3m7kyg8yps7e40/van+demark+getting+started+with+WALANT+in+your+hospital.mp4/file

CHAPTER 13

PERFORMING YOUR FIRST
CASES WITH WALANT

Andrew W. Gurman, Robert E. Van Demark, Jr., Günter Germann, Jason Wong, and Donald H. Lalonde

SUGGESTIONS ON GETTING STARTED

There are a number of wonderful descriptions in this book about WALANT and its use in some very complex surgical procedures. Chapter 4 and Chapter 5 offer clear descriptions and videos of exactly where and how to inject local anesthetic. Patients express greater overall satisfaction when you perform their procedure with the minimal pain injection methods outlined in Chapter 5. This is an important preliminary reading and/or video watching.

DO SOME HOMEWORK

There are several excellent articles published describing the WALANT technique and medication dosages.[1,2,3,4] They are well worth your time to read, but their material is contained in greater detail in this book.

TAKING THE FIRST STEPS

- Perhaps the biggest obstacle to starting WALANT surgery is taking the first step. If you started practice before 2005. You probably have done most of your ambulatory surgery cases with a combination of intravenous regional anesthesia, local with sedation, and/or general anesthesia. Usually this has worked well, except for the patients who had tourniquet pain and narcotic hangovers with nausea and vomiting. That is no longer the case when you perform the surgery with local injection only of 1% lidocaine with 1:100,000 epinephrine.

- Consider visiting someone who uses the technique or at least watch videos in this book.

- Read Chapter 2 to understand and discuss advantages with your patients and colleagues.

- Choose your first cases carefully. Start small: trigger fingers, carpal tunnel releases, first dorsal compartments, simple masses, and skin lesions. Don't do a Dupuytren's fasciectomy as your first WALANT case. You will find the bleeding there troubling if you have only operated with a tourniquet.

- Choose your first patients carefully. Choose sensible, balanced patients who do not require sedation if they have a dental procedure.

- Patients can have breakfast and can continue their preoperative medications (including blood thinners).

- Put a tourniquet on the arm for your first few cases. You will not use it, but it is comforting to have it in place until you see for yourself how well this works. As a corollary, you can place the tourniquet for more complex surgeries and only inflate it for very brief periods when needed.

- We still use a Penrose drain as a digital tourniquet for digital mucous cysts and nail bed cases. Patients do not feel it with a good digital block (see Chapter 1).

- Stay in your comfort zone. It takes a while to get comfortable with WALANT for some cases. If you have any doubts about a particular case, have the appropriate anesthesia personnel available in case you need to convert to general anesthesia. The numbness provided by lidocaine with epinephrine lasts an average of 5 hours in the hand[4] when we use median and ulnar nerve blocks as part of the tumescent local anesthesia. Numbness lasts an average of 10 hours as a digital block with epinephrine.[5] We inject one or two patients ahead of the one we are operating on so the lidocaine and epinephrine have at least 26 minutes to take effect (see Chapter 14).

- Avoid making an incision immediately after injection. We inject our patients in rooms outside the operating room. We do this so that it will bleed less when we make the first incision. It takes an average of 26 minutes for maximal vasoconstriction to peak after 1:100,000 epinephrine injection in humans.[6] Lidocaine also increases its numbing effect over that time.

- In the first cases, we did not wait long enough after injection of the local anesthetic. Patients had residual pain and the bleeding was annoying. Since we started waiting 30 minutes, we have not encountered this problem.

- Initially, we were not generous enough with the volume of local anesthetic. Changing that early in our practice eliminated patient discomfort and inevitable "top-up" injection of additional local anesthesia.

- Don't force this approach on patients who are reluctant.

- This may not be a good technique for you if you do not have a gentle, kind approach and if don't like talking to patients.

START WITH LOCAL ANESTHESIA WITHOUT TOURNIQUET IN CONJUNCTION WITH GENERAL ANESTHESIA

- Injection of lidocaine and epinephrine improves the patient's experience when they also get general anesthesia. Anesthesiologists can administer less nausea-producing medication.

- Apply the tourniquet but do not inflate it. Inject the patients as soon as they are asleep before you prep and drape and wash your hands so the epinephrine can get as close to 26 minutes of working time as possible.

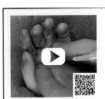

Video 13.1 Injection of lidocaine with epinephrine as soon as the patient is asleep with general anesthesia for no tourniquet surgery.

FOLLOW THE RULES

The published literature and this book describe the WALANT technique and local doses nicely: Do not try to innovate or create a new protocol in your early experience with the technique. When you use 1:100,000 epinephrine, the maximal vasoconstriction occurs approximately 26 minutes after the injection.[6] If you try to cut the waiting time short, you will be disappointed. That is why it is important to do the local injection in a preoperative holding area. Make certain you do the injection with the patient supine. This will help to minimize the vasovagal (fainting) events. Remember that the wound will not be completely dry. Although this will not be a significant problem, the wound will ooze somewhat initially.

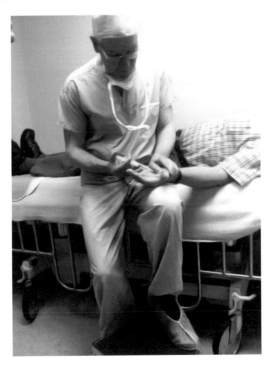

Fig. 13.1 Injecting patients outside the main operating room in the patient holding area or in the recovery room lying down on a stretcher helps to decrease the risk of the patient's fainting (see Chapter 6) and gives the lidocaine and epinephrine 26 minutes or more to work.

DO NOT BE AFRAID TO INJECT PHENTOLAMINE IF THE WHITE FINGER SCARES YOU IN THE BEGINNING

After you inject phentolamine once (see Chapter 3), you will no longer be afraid of the white or bluish finger. This is the same as getting rid of the fear of apnea with morphine by injecting naloxone. It will also reassure the nurses who are used to seeing post-tourniquet bright red hyperemic fingertips. They have to get used to seeing the normal epinephrine effect.

WORST CASE SCENARIO

The unlikely worst case scenario could be that you need to abandon WALANT because the patient is unable to tolerate it, or you run into unforeseen problems intraoperatively. If it happens, we would simply cover the wound with a bandage or close the skin and finish the operation later with the patient under general anesthesia. This is not a terrible fallback position that has still not happened to us.

HEMOSTASIS

- We seldom use a cautery for WALANT surgery, but we have it available. At a concentration of 1:100,000, epinephrine produces very good hemostasis. Setting up a cautery with every case is a waste of time and money.

- If we encounter a larger vein, we clamp it with a hemostat and leave it to clot for a few minutes or tie it off.

- The higher the concentration of epinephrine, the better the hemostasis, and the longer the vasoconstriction will last.[7] However, 1:400,000 to 1:1,000,000[8] concentrations provide enough hemostasis so that cautery is not required for most cases.

- Simply ignore the small amount of bleeding after the incisions and it will dry up. The time you will save by not having to cauterize bleeders after letting down a tourniquet will be worth it.

References

1. Lalonde DH, Wong A. Dosage of local anesthesia in wide awake hand surgery. J Hand Surg Am 2013;38(10):2025–2028
2. Lalonde D, Martin A. Tumescent local anesthesia for hand surgery: improved results, cost effectiveness, and wide-awake patient satisfaction. Arch Plast Surg 2014;41(4):312–316
3. Lalonde D. Minimally invasive anesthesia in wide awake hand surgery. Hand Clin 2014;30(1):1–6
4. Chandran GJ, Chung B, Lalonde J, Lalonde DH. The hyperthermic effect of a distal volar forearm nerve block: a possible treatment of acute digital frostbite injuries? Plast Reconstr Surg 2010;126(3):946–950

5. Thomson CJ, Lalonde DH. Randomized double-blind comparison of duration of anesthesia among three commonly used agents in digital nerve block. Plast Reconstr Surg 2006;118(2):429–432

6. McKee DE, Lalonde DH, Thoma A, Glennie DL, Hayward JE. Optimal time delay between epinephrine injection and incision to minimize bleeding. Plast Reconstr Surg 2013;131(4):811–814

7. Fitzcharles-Bowe C, Denkler K, Lalonde D. Finger injection with high-dose (1:1,000) epinephrine: does it cause finger necrosis and should it be treated? Hand (N Y) 2007;2(1):5–11

8. Prasetyono TO, Biben JA. One-per-mil tumescent technique for upper extremity surgeries: broadening the indication. J Hand Surg Am 2014;39(1):3–12.e7

CHAPTER 14

HOW TO SCHEDULE 15 OR MORE HAND SURGERY CASES PER DAY WITH ONE NURSE

Donald H. Lalonde

HOW TO BOOK 15 OR MORE ELECTIVE CASES IN A DAY

With good planning and coordination with staff, it is possible to schedule 15 or more elective cases per day that one surgeon, one nurse, and one receptionist can perform in the office or hospital minor procedure room outside of the main operating room.

- For the first three cases, schedule simple procedures such as carpal tunnel or trigger fingers. Ask the patients to come at 7:45 AM, 7:50 AM, and 7:55 AM.

- Schedule all the left carpal tunnels in a group and then schedule all the right hands in a second group to avoid wasting time changing the arm board position.

- Schedule longer cases and trauma cases with less predictable lengths later in the day in case those procedures run overtime.

- Inject the first three patients with local anesthetic.

- Inject patients while they are lying down on a stretcher. They are less likely to faint (vasovagal reaction) if they are lying down (see ▶ Video 6.1 on managing the fainting patient).

- As soon as patients feel well after the injection, they can be asked to sit in a chair to liberate the stretcher so you can inject another patient. Two stretchers and an operating table to inject patients are ideal in the event you encounter a patient who faints and needs to remain lying down for a while. However, if necessary, one stretcher and one operating table will suffice for local anesthetic injections.

- After you inject the first three patients, complete their paperwork.

- While you inject the first three patients and do their paperwork, the nurse sets up the first patient on the operating table and opens the tray of surgical instruments.

- We perform most clinic and office surgeries safely with field sterility, which increases efficiency (see Chapter 10).

- After you finish the first operation, inject the fourth patient and do paperwork while the nurse sets up the tray for the second case and brings the second patient into the minor procedure room.

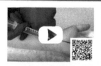

Video 14.1 Patient education during painless carpal tunnel injection: part 1.

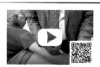

Video 14.2 Patient education during second half of painless carpal tunnel injection.

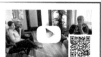

Video 14.3 Four patients waiting for local anesthesia to work while reading postoperative instructions.

- The nurse can put on a pair of gloves and perform retraction if needed during part of the surgery. The rest of the time, the nurse circulates. You get your own instruments off the tray. Having a very simple tray of instruments as described in Chapter 16 is helpful.

- Always try to inject one or two patients ahead of the one you are operating on so the lidocaine and epinephrine have at least 30 minutes to work optimally. It takes an average of 26 minutes for maximal vasoconstriction to peak after 1:100,000 epinephrine injection in humans.[1] The carpal tunnel mixture of 20 mL of 1% lidocaine with 1:100,000 epinephrine described in Chapter 26 will last at least 2 hours without having to reinject.

- Do not inject the patient and make an incision immediately after. The site will bleed less if you organize your time as described above to allow an adequate interval for the epinephrine to work. The lidocaine component also increases its effect over 30 minutes.

- You can educate the patient to decrease complications while you inject the local anesthetic if you inject painlessly as described in Chapter 5.

- If you are working with medical students or residents, first teach them how to give local anesthetic injections in a minimally painful fashion (have them read Chapter 5 and look at the videos first), and have the patients score their injection technique. When they amaze patients with minimal pain injections, the patients will be much more comfortable about allowing them to participate in the surgery under your direction.

INTEGRATING PATIENT CONSULTATIONS FROM THE EMERGENCY DEPARTMENT AND TRAUMA SURGERY IN A HOSPITAL MINOR PROCEDURE ROOM

- We schedule our emergency department consultations to come to the hand surgery clinic in the hospital in the mornings of Mondays and Fridays, where we triage them and operate on those who need surgery in minor procedure rooms in the clinic (see hospital setup videos in Chapter 16).

- When we see a list of patients who arrive from the emergency department for consultation, we do not know which ones will need surgery. When we evaluate a patient who needs surgery, we go ahead and inject that patient at the end of the consultation. If necessary, he or she can wait for 1 or 2 hours after we inject the local anesthetic, and it will not wear off. After we finish our nonsurgical consultations, we perform surgeries on those patients who need it.

- If we know ahead of time that there are trauma patients requiring surgery who are coming to our clinic, we schedule them to come an hour before the end of the clinic consultation patients. This allows the surgical patients an hour in which the local anesthetic can take effect before we perform their surgery. In the meantime, we can finish seeing our clinic consultation patients.

Reference

1. McKee DE, Lalonde DH, Thoma A, Glennie DL, Hayward JE. Optimal time delay between epinephrine injection and incision to minimize bleeding. Plast Reconstr Surg 2013;131(4):811–814

CHAPTER 15

INTEGRATING HAND THERAPISTS INTO WALANT

Amanda Higgins, Lisa Flewelling, Susan Kean, and Donald H. Lalonde

INCORPORATING HAND THERAPISTS INTO YOUR HAND SURGERY CLINIC

If you do not presently have hand therapists seeing patients with you before and after their complex surgery in your hand surgery clinic, you should think about making that happen for at least a few hours per week. There are many advantages to this[1]:

- You can educate each other so you both enhance your skills.

- Verbal communication between you and the hand therapists will produce better patient outcomes in complex problems such as flexor tendon repair and reconstruction.

- The patient will see that you are a team and will want to become an active participant in your efforts to produce the optimal outcome.

- The patient will see that you value the therapist's opinion and thus will be more likely to listen to the therapist and comply with instructions.

- In some systems such as ours, therapists can take over patient care from the surgeon and complete the care for many hand problems. This frees up the surgeon's time, and the therapist can provide excellent ongoing one-on-one care.

- If you begin performing WALANT hand surgery in your minor procedure room outside of the main operating room, therapists can watch the surgery and assess the patients. In addition, therapists can educate the patient between the time of local anesthetic injection and surgery, as well as during the surgery itself. ▶ Video 15.1 shows hand therapists engaging in preoperative therapy consultation between injection of local anesthetic and surgery for a flexor tendon repair in a 10-year-old girl.

- Therapists will avoid wasting time and making judgment errors based on inadequate information because they could not communicate with the surgeon.

- It will be easier for you to start doing early protected movement for K-wired finger fractures if the therapists see patients with you in the clinic (see Chapter 41).

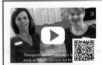

Video 15.1 Hand therapists in preoperative and intraoperative therapy consultation for a 10-year old with flexor tendon repair.

HOW TO INTEGRATE HAND THERAPISTS INTO YOUR CLINICS AND WALANT PROCEDURES

- The surgeon must start the effort to integrate therapists into the clinic because no one else will do it. You can begin by making appointments with the hospital and therapy administrators, one at a time, to get this process off the ground.

- Arrange to talk to the key hospital administrators, one at a time instead of having the first approach at the committee level. (That comes after you convince them one at a time.) Convince them that you need a hand therapist to come to your clinic for 1 hour once a week so you can see patients with complex hand conditions together. You can schedule those patients to arrive when the therapist is there so that no time is wasted. We began this at our hospital 30 years ago. One hour became 2 hours; once a week became twice a week; one therapist became two therapists. We now have two or three therapists for 4 hours 3 days a week.

- We perform our WALANT hand/finger fractures and tendon repairs in minor procedure rooms in the clinic while the therapists are working in another clinic room where they make orthoses (splints) and see patients (see ▶ Video 16.1 for the clinic setup in Saint John, Canada).

- We ask the therapists to come into the clinic procedure rooms to observe parts of appropriate operations. They perform intraoperative patient assessment and education as required (see ▶ Video 15.2 that follows) in between their splinting and consultation duties.

- Point out anatomic structures to the therapists, as you would do with a medical student or resident. Demonstrate how reconstructed tendons and bones move or function during the surgery.

- Hand therapists start to engage with the patient even before the surgery. They can start patient education in the time after the local anesthetic injection while the surgeon is seeing other patients and waiting for the local anesthetic to take optimal effect. When they are familiar with your techniques, they can do a better job of educating your patients about what to expect after surgery. This will be even easier for them if they have seen you perform the surgery.

- Do not forget that the hand therapist is in the procedure room! Talk with the therapist about what you are seeing or doing. This will help him or her to determine the best postoperative care.

SURGEONS AND THERAPISTS MAKE A THERAPY PLAN TOGETHER DURING THE SURGERY

- The surgeon and therapist can examine the state of the tendon repair, pulley venting, and full range of motion before the skin is closed. They do the same for K-wired finger fracture stability with full range of motion at the end of the case.

- Hand surgeons with therapists determine safely repaired tendon or K-wired fracture positions the reconstructions can endure postsurgery (orthosis design).

- Hand surgeons with therapists can determine what kind of safe early active tendon glide the repair can endure postsurgery.

- Pain-guided therapy starts early after a pause to let bleeding stop, swelling settle, and patients to get off pain medication.

- It is ideal to start early active tendon glide of a repaired tendon as soon as safely possible to avoid scar adhesions which can limit the range of motion of the finger.

- We immobilize and elevate the operated hand for 3 to 5 days to permit internal bleeding to stop and swelling to subside.

- This delay also lets patients get off all pain medication so they can start pain-guided therapy and not do what hurts to avoid complications.

- Collagen formation does not start until day 3 so scar adhesions do not happen in the first couple of days. Movement in the first two days can generate internal bleeding which turns to clot and then more scar.

ADVANTAGES FOR HAND THERAPISTS IN GENERAL

- They see live tissue and how it functions with active movement during surgery.

- They understand surgical technique because they have seen it firsthand, not just from hearing or reading about it.

- They can assess patient compliance and reliability before, during, and after the operation.

- There is real-time interaction between the surgeon and therapist, avoiding miscommunication about the outcome and treatment plan.

- This establishes the therapist in the "role of coach" to the patient.

ADVANTAGES FOR THE PATIENT

- An educated patient who has undergone wide awake hand surgery is aware of what happened during surgery and what he or she needs to do for a successful recovery.

- See ▶ Video 19.TT9 for an example of a patient who sees his repair at surgery and cooperates fully through rehabilitation with a relative motion flexion splint to help get his flexor digitorum profundus (FDP) out of scar to end with a good result without tenolysis.

- From the start, the patient becomes an active participant in the rehabilitation team with the surgeon and the therapist.

- The patient's intraoperative interaction places ownership for postoperative care squarely on his or her shoulders.

ADVANTAGES FOR HAND THERAPY IN FLEXOR TENDON REPAIR

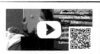

Video 15.2
Intraoperatively, the surgeon and therapist teach the patient about postoperative care.

- See Chapter 19 for extensive discussions in both video and text on post-operative therapy tips of flexor tendon repair.

- In ▶ Video 15.2 the surgeon and therapist teach the patient about the Saint John's postoperative protocol[2] during flexor tendon surgery.

- Therapists can see intraoperative, full-fist active flexion and extension testing of tendon integrity (no gapping) and glide-through pulleys at the time of surgery.

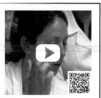

Video 15.3
Allowing wrist extension and active flexion after flexor tendon repair.

- The therapist can initiate communication regarding repair and the treatment protocol with the surgeon and patient before, during, and immediately after the surgery.

- When therapists see full-fist flexion and extension without gapping at surgery, they know that 3 days later the patient is unlikely to have gap-ping and rupture if he or she limits movement to half a fist. This helps therapists gain the increased confidence to move the repaired tendon early with true active movement for better results with less potential for rupture and tenolysis.[3] (See Chapter 19 for many videos with ther-apy tips including "up to half a fist" of true active movement.)

ADVANTAGES FOR HAND THERAPY IN EXTENSOR TENDON REPAIR

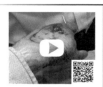

Video 15.4
Relative motion extension splinting for extensor tendon repair.

- Seeing no gap at surgery with intraoperative testing of the repair with sim-ulated relative motion extension splinting assures the surgeon and thera-pist that they can allow the patient an earlier return to work (as early as 3 to 5 days postoperatively) wearing a relative motion extension splint.[4,5]

- Watching the repaired hand move during surgery helps therapists decide whether they should incorporate the wrist component of rela-tive motion extension splinting or not.

- Therapists can see and assess the stress placed on the repair when they start early protected movement (see Chapter 35 for many therapy tips on relative motion splinting for extensor tendon repair of the finger).

ADVANTAGES FOR HAND THERAPY IN FINGER FRACTURES

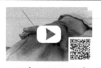

Video 15.5 Early protected active motion after K-wired repair of finger fractures decided with the therapist during surgery.

- Therapists and surgeons are able to see how stable the reduced finger fractures are when they move after K-wire insertion at surgery. This increases confidence for both the surgeon and therapists to begin early protected active movement protocols after fixing finger fractures with K-wires[6,7] (Chapter 41).

- See Chapter 41 for extensive discussions in videos and text on early pro-tected movement with hand therapy tips after K-wiring finger fractures. You should move K-wired fingers early, as you do with flexor tendon repairs.

- Watching active movement during surgery lets therapists and surgeons know whether K-wire placement interferes with joint motion.

- Seeing active movement during the surgery helps the surgeons and therapists decide what kind of splint to use to protect the fracture after surgery.

Video 15.6
Therapist teaching early protected movement 3 days after K-wiring finger fractures with patient off all pain killers and performing pain-guided therapy (see Therapy Tips in Chapter 19 and Chapter 41).

References

1. Lalonde D. How the wide awake approach is changing hand surgery and hand therapy: inaugural AAHS sponsored lecture at the ASHT meeting, San Diego, 2012. J Hand Ther 2013;26(2):175–178
2. Higgins A, Lalonde DH. Flexor tendon repair postoperative rehabilitation: the Saint John Protocol. Plast Reconstr Surg Glob Open 2016;4(11):e1134
3. Higgins A, Lalonde DH, Bell M, McKee D, Lalonde JF. Avoiding flexor tendon repair rupture with intraoperative total active movement examination. Plast Reconstr Surg 2010;126(3):941–945
4. Merritt WH. Relative motion splint: active motion after extensor tendon injury and repair. J Hand Surg Am 2014;39(6):1187–1194
5. Merritt WH, Wong AL, Lalonde DH. Recent developments are changing extensor tendon management. Plast Reconstr Surg 2020;145(3):617e–628e
6. Jones NF, Jupiter JB, Lalonde DH. Common fractures and dislocations of the hand. Plast Reconstr Surg 2012;130(5):722e–736e
7. Gregory S, Lalonde DH, Fung Leung LT. Minimally invasive finger fracture management: wide-awake closed reduction, K-wire fixation, and early protected movement. Hand Clin 2014;30(1):7–15

CHAPTER 16

MINOR PROCEDURE ROOM SETUP

Donald H. Lalonde and Geoffrey Cook

WE HAVE MOVED MOST OF OUR HAND SURGERY OUTSIDE OF THE MAIN OPERATING ROOM THEATER

With the advent of WALANT and field sterility, we perform most of our hand surgery in minor procedure rooms outside of the main operating room (OR). In this chapter, we provide videos and descriptions of the minor procedure room setup in two hospitals and one surgeon's office where we perform these procedures at Saint John, New Brunswick, Canada.

PHYSICAL SPACE

A reception area with seating and a receptionist to manage this area is essential. After you inject patients with local anesthetic, most can go back to sit in the reception area to wait for their procedure with their families. This allows a half hour between the injection of the local anesthetic and the onset of optimal numbing and epinephrine vasoconstriction.[1]

OUR FACILITIES AT SAINT JOHN, NEW BRUNSWICK, CANADA

We have performed wide awake hand surgery for more than 30 years in our facility with a relatively modest investment of money, space, equipment, and staffing in our accredited minor procedure rooms.

Video 16.1 Clinic consultation and minor procedure room setup at the Saint John Regional Hospital.

Video 16.2 Clinic consultation and minor procedure room setup at St. Joseph's Hospital.

Video 16.3 Minor procedure accredited operating room at Dr Lalonde's office.

135

MINOR PROCEDURE ROOMS

- Our office minor procedure room in Canada is accredited by the Canadian Association for Accreditation of Ambulatory Surgical Facilities (CAAASF), *http://caaasf.org*, for pure local anesthesia (no sedation).

- In the United States, as in Canada, you can have a minor procedure room in your office accredited for pure local anesthesia (no sedation) by the American Association for Accreditation of Ambulatory Surgery Facilities (AAAASF), *http://www.aaaasf.org*, more easily and with much less cost than you would need for accreditation for performing procedures with sedation or general anesthesia.

- It is ideal to have two or more stretchers in addition to the procedure table on which to inject lying-down (supine) patients, but one is sufficient. We do injections with the patient lying down instead of sitting up to decrease the risk of fainting (see Chapter 6).

- In one of our hospitals, we have access to only one procedure room most of the time. In this situation, we inject patients on stretchers in other rooms down the hall. After we inject the local anesthetic, most patients can then sit with their relatives for 30 minutes or more before surgery while the local anesthetic achieves optimal numbing and vasoconstriction. If patients need to remain lying down because of fainting or other issues, we let them lie on their stretcher until we move them to the procedure room.

- All you really need in a procedure room is a stretcher that can be adjusted to the Trendelenburg position (head down, feet up), an arm board, and a good light (fixed or portable). All hospitals have these facilities.

- Cleaning staff wash the minor procedure room floors in the evening, but not between cases, unless there is an infection issue such as abscess drainage or a patient who has been identified as having a methicillin-resistant *Staphylococcus aureus* (MRSA) infection.

- Specialized air systems are not required for minor hand surgery procedures.[4]

PERSONNEL

- In addition to the receptionist, only one nurse is required to help the surgeon for most simple cases such as carpal tunnels and trigger fingers to perform up to 15 procedures per day (Chapter 15).

- The nurse both circulates and assists. She puts on gloves only to hold retractors if and when necessary. The surgeon gets his or her own instruments off the tray. We get a second assistant when required for complex cases, such as fracture reduction.

- No recovery room or recovery personnel are required, since no sedation is given, which would require recovery. Patients just sit up and go home after the surgery like at the dentist.

EQUIPMENT

SURGICAL EQUIPMENT IN OUR MINOR PROCEDURE ROOM

- For minor hand surgery procedures such as carpal tunnel surgery, we use small drapes with a hole, or small sterile towels.

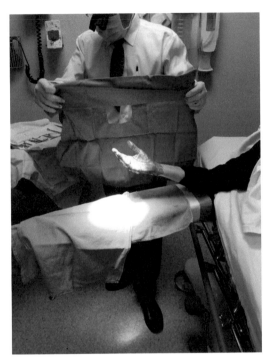

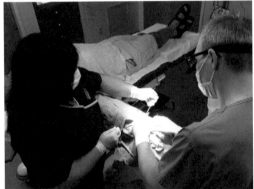

Fig. 16.1 and Fig. 16.2 A typical Canadian minor procedure room setup with field sterility (see Chapter 10) for performing carpal tunnel surgery with one surgeon and one nurse assistant. The nurse puts on gloves only to hold retractors if and when necessary. The nurse both circulates and assists. The surgeon takes his or her own instruments off the tray. This is the way most Canadian carpal tunnel surgery is performed.[2]

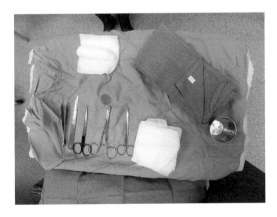

Fig. 16.3 A basic instrument tray for carpal tunnel surgery includes scalpel handle, forceps, suture scissors, dissecting scissors, a needle holder, and a cup to hold the sterilizing liquid.

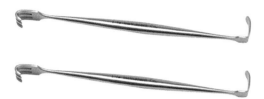

Fig. 16.4 Two Senn retractors for carpal tunnel procedures. We open the Senn retractors separately.

- We use Desmarres (vein) retractors wrapped separately for trigger fingers and De Quervain's surgery (see Chapter 17 for a photo of Desmarres retractors).

- Also wrapped separately, we keep periosteal elevators, skin hooks, hemostats, rongeurs, towel clips to reduce fractures, K-wires, curettes, and army-navy retractors for lacertus tunnel release.

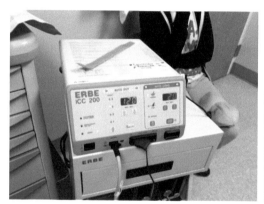
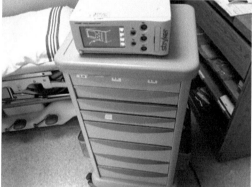

Fig. 16.5 and Fig. 16.6 We have a cautery machine available in the minor procedure room but seldom use it. We also have an electric K-wire driver.

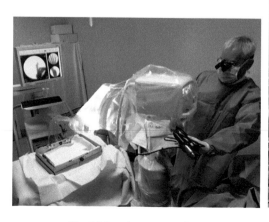
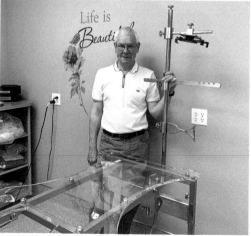

Fig. 16.7 and Fig. 16.8 A low-radiation C-arm (such as the Hologic Fluoroscan InSight-FD Mini C-arm) is very valuable for diagnostic and therapeutic procedures. A radiation technologist is not required because of the low radiation produced by these types of devices.[3] Dr Lalonde has a universal hand table in his office; thanks to Olivier Koronowski.

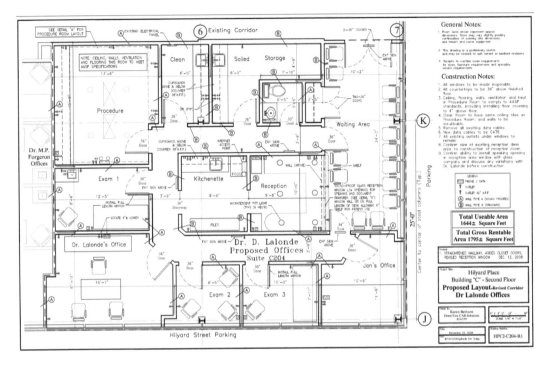

Fig. 16.9 Blueprint of Dr Lalonde's current office conceived in 2008. We would make the procedure room bigger than the current 13 by 16 feet if we did it again. Also, the exam 1 room served as a second procedure room in 2020 because Dr Lalonde no longer uses an overhead light and only a headlight for office and hospital minor procedure room surgery. Clearly, we would make the second procedure room larger than the current 12 by 8 feet if we did it over again. However, you can easily do WALANT safely in a room that small.

- We have sterile gowns and large drapes available when we choose to have augmented field sterility for cases such as open finger and hand fractures, and flexor tendon repairs. Sterile C-arm drapes are also available such as in ▶ Fig. 16.7 when we open fractures.

- We do have a tourniquet but seldom use it. We use a sterile 0.25-inch Penrose drain for a tourniquet for some finger procedures such as nail bed work, schwannoma, or giant cell tumor excision.

- We now have a portable ultrasound machine which is also very helpful for diagnostic and therapeutic purposes (see Chapter 49).

HAND TRAUMA

- In many Canadian cities, most trauma surgery, such as K-wiring fractures and repairing lacerated tendons and nerves, happens in clinical minor procedure rooms. We operate at our convenience in daytime hours with field sterility (see Chapter 10). In Calgary, wide awake hand surgery trauma minor procedure rooms are available to surgeons on weekends as well (▶ Fig. 16.10).

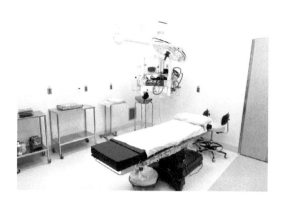

Fig. 16.10 Minor procedure room at Foothills Medical Centre, Calgary where WALANT hand trauma surgery (including plates and screws) is performed 7 days a week.

- Our typical telephone discussion with the emergentologists at Saint John is like this: "Thank you for your (Saturday night) call. I would be so grateful if you would kindly wash it out, close the skin, and we will be delighted to see the patient in the clinic Monday/Friday morning."

- It is ideal to have a clinic with a WALANT minor procedure room adjacent to the emergency department (ED) as they do in Ottawa, Canada. Hand trauma patients go directly from the ED to the WALANT room at the Ottawa Civic Hospital.

- At Saint John, our emergentologists refer most hand trauma patients to the hand surgery clinics four mornings a week. There we triage them into those who need surgery and those who do not. Patients requiring surgery can have it done right there in the minor procedure rooms the morning we see them.

HAND THERAPISTS TREATMENT ROOM NEAR THE MINOR PROCEDURE ROOMS

- It is ideal to have the hand therapists working in a room nearby (see ▶ Video 16.1) so we can invite them into our minor procedure rooms to witness tendon and fracture surgery, educate patients during the surgery, and fabricate splints before or after the surgery (see Chapter 15).

PROCEDURES NOT PERFORMED IN MINOR PROCEDURE ROOMS

- For some procedures, we prefer doing WALANT in a formal OR environment for full sterility or vital sign monitoring of the patient.

- Full sterility may also be desirable when inserting foreign bodies such as joint implants. We also use main OR full sterility for long procedures in relatively avascular areas, such as thumb basal joint arthroplasty, extensive tendon transfers, or secondary tendon reconstruction.

- If a patient has cardiac issues and monitoring is desirable, we use monitors for WALANT patients in the main OR. We can also decrease the concentration of epinephrine to 1:400,000. It washes out faster and bleeds a little more but still provides excellent visualization.

References

1. McKee DE, Lalonde DH, Thoma A, Glennie DL, Hayward JE. Optimal time delay between epinephrine injection and incision to minimize bleeding. Plast Reconstr Surg 2013;131(4):811–814
2. Leblanc MR, Lalonde J, Lalonde DH. A detailed cost and efficiency analysis of performing carpal tunnel surgery in the main operating room versus the ambulatory setting in Canada. Hand (N Y) 2007;2(4):173–178
3. Thomson CJ, Lalonde DH. Measurement of radiation exposure over a one-year period from Fluoroscan mini c-arm imaging unit. Plast Reconstr Surg 2007;119(3):1147–1148
4. Yu J, Ji TA, Craig M, McKee D, Lalonde DH. Evidence-based sterility: the evolving role of field sterility in skin and minor hand surgery. Plast Reconstr Surg Glob Open 2019;7(11):e2481

Section III

DETAILS OF HOW TO DO WALANT WITH THERAPY
TIPS FOR THE UPPER EXTREMITY

CHAPTER 17

TRIGGER FINGER

Donald H. Lalonde and Thomas Apard

ADVANTAGES OF WALANT VERSUS SEDATION AND TOURNIQUET IN TRIGGER FINGER SURGERY

- All of the general advantages listed in Chapter 2 apply to both the surgeon and the patient (no nausea, no tourniquet pain[1] or let-down bleeding, decreased cost[2,3,4,5] without sedation in minor procedure room, safer surgery without sedation, etc.).

- Patients are able to see that the triggering action is gone as they watch themselves moving their fingers through a full range of motion during the surgery.

- You only need to divide the part of the pulley that is required to solve the problem as seen by active flexion, not the entire A1 pulley.

- After you release the pulley, you will occasionally see a band of fibrous tissue proximal to the pulley still causing triggering when the patient makes a fist during the surgery. You can release it to make sure you have solved the problem with full active flexion.

- A major advantage of eliminating sedation for trigger finger surgery is that you do not need to perform the procedure in the main operating room. We perform all trigger finger procedures in minor procedure rooms in the clinic outside the main operating room with field sterility (see Chapter 10).

- You can easily perform 15 or more carpal tunnel releases mixed with trigger finger procedures in 1 day with only one nurse with field sterility in the office or clinic. You can also see consultation and recheck patients between operations (see Chapter 14).

- You do not need cautery, particularly if you inject the lidocaine–epinephrine solution half an hour before you make an incision. We have not opened a cautery for 35 years for trigger fingers, and hematoma has not been a problem, even in patients receiving anticoagulants.

- WALANT trigger finger release is also easily accomplished in children[6] (also see ▶ Video 9.5, Chapter 9).

- See Chapter 49 for ultrasound-guided trigger finger release with WALANT.

Video 17.1
Explaining to patients that many trigger fingers get better without treatment and how WALANT surgery is done (Lalonde, Canada).

- As 50% of trigger fingers and thumbs resolve by 8 months after consultation with no treatment whatsoever, many do not need surgery or steroid injection if they do not bother the patients very much[7] (see ▶ Video 17.1 for explanation of how to tell patients this).

WHERE TO INJECT THE LOCAL ANESTHETIC FOR TRIGGER FINGER AND TRIGGER THUMB

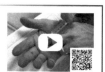

Video 17.2
Injection of local anesthesia for trigger finger surgery (Lalonde, Canada).

Video 17.3
Injection of local anesthesia for trigger thumb surgery in supine position (Lalonde, Canada).

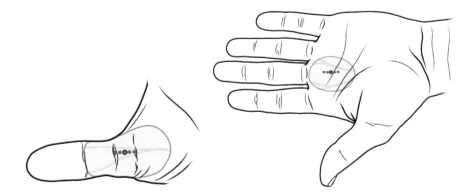

Fig. 17.1 and Fig. 17.2 Inject 4 mL of 1% lidocaine with 1:100,000 epinephrine (buffered with 10 mL lido/epi: 1 mL of 8.4% sodium bicarbonate) under the skin in the fat at the red injection dot site. Do NOT inject in the sheath! It hurts unnecessarily. Let the local anesthesia diffuse into the sheath over 30 minutes or more.

SPECIFICS OF MINIMALLY PAINFUL INJECTION OF LOCAL ANESTHETIC FOR TRIGGER FINGER SURGERY

- Local anesthesia injection should barely hurt at all if you follow the simple rules of Chapter 5 for hints to minimize injection pain. The patients will think you are magical.

- We always inject all patients while they are lying down to decrease the risk of their fainting (see Chapter 6).

- Inject just under the skin. The local anesthetic will diffuse into the sheath over 30 minutes. There is no need to inject into the sheath; this adds a lot of unnecessary pain.

- If you inject into the sheath, the local anesthetic will diffuse up the sheath into the whole finger or thumb. With enough pressure, the sheath will "explode" or burst. This will cause pain and send the epinephrine and lidocaine to the very end of the digit. This can cause a white fingertip. As with almost all white fingertips, it will eventually pink up. However, phentolamine can be injected to reverse accidental intrasheath white finger vasoconstriction (see ▶ Video 3.3, Chapter 3).

- Inject the anesthetic solution a minimum of 30 minutes before surgery to allow the epinephrine to take optimal effect and provide an adequately dry working field,[8,9] as outlined in Chapter 4 and Chapter 14.

Video 17.4
Injecting in the sheath hurts a lot more than in the fat. It also results in white finger (Lalonde, Canada).

TIPS AND TRICKS FOR PERFORMING TRIGGER THUMB OR FINGER SURGERY WITH THE WIDE AWAKE APPROACH

- The patient needs to look at the fingers to get them to move, since he or she cannot feel the numbed digit. Although most patients don't mind looking at the wound, you can cover the wound with a towel as the patient flexes all fingers together while looking at them.

- Close the skin with buried intradermal simple interrupted 5-0 Monocryl sutures as shown in detail for carpal tunnel closure in ▶ Video 26.8.

- Many patients are interested in looking at the tendon to understand the nature of their problem. Offer patients a guided tour of their trigger finger surgery. Many will accept and be delighted that they were given the opportunity to experience seeing the inside of their hand. You can put a mask on the patient, show him or her the tendon and have him or her watch it move. Many patients love this. Some patients have told others it is something they need to put on their bucket list!

- Outside the operating room, inject two to four patients who will undergo straightforward procedures such as trigger finger or thumb release, carpal tunnel release, and excision of a ganglion cyst before operating on the first patient. This gives at least half an hour for the local anesthetic to work both for lidocaine numbing and for epinephrine vasoconstriction. It takes 26 minutes to achieve peak vasoconstriction in humans after 1:100,000 epinephrine injection (level I evidence).[8,9]

- After you inject the first patient, most of them usually feel well enough to go sit in the waiting area for their surgery. You can then inject the second patient, then the third one. Next you can perform the surgery on the first patient. While the nurse turns over the room after the first one, you can inject the fourth patient.

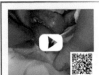

Video 17.5 Trigger thumb surgery in supine position (Lalonde, Canada).

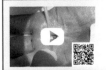

Video 17.6 Trigger finger surgery (Lalonde, Canada).

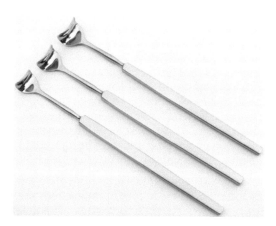

Fig. 17.3 We use Desmarres or vein retractors, which help to keep the fat out of the way and show the sheath (see ▶ Video 17.6).

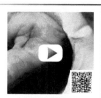

Video 17.7 Prone position for trigger thumb local injection (patient lying on abdomen) (Lalonde, Canada).

Video 17.8 Prone position for trigger thumb surgery and skin closure with buried dermal interrupted Monocryl so that there are no sutures to remove (Lalonde, Canada).

Video 17.9 Percutaneous needle trigger finger release with ultrasound guidance (Apard, France).

- Have your assistant push down on the Desmarres retractors to keep the fat out of the way and decrease the small amount of bleeding that sometimes occurs, especially if the patient is hypertensive or receiving anticoagulants.

- Patients who are comfortable lying on their abdomen can have trigger thumb local anesthesia injection or surgery in the prone position. This makes seeing the tendon sheath easier than when they are lying on their back.

- Buried simple interrupted sutures of absorbable monofilament Monocryl mean that there are no sutures to remove. It also makes it much easier for patients to take their bandage off and get in the shower the day after surgery when there are no sutures sticking out of the skin. We let all our trigger finger and carpal tunnel patients get in the shower with a naked hand the day after surgery.

- You can educate the patient during the local anesthetic injection (3 minutes) and during the surgery and bandage application (10 minutes). This gives you 13 minutes of patient education time, which will serve to decrease your complication rate and decrease the time you would spend educating the patient in the office (see ▶ Video 9.5 on good intraoperative advice on postoperative activity, pain medicine, pain-guided healing, and showering in an 8-year-old with trigger thumb with her mother in the minor procedure room in Dr Lalonde's office).

- You can also release the trigger finger with a needle and ultrasound guidance as shown in ▶ Video 17.9. You can learn much more about ultrasound in the hand and ultrasound-guided surgery in Chapter 49 and Chapter 50.

References

1. Gunasagaran J, Sean ES, Shivdas S, Amir S, Ahmad TS. Perceived comfort during minor hand surgeries with wide awake local anaesthesia no tourniquet (WALANT) versus local anaesthesia (LA)/tourniquet. J Orthop Surg (Hong Kong) 2017;25(3):2309499017739499

2. Kazmers NH, Stephens AR, Presson AP, Yu Z, Tyser AR. Cost implications of varying the surgical setting and anesthesia type for trigger finger release surgery. Plast Reconstr Surg Glob Open 2019;7(5):e2231

3. Codding JL, Bhat SB, Ilyas AM. An economic analysis of MAC versus WALANT: a trigger finger release surgery case study. Hand (N Y) 2017;12(4):348–351

4. Burn MB, Shapiro LM, Eppler SL, Behal R, Kamal RN. Clinical care redesign to improve value for trigger finger release: a before-and-after quality improvement study. [published online ahead of print] Hand (N Y) November 5, 2019;1558944719884661. 10.1177/1558944719884661

5. Far-Riera AM, Pérez-Uribarri C, Sánchez Jiménez M, Esteras Serrano MJ, Rapariz González JM, Ruiz Hernández IM. Estudio prospectivo sobre la aplicación de un circuito WALANT para la cirugía del síndrome del túnel carpiano y dedo en resorte [Prospective study on the application of a WALANT circuit for surgery of tunnel carpal syndrome and trigger finger]. Rev Esp Cir Ortop Traumatol 2019;63(6):400–407

6. Wang HC, Lin GT. Percutaneous release for trigger thumb in children under general and local anesthesia. Kaohsiung J Med Sci 2004;20(11):546–551

7. McKee D, Lalonde J, Lalonde D. How many trigger fingers resolve spontaneously without any treatment? Plast Surg (Oakv) 2018;26(1):52–54

8. McKee DE, Lalonde DH, Thoma A, Glennie DL, Hayward JE. Optimal time delay between epinephrine injection and incision to minimize bleeding. Plast Reconstr Surg 2013;131(4):811–814

9. Mohd Rashid MZ, Sapuan J, Abdullah S. A randomized controlled trial of trigger finger release under digital anesthesia with (WALANT) and without adrenaline. J Orthop Surg (Hong Kong) 2019;27(1):2309499019833002

CHAPTER 18

DE QUERVAIN'S RELEASE

Donald H. Lalonde, Xavier Gueffier, and Alistair Phillips

ADVANTAGES OF WALANT VERSUS SEDATION AND TOURNIQUET IN DE QUERVAIN'S RELEASE

- All of the general advantages listed in Chapter 2 apply to both the surgeon and the patient (no nausea, no tourniquet pain or let-down bleeding, decreased cost without sedation in minor procedure room, safer surgery without sedation, etc.).

- You can see active movement differentiating the abductor pollicis longus (APL) and the extensor pollicis brevis (EPB) so you can identify and release both compartments.

- A major advantage of eliminating sedation for trigger finger surgery is that you do not need to perform the procedure in the main operating room. We perform all trigger finger procedures in minor procedure rooms in the clinic outside the main operating room with field sterility (see Chapter 10).

- You can easily perform 15 or more carpal tunnel releases mixed with trigger finger procedures in 1 day with only one nurse with field sterility in the office or clinic. You can also see consultation and recheck patients between operations (see Chapter 14).

- Active movement can ensure the lack of tendon subluxation after the compartment release. Reconstruction can be performed as shown in ▶ Video 18.3 if this occurs.

WHERE TO INJECT THE LOCAL ANESTHETIC FOR DE QUERVAIN'S RELEASE

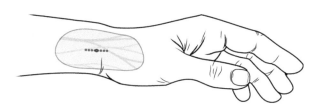

Fig. 18.1 Inject 10 mL of 1% lidocaine with 1:100,000 epinephrine (buffered with 10 mL lido/epi: 1 mL of 8.4% sodium bicarbonate) subcutaneously in the center of the incision area. **Do NOT inject in the sheath!** It hurts unnecessarily. Let the local anesthesia diffuse into the sheath over 30 minutes or more.

- See Chapter 1, Atlas, for more illustrations of the anatomy of diffusion of tumescent local anesthetic in the forearm, wrist, and hand.

SPECIFICS OF MINIMAL PAIN INJECTION OF LOCAL ANESTHETIC IN DE QUERVAIN'S RELEASE

- Local anesthesia injection should barely hurt at all if you follow the simple rules of Chapter 5 for hints to minimize injection pain. The patients will think you are magical.

- Inject just under the skin. **There is no need to inject into the sheath; this would only add unnecessary pain.** The local anesthetic will diffuse into the sheath if you wait half an hour.

- Since the skin on the radial wrist is thin and elastic, you can pinch it proximal to the needle insertion site and lift the skin into the needle to add the sensory "noise" of pressure to decrease the pain from the first needle insertion.

- There is no need to move the needle from the initial placement site under the skin. The local anesthetic will go everywhere it needs to go. Think of it as an extravascular Bier block injected only where you need it.

- We inject the anesthetic solution a minimum of 30 minutes before surgery to allow the epinephrine to take optimal effect and provide an adequately dry working field, as outlined in Chapter 4 and Chapter 14.

- We inject supine patients lying down on stretchers in a waiting area to decrease the risk of their fainting (see ► Video 6.1).

Video 18.1
Injection of local anesthesia for De Quervain's release (Lalonde, Canada).

TIPS AND TRICKS FOR PERFORMING DE QUERVAIN'S RELEASE WITH THE WIDE AWAKE APPROACH

- The patient probably needs to look at the thumb to get it to move because it is numb. Although most patients do not mind looking at the wound, you can partly cover the wound with a towel as the patient flexes and extends the thumb.

- Many patients are interested in looking at the tendon to understand the nature of their problem. You can put a mask on them, then show them the tendon and watch it move. Many patients love this. Some will tell others it is something they need to put on their bucket list!

- Desmarres or vein retractors help to keep the fat away and show the sheath.

- ▶ Video 18.2 has other tips and tricks by Lalonde for De Quervain's release.

- Although Lalonde prefers simple decompression of De Quervain's canal, Gueffier from France shows ancillary synovectomy techniques and ultrasound images in ▶ Video 18.3.

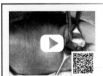

Video 18.2
Surgery for De Quervain's release (Lalonde, Canada).

Video 18.3
Surgery for De Quervain's release (Gueffier, France).

CHAPTER 19

FLEXOR TENDON REPAIR OF THE FINGER

*Jin Bo Tang, Shu Guo Xing, Jason Wong,
Amanda Higgins, Lisa Flewelling, Egemen Ayhan,
Thomas Apard, Geoffrey Cook, Paul Sibley, Asif Ilyas,
Xavier Gueffier, Duncan McGrouther, Ian Maxwell,
Amir Adham Ahmad, and Donald H. Lalonde*

ADVANTAGES OF WALANT VERSUS SEDATION AND TOURNIQUET IN FLEXOR TENDON REPAIR OF THE FINGER

- All of the general advantages listed in Chapter 2 apply to both the surgeon and the patient (no nausea, no tourniquet pain or let-down bleeding, decreased cost without sedation in minor procedure room, safer surgery without sedation, etc.).

DECREASE RUPTURE RATES BY ALLOWING YOU TO SEE AND REPAIR GAPS CAUSED BY THE FORCES OF ACTIVE MOVEMENT WITH INTRAOPERATIVE PATIENT ACTIVE FULL-FIST FLEXION AND EXTENSION TESTING

- You are less likely to have to perform a secondary surgery for rupture repair if you test the repair intraoperatively by having the patient take the fingers through a full range of flexion and extension before skin closure.[1,2]
- If you see the repair gapping after you ask the patient to make a full fist and completely straighten the fingers, you can repair the gap with more sutures, retest the repair to confirm that it is reliable with intraoperative flexion testing, and then close the skin. This is like testing blood flow through a microvascular anastomosis to avoid failure.[4]

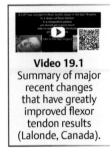

Video 19.1
Summary of major recent changes that have greatly improved flexor tendon results (Lalonde, Canada).

- Detecting a gap that would cause rupture is easy in WALANT patients. Get them to fully flex and extend the fingers or thumb several times to reveal sutures that are too loose and would go onto gap and rupture.

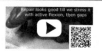

Video 19.2a
Avoiding rupture by testing repair with full-fist active flexion and extension and repairing gaps that would rupture (Lalonde, Canada).

Video 19.2b A second beautiful six-strand flexor pollicis longus (FPL) repair pulled apart by the hard edge of a pulley with active movement testing. We redid the repair after cutting the pulley. This would have ruptured but WALANT showed us the problem and we fixed it (Lalonde, Canada).

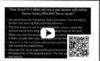

Video 19.3a How to fix gaps and avoid rupture (Lalonde, Canada).

Video 19.3b Avoiding tenolysis with full-fist flexion and extension testing leading to complete venting of A1 and A2 pulleys with no clinically significant bowstringing on the table or after surgery (Lalonde, Canada).

How to Fix a Gap that Appears with Active Movement Testing of the First Suture of a Repaired Tendon at Surgery to Avoid Rupture (see ▶ Video 19.3a)

- Do not remove the first suture that is too loose. This will add to tendon end scarring that promotes adhesion.

- The first thing is to put in a second tighter suture. Leave the second suture ends long instead of cutting them short at the knot.

- Make sure that the second tighter suture holds the repair and that it does not gap when you test it with full-fist flexion and extension.

- Now pull on the first loose suture knot until the first suture is tight enough and holding the repair firmly.

- Now take the loose exposed thread and knot of the first tightened suture and tie it to the long ends of the second suture. The first suture is now tight enough and secure. You now have a four-strand repair.

WALANT CAN DECREASE TENOLYSIS RATES BY MAKING SURE THE REPAIRS FIT THROUGH THE PULLEYS WITH ADEQUATE PULLEY VENTING TESTED WITH ACTIVE PATIENT FULL-FIST FLEXION AND EXTENSION BEFORE YOU CLOSE THE SKIN

- A lot of unnecessary tenolysis is performed because the flexor tendon repair cannot fit through unvented A2 or A4 pulleys. You are less likely to have to come back for tenolysis if you see the patient take the fingers through a full range of motion before you close the skin. See ▶ Video 19.4a and section Tips and Tricks of Pulley Venting later in this chapter.

- You can also avoid many cases of tenolysis with relative motion extension splinting to get the flexor digitorum profundus (FDP) out of scar instead of unnecessary surgery (see ▶ Video 19.TT9) in Therapy Tips after Zones 1 and 2 Flexor Tendon Repair below).

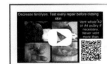

Video 19.4a
Avoiding tenolysis with full-fist flexion and extension testing (Lalonde, Canada).

WALANT HELPED US DEVELOP AN ELEGANT NEW SOLUTION TO A 2-MONTH-OLD JERSEY FINGER PROBLEM

- When we completely separated FDS from FDP in a 2-month-old Jersey finger, the profundus easily reached the distal phalanx and allowed full active extension after reinsertion to the bone. It may be the adhesions between profundus and superficialis that "hold FDP too short" in neglected Jersey fingers.

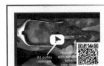

Video 19.4b
Elegant new solution to 2-month-old jersey finger (Maxwell and Lalonde, Canada).

SEEING THE PATIENT MAKE A FULL FIST AND COMPLETELY STRAIGHTEN OUT THE FINGERS WITHOUT GAPPING AT SURGERY GIVES THE SURGEON FULL CONFIDENCE TO ALLOW UP TO HALF A FIST OF PAIN-GUIDED TRUE ACTIVE MOVEMENT 3 TO 5 DAYS LATER

- Like others, we have abandoned the use of Kleinert rubber bands as well as "full-fist, place-and-hold" active extension and passive flexion in favor of true active movement in our postoperative regimen[6,9,10] (see Therapy Tips after Zones 1 and 2 Flexor Tendon Repair at the end of this chapter).

- We feel that up to half a fist of true active pain-guided finger flexion and full finger phalangeal joint extension has improved the results of our repair. We allow full wrist extension, up to half a fist of active flexion (45 degrees of active metacarpophalangeal [MP] extension, and up to 45 degrees of active proximal interphalangeal [PIP] and distal interphalangeal [DIP] flexion), providing it does not hurt and that the patient is off all pain medication.

- The greatest risk of rupture is in the last half of a fist.[6]

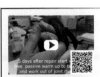

Video 19.5 Start up to half a fist of pain-guided true active movement 3 to 5 days after flexor tendon repair (Higgins, Canada).

- We only need up to half a fist of finger movement to consistently provide 5 to 15 mm of profundus glide.[7]

Video 19.6 Seeing no gap with full fist flexion and extension at surgery gives surgeon confidence to start up to half a fist of flexion at 3 to 5 days after surgery (Lalonde, Canada).

Video 19.7a Intraoperative patient education in unsedated patients who remember everything will decrease postoperative complications such as rupture and tenolysis (Lalonde, Canada).

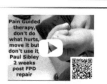

Video 19.7b Intraoperative patient education in unsedated patients leads to good pain-guided therapy (don't do what hurts, move it but don't use it) (Sibley, USA).

Video 19.7c Intraoperative patient education to avoid rupture and tenolysis (Lalonde, Canada).

INTRAOPERATIVE PATIENT EDUCATION DECREASES THE RISK OF POSTOPERATIVE RUPTURE AND THE NEED FOR TENOLYSIS

- The ability to educate the patient intraoperatively during a WALANT flexor tendon repair decreases rupture and tenolysis rates because the patient sees it all and remembers the consequences of moving versus using the hand after surgery.

- You get the chance to hear what activities your patient HAD planned the week after the surgery. A flexor tendon repair will certainly change the patient's life plan for a while. You can help the patient think through this as you discuss safe activities during the surgery.

- When patients leave the operating room, they know exactly what they need to do to get a good result. What is more important, they know what they must *not* do. They know they can *move* the fingers, but that they cannot *use* the fingers or they will lose the good result.

- WALANT allows you and the hand therapist (see Therapy Tips after Zones 1 and 2 Flexor Tendon Repair below) to assess patients and educate them for up to 60 uninterrupted minutes during the surgery. We know this has been very important in improving our results.

- You and the hand therapist can get to know patients during the surgery and decide whether you can trust them with early protected movement (see ▶ Video 15.1).

- For a clip on a surgeon and therapist explaining the Saint John postoperative flexor tendon repair protocol to a patient during surgery, see ▶ Video 15.2.

- Patients get to see that the repaired tendon works as they watch themselves moving the fingers through a full range of motion before the skin is closed. They know that their finger will function well once they get past the postoperative discomfort and stiffness if they put the effort into therapy.

- Patients start their therapy at 3 to 5 days with up to half a fist of true active movement knowing that they must be off all pain medicine, that they must not do what hurts in therapy (pain-guided therapy), and that they can move their hand but they cannot use it.

WALANT ALLOWS YOU TO DETERMINE WHETHER SUPERFICIALIS REPAIR IS APPROPRIATE

- You can repair one or both slips of superficialis and see how this affects the full range of active movement during the surgery. If superficialis repair downgrades the movement, you can resect one of the slips or take down the whole superficialis repair to get the best possible active movement before you end the operation (see ▶ Video 19.8).

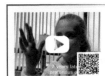

Video 19.8
Deciding whether or not to repair superficialis by what you see moving at surgery after the repair in a 6-year-old—7-year follow-up (Lalonde, Canada).

YOU CAN RECONSTRUCT THE PULLEY AT THE TIME OF FLEXOR TENDON REPAIR IF YOU SEE CLINICALLY SIGNIFICANT BOWSTRINGING WITH ACTIVE MOVEMENT

- Primary pulley reconstruction with a graft during wide awake flexor tendon repair is helpful as demonstrated in ▶ Video 19.9. You can also use the superficialis tendon with its insertion intact to create a very solid pulley as we did in ▶ Video 19.4b.

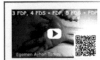

Video 19.9
Primary pulley reconstruction at the time of flexor tendon repair (Ayhan, Turkey).

PRONE SURGERY CAN EASILY FACILITATE FLEXOR POLLICIS LONGUS (FPL) REPAIR IN WALANT PATIENTS WHO ARE COMFORTABLE LYING ON THEIR ABDOMEN

- Start by asking the patients if they are comfortable sleeping on their stomach.
- If they are, thumb flexor tendon surgery is easier in this position (see trigger thumb surgery in ▶ Video 17.7).

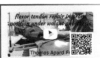

Video 19.10 Flexor pollicis longus (FPL) repair is easier in the prone position which is easy with WALANT (Apard, France).

IF A DELAYED TENDON REPAIR HAS MADE FDP TOO SHORT, WALANT ENABLES FDP FRACTIONAL LENGTHENING IN THE FOREARM IN DELAYED REPAIR OF FINGER FLEXOR LACERATIONS WITH ACCURATE TENSIONING

- We used to think that you cannot perform primary repair of tendons after 3 weeks post injury. Wide awake surgery has repeatedly shown us that you can (see ▶ Video 19.25 and Video 19.26 for examples). Patients can stretch them out over a year or two in some cases even if they are too tight.

- If the tendon is really too short, you can lengthen it as shown in ▶ Video 19.11.

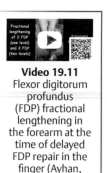

Video 19.11
Flexor digitorum profundus (FDP) fractional lengthening in the forearm at the time of delayed FDP repair in the finger (Ayhan, Turkey).

OTHER ADVANTAGES OF WALANT VERSUS SEDATION AND TOURNIQUET

- A major advantage of eliminating sedation and the tourniquet for flexor tendon repair is that you do not need to perform the procedure in the main operating room. Some of us (Lalonde) do all tendon repairs in minor procedure rooms in the clinic outside the main operating room Monday to Friday, 8 AM to 4 PM (see Chapter 16). This means we no longer do these procedures at night. We know that we do better tendon repairs at 2 PM when we are fresh and awake than at 2 AM, when we are tired and sleepy.

- We perform the surgery with field sterility or add gowns and drapes for augmented field sterility (see Chapter 10).

- Working outside the main operating room also allows our hand therapists to be there to teach patients during the surgery and see the repair (see Chapter 15 and Therapy tips after Zones 1 and 2 Flexor Tendon Repair below).

- We no longer have to admit patients because of their medical comorbidities, which are only a problem when we sedate them.

WHERE TO INJECT THE LOCAL ANESTHETIC FOR FLEXOR TENDON REPAIR OF THE FINGER

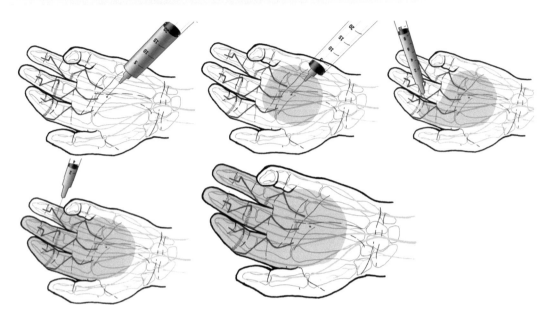

Fig. 19.1 (a, b) Inject 10 mL of 1% lidocaine with 1:100,000 epinephrine buffered with sodium bicarbonate (1 mL of 8.4% bicarbonate for each 10 mL of 1% lidocaine with 1:100,000 epinephrine) in the most proximal injection point. The first few milliliters go under the skin, and the rest is injected under the superficial palmar fascia without moving the needle. Wait 30 minutes for the local anesthesia to numb the common digital nerves, and then inject the distal palm (3 mL at each finger base) and fingers for the epinephrine effect. **(c–e)** Inject 2 mL in the fat just below the skin between the two digital nerves in each of the proximal and middle phalanges. Inject 1 mL of the same solution in the subcutaneous fat in the middle of the distal phalanx just past the crease if you feel you will need to dissect in the distal phalanx. (Reproduced with permission from Lalonde DH, Kozin S. Tendon disorders of the hand. Plast Reconstr Surg 128:1e, 2011.)

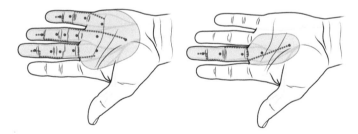

Fig. 19.2 (a, b) Alternative rectangular flap incisions are shown, which cover the tendon more effectively if the wounds dehisce. Some surgeons prefer to use only parts of the possible incisions illustrated.

SPECIFICS OF MINIMALLY PAINFUL INJECTION OF LOCAL ANESTHETIC IN FLEXOR TENDON REPAIR OF THE FINGER

Video 19.12 How to inject local anesthetic for one finger flexor tendon repair (Lalonde, Canada).

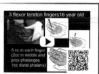

Video 19.13 How to inject local anesthetic for three fingers flexor tendon repair (Lalonde, Canada).

- Inject local anesthetic into the hand in the waiting area 30 or more minutes before surgery, as outlined in Chapter 4, Chapter 5, and Chapter 14. This allows the epinephrine to take effect and provides an adequately dry working field.[3]

- Local anesthesia injection should barely hurt at all if you follow the simple rules of Chapter 5 for hints to minimize injection pain. The patients will think you are magical. We always inject all patients while they are lying down to decrease the risk of their fainting (see ▶ Video 6.1).

- Start by injecting 10 mL with a 27-gauge needle into the most proximal location that you are likely to find the proximal tendon stumps. For finger tendon lacerations, this usually means the proximal palm at the level at which the median nerve begins branching. If the injury disrupted the vincula and the proximal tendon flips proximally with great force out of the sheath and into the palm, you can retrieve it easily from the numbed palm.

- Inject the first 0.5 mL until it is visible below the skin, then pause. The first bleb must be visible or palpable under the skin to properly numb the needle insertion site. Wait 15 to 45 seconds until the patient tells you that the sting is gone. Then inject the rest of the 10 mL infiltration very slowly (over 2 to 3 minutes) without moving the needle.

- There is no need to move the needle distally as you inject. If you keep your needle in one place and continue to inject slowly, you will see and palpate the local anesthetic going everywhere in the palm. You want the area you will dissect to become a little firm with visible and palpable local anesthetic. You will not cause a palmar compartment syndrome. As soon as you incise the skin, the pressure will come down as the local anesthetic leaks out.

- If you inject 10 to 20 mL into the palm, where is it going to go? Everywhere! It is like an extravascular Bier block, but only where you need it.

- The goal of the injection is to bathe visible and palpable local anesthetic 2 cm beyond wherever you think you have even a small chance of dissecting.

- Wait 30 or more minutes, if possible, to let the palm's common digital nerves become completely numb. Then inject the distal palm with 3 mL at the base of each finger you are going to dissect. After this, inject each proximal and middle phalanx with only 2 mL of buffered lidocaine and epinephrine in the subcutaneous fat between both digital nerves. The distal phalanges only get 1 mL between the digital nerves if dissection will be needed there. These finger injections are for the epinephrine effect.

- Only reinsert the needle into clearly numb areas to avoid pain after the first injection (see ▶ Video 5.3).

TIPS AND TRICKS FOR PERFORMING FLEXOR TENDON REPAIR OF THE FINGER WITH THE WIDE AWAKE APPROACH

TIPS AND TRICKS OF PULLEY VENTING

- We used to believe that you could not vent the A2 or A4 pulleys. This rule gave us 50 years of unnecessary rupture and tenolysis. The new rule is **"Do not vent more than a total of 1.5–2.0 cm pulley to avoid clinically significant bowstringing."**[6,8]

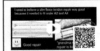

Video 19.14 On how and why vent pulleys to get good results (Lalonde, Canada).

- After the first core suture, you incrementally vent only the amount of pulley that you need in order to permit active full-fist flexion and extension of the fingers or thumb by the awake patient.

- You can vent the entire A4 pulley or a part or even the entire A2 pulley if you need in order to get full-fist flexion and extension, but not both the A2 and A4 at the same time. You can vent A3 and A4 at the same time if necessary. In the majority of patients, venting a part (not entire) of A2 pulley is sufficient, because you always can vent adjacent sheath with the part of the A2 pulley. Occasionally venting of the entire A2 pulley is necessary and reports (and ▶ Videos like 19.3b) show there are no adverse consequences.[8] A small amount of bowstringing is often not clinically significant if it does not impair a full range of motion, which is easily assessed in the awake patient.

Video 19.15 Another example of A4 pulley venting with no clinically significant bowstringing postoperatively (Ayhan, Turkey).

- As noted above, you can reconstruct pulleys if you get clinically significant bowstringing with active movement at the time of repair (see ▶ Video 19.19).

TIPS AND TRICKS OF PROXIMAL TENDON RETRIEVAL

- When you are pulling the proximal tendon stump distally, an awake patient may find it hard to relax and may pull the tendon away from you. Ask the patient to extend the fingers while you passively flex the wrist and MP joints. Active extension of the fingers causes a spinal reflex relaxation of the finger flexors to help you deliver the tendon without extra incisions.

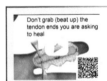

Video 19.16a Tips on how to retrieve the proximal tendon ends (Lalonde, Canada).

- You must take down barrier sheets and let the patient see his or her fingers if you want him or her to move them the way you would like. Patients need to look at their fingers to know whether they are moving because they cannot feel them. However, if patients look, they can move just as they wish. Although most patients do not mind looking at the wound, you can cover it with a towel as they flex their fingers if they do not want to see the open wounds.

Video 19.16b
Separate incision in the palm to retrieve tendon permits shorter finger incision to reduce finger scarring and postoperative swelling and stiffness (Tang, China).

- Consider accessing the tendon through a proximal sheathotomy where you can see it through the sheath. Leave the tendon in the sheath and push it with two Adson forceps like pushing a rope in a tube (see ▶ Video 19.16b). You avoid having the forceps crush the severed tendon ends you are trying to heal.

- You are more likely to keep the FDP between the two slips of the flexor digitorum superficialis (FDS) if you push it from proximal to distal than if you pass a red rubber catheter proximally and blindly down the sheath from the laceration site. However, even when you push the tendon from a proximal sheathotomy, it may not end up between the superficialis slips. Be sure you have restored that normal anatomy before you suture the tendon.

- We prefer less invasive exposure of the flexor sheath in the finger. Instead of a long incision in the finger, which creates more scarring, make a separate incision in the palm and possibly advance the tendon from there using a pediatric feeding tube or push it with Adson forceps.[5]

- We prefer retrieval of the retracted FDP tendon through making a separate incision in the palm to find the FDP tendon and push the FDP tendon distally with two forceps. This will not damage the FDP tendon ends and also minimize the length of incision at the site of tendon repair (▶ Fig. 19.3).

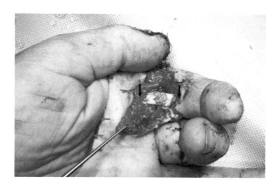

Fig. 19.3 Very limited (usually <2 cm) extension of the cut wounds in the finger to expose the distal flexor digitorum profundus (FDP) tendon stump with the distal interphalangeal (DIP) joint flexed. This decreases finger scarring. The retracted proximal FDP tendon is pushed with two forceps through a separate transverse incision in the palm (indicated with blue arrows). The length of the sheath-pulley venting is 1.5 to 2 cm, which fits exactly to the length of skin incision (two black arrows). In this patient, also seen post-op in ▶ Fig. 19.4 and ▶ Fig. 19.5, the distal half of the A2 pulley with 1 cm of the sheath distal to the A2 pulley was vented in the index finger. The FDP tendon was repaired with six-strand M-Tang repair plus a sparse running peripheral suture. (Copyright of Jin Bo Tang, MD.)

TIPS AND TRICKS OF TESTING THE REPAIR WITH FULL-FIST ACTIVE FLEXION AND EXTENSION

- After the repair, ask the patient to make a full fist and extend the fingers completely. This is an important test to verify that the repair is strong and can tolerate early active motion. The three parts of the digital extension–flexion test are:

  – Full active extension to verify no gapping between the tendon ends.

- Smooth active flexion to verify smooth gliding of the repair site.
- Total active flexion to verify that none of the pulleys prevents tendon gliding.

- Do not be afraid to test full-fist flexion and full extension of the fingers and thumb. Your sutures need to be strong enough to take it. If they are not, you need to reinforce them. Repeated evaluation of total active movement is important to verify that the repair is strong and enough pulley has been vented.

- If the extension–flexion test creates a visible gap between the two tendon ends during finger extension, the suture is usually not tight enough and needs repair with additional tighter sutures with proper tension to avoid rupture. You can remove, tighten, or leave the previously loose suture, as appropriate (▶ Video 19.3a). Slightly tensioning the repair is very important to prevent gapping.

- See ▶ Video 19.3a for how to repair a gap when you see one after full-fist flexion and extension testing.

WE ONLY CUT AS MUCH SHEATH AS WE NEED TO. WALANT CAN ACTUALLY HELP PRESERVE MORE SHEATH IF IT DOES NOT IMPAIR MOVEMENT. YOU CAN REPAIR THE TENDON INSIDE THE SHEATH WITH SHEATHOTOMIES

- You can suture the tendon inside the flexor sheath through sheathotomies to get a 1-cm bite without having to cut long segments of sheath when the patient is wide awake (see ▶ Video 19.17 and Video 19.18). You can do this because you can then test active flexion to prove that you have not caught your needle and suture inside the sheath.

- Retrieve the proximal tendon by performing a sheathotomy where you can see it through the sheath. Do not grab and crush the tendon ends you want to heal. Push the tendon forward in small increments by grabbing the tendon on the sides with two Adson forceps. Repair the tendon through sheathotomies. Verify that you have not caught your needle with active flexion and extension. Repair the sheathotomies with an absorbable suture.

Video 19.17
Intraoperative flexor pollicis longus (FPL) flexion and extension testing after the repair (Lalonde, Canada).

Video 19.18
Full-fist flexion and extension testing, repairing the tendon inside the sheath, and more tips on WALANT flexor tendon repair (Lalonde, Canada).

Video 19.19
Preserving sheath by suturing through sheathotomies (Lalonde, Canada).

DISCUSS THE ALTERNATIVES OF TREATMENT WITH THE PAIN-FREE NUMBED PATIENT WHEN YOU HAVE SEVERE FINGER DAMAGE

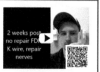

Video 19.20
After a good discussion, this patient opted to have a superficialis finger instead of an amputation (Lalonde, Canada).

- A superficialis finger is a good finger. Sometimes it is better to not even try to repair a profundus tendon as illustrated in ▶ Video 19.20.

- The awake pain-free numbed patient is in a much better position to understand the alternatives of treatment and make a wiser choice with fewer regrets.

YOU DON'T NEED CAUTERY TO REPAIR FLEXOR TENDONS

- We do not worry about minor bleeding when we cut the skin, because most of the little bleeders will stop spontaneously by the time we sew the flaps to the dorsal skin for exposure. We no longer use cautery for most cases. We occasionally leave a hemostat on bigger veins for a few minutes till they stop bleeding without tying them off.

- By the time the flexor repair is done, all of the bleeding will have subsided. The well-informed awake patient then quietly elevates the hand above the heart and keeps it there for the next 3 to 5 days till we see him or her again to start early protected pain-guided therapy.

TIPS ON ZONE 1 INJURIES

Video 19.21
How not to get numbness when exposing the distal tendon stump for suture in zone 1 (Lalonde, Canada).

- To avoid numbness in the fingertip after dissection in zone 1 flexor tendon injuries, remember that 90% of the digital nerve goes to the fingertip. You want to make incisions midline in the volar pulp of the fingertip only as far as the center of the whorl of the fingerprint. Spread with scissors proximal to distal to the center of the whorl to avoid damaging the "leaves of the tree" of the digital nerves.

- When there is distal stump to sew to, we prefer primary repair as advocated by Jin Bo Tang. Sewing into the volar plate can be helpful when there is no stump (see ▶ Video 19.22).[11]

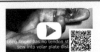

Video 19.22 Jersey fingers with and without stump sewn to stump and distal end of volar plate (Lalonde, Canada).

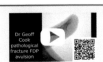

Video 19.23 Jersey fingers with bony block. Two cases from Canada and France (Cook, Canada; Apard, France).

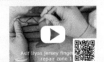

Video 19.24 Jersey finger flexor tendon repair in zone 1 (Ilyas, USA).

OTHER APPLICATIONS OF WALANT FLEXOR TENDON REPAIR

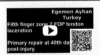

Video 19.25 Primary repair at 40 days after injury can deliver a good result, even in the little finger (Ayhan, Turkey).

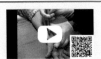

Video 19.26 Primary repair of flexor pollicis longus (FPL) at 5.5 weeks after injury can deliver a good result (Lalonde, Canada).

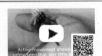

Video 19.27 Active movement shows you that you can preserve small bits of important pulley (Ahmad, Malaysia).

Video 19.28 The hand surgeon finds the exact location of the two ends of the finger flexor tendon with ultrasound before surgery. This video includes local anesthesia injection and surgery (Gueffier, France).

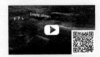

Video 19.29 Ultrasound video of flexor pollicis longus (FPL) repair including pre-op ultrasound (Gueffier, France).

THERAPY TIPS AFTER ZONES 1 AND 2 FLEXOR TENDON REPAIR

THE NANTONG/SAINT JOHN PROTOCOL

- Eliminating any gap with full-fist flexion and extension testing during the surgery gives us the confidence to move away from full-fist, place-and-hold to true active movement as advocated by Tang,[6] Higgins,[13] and Lalonde.[14]

- WALANT has taught us to avoid full-fist, place-and-hold movement in a full-fist position exercise.[12]

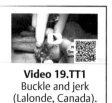

Video 19.TT1
Buckle and jerk
(Lalonde, Canada).

- ▶ Video 19.TT1[12] explains why we do up to half a fist of true active movement instead of full-fist, place-and-hold. True active movement has nice normal gliding motion. WALANT frequently reveals that full-fist, place-and-hold movement has the tendon stop moving with passive flexion at half a fist and then jerk into the rest of full-fist flexion when we ask the patient to hold the fist in flexion. Jerking a freshly repaired tendon could lead to rupture.

FIRST 4 DAYS POSTSURGERY

- The hand is placed in a dorsal block orthosis (splint) with interphalangeal (IP) joints of all fingers in full extension, MP joints in 30 degrees of flexion, and wrist in comfortable extension.[15]

- Patient is taught to keep the hand elevated above the level of the heart all the time either by resting the hand on the opposite shoulder or with the use of pillows.

- The hand is kept at rest. No exercise is taught at this time. This will allow for the bleeding at the repair site to stop, and for patients to get off all pain medicine, listen to their body, and follow pain-guided therapy by not doing what hurts. Less blood clot in and around the repair area means less scar formation.

4 DAYS POSTSURGERY TO 10 DAYS POSTSURGERY (FIRST WEEK)

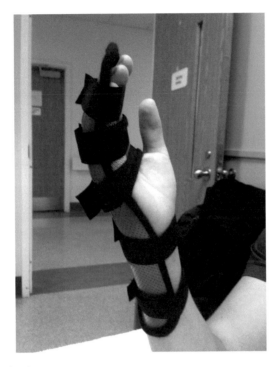

Fig. 19.TT1 Dorsal block splint.

The patient is retaught what positions the hand and wrist need to avoid to protect the tendon repair 4 to 10 days after the surgery.

- The patient should now be off ALL pain medication. He or she is taught to safely remove the orthosis and bandages over the wound. We teach him or her how to safely wash the wound with tap water and mild soap, without putting the hand and wrist in dangerous positions. We show him or her how to dress the wound with a light layer of Vaseline and gauze dressing.

- Patient is instructed to wear the dorsal block orthosis all the time, except when performing wound care or when performing certain exercises.

- Patients can complete their exercises in or out of the orthosis: this is a clinical decision made by the therapist.

- A discussion is had with our surgeons about whether to begin our protocol in a Manchester short splint.

- Patient is not able to use the hand for any heavy lifting, tugging, torqueing, or twisting activity.

- Coban or compression wrap may be applied to repaired finger to help cover the wound and control edema. The patient is taught how to apply this dressing without compromising the tendon repair. We do not remove the Coban to do the exercises.

Video 19.TT2a
Passive finger
flexion and active
extension within
dorsal block splint
(Higgins, Canada).

Video 19.TT2b
Tuna and Ayhan
start three finger
blocking active
flexion at 4 days
after surgery
(video by Zeinep
Tuna) (Ayhan,
Turkey).

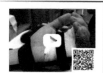

Video 19.TT3
Active modified
tuck exercise
no more than
half a fist within
dorsal block splint
(Higgins, Canada).

- Exercise #1: Passive composite flexion exercises to all fingers. This exercise is used as a "warm-up" to take tension out of the joints. Each finger can be held for 30 seconds each hour, until full passive range of motion is achieved with ease.
- Exercise #2: Active tendon glide of all the fingers up to a half fist position or a modified tuck position. The aim is to have flexion of the DIP and PIP joints while the MP joints maintain a 30-degree flexed position (similar to our orthosis positioning). We do not want a full-fist position. This movement should be gentle, pain-free, and without forceful pulling or force on the repaired tendon. This is our most important exercise.
- Exercise #3: Active IP joint extension with the MP joint held in flexion. Keeping the MP joint in a flexed position will help to encourage full PIP joint extension. If this exercise is taught with splint, patients can be encouraged to touch to the roof of the orthosis. If this is taught early enough, PIP joint flexion contractures can be avoided.
- Exercises 2 and 3 can be done 10 times every hour patients are awake during the day. Patients actively hold each repetition for 10.

- Patients perform active tendon glide of all the fingers within the dorsal block orthosis. They try to actively flex to a half fist position or a modified tuck position. The aim is to have flexion of the DIP and PIP joints while the MP joints maintain a 30-degree flexed position within the dorsal block splint. We do not want a full-fist position. This movement should be gentle, pain-free, and without forceful pulling or strenuous force on the repaired tendon.
- Jin Bo Tang has regularly performed out-of-splint, early active motion from the first week after surgery.[6] The motion of early active motion is the same as described above, i.e., half a fist active flexion and full active extension, after passive motion of the repaired fingers (examples in ▶ Fig. 19.4 and ▶ Fig. 19.5).

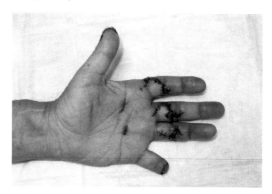

Fig. 19.4 This is the view of the hand with repaired flexor digitorum profundus (FDP) tendons of the index and ring fingers at day 6 after surgery of the patient in ▶ Fig. 19.3 and ▶ Fig. 19.5. Because the FDP tendons were retrieved from separate incisions in the palm and the incisions for FDP tendon repairs were very limited (operative picture shown earlier), the edema of the fingers are quite mild. Out-of-splint, early active motion can be performed easily. The picture shows that Dr Tang permits full active extension of the finger at 6 days after surgery. (Copyright of Jin Bo Tang, MD.)

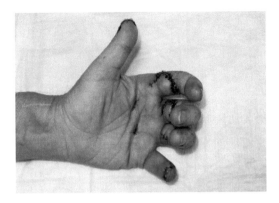

Fig. 19.5 Half a fist early active flexion exercise at 6 weeks postoperatively of the patient in ▶ Fig. 19.3 and ▶ Fig. 19.4. The range of active flexion is increased gradually over the next 3 to 4 weeks, with the full active flexion at week 4 or 5. (Copyright of Jin Bo Tang, MD.)

11–14 DAYS (SECOND WEEK POST REPAIR)

- Continue with edema management using Coban or compression wrap until there is no more swelling.

- At the 2-week mark, the dorsal block orthosis is changed to the Manchester short splint if they did not start their therapy in this orthosis.[15] This splint allows the wrist to fully flex, but limits wrist extension to 40 to 45 degrees. Fingers are still kept in the same position as described above. Splint is still worn full time except for hand cleaning. Note that Dr Tang lets his patients do most of exercises carefully outside the splint.

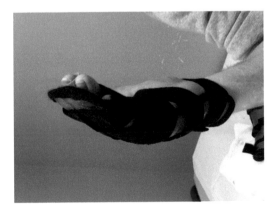

Fig. 19.TT2 Manchester short splint.

Video 19.TT4
Passive flexion
active extension
exercise within
Manchester short
splint (Higgins,
Canada).

Video 19.TT5
Active modified
tuck at three-
fourths or near-full
fist position within
Manchester short
splint (Higgins,
Canada).

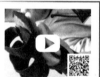

Video 19.TT6
Synergistic
movement within
Manchester short
splint (Higgins,
Canada).

- The patient continues to work on full passive composite flexion of all fingers and active extension of each finger in the orthosis.

- To really work on PIP joint extension, patients are reminded to try and passively block MP joint down into flexion during the active extension exercise.

- The patient continues to work on gentle active tendon glide trying to achieve a three-fourths or near-full fist position, with all the flexion concentrated at the DIP and PIP joints. Again, the patient is taught to avoid forceful jerking movements.

- A new exercise is introduced involving active synergistic movement of the wrist and fingers. With Manchester short splint on, patients are taught to flex wrist while extending fingers, hold for 5 seconds count, and then extend wrist (up until the block) while curling fingers into a tuck position. Everything is done in a smooth, controlled, and gentle fashion. This helps to promote differential glide of the FDS and FDP tendons.

- This should be done frequently throughout the day, every waking hour, 10 repetitions, holding for 10 seconds each time.

- If the patient is following the program, and the repair involves only the ring or small finger, the patient is taught how he/she can remove the index finger from the protective straps of the Manchester short splint to allow the patient to use the thumb and index finger to start some light activities (e.g., zippering winter jackets, opening purse or book bag, pulling up pants).

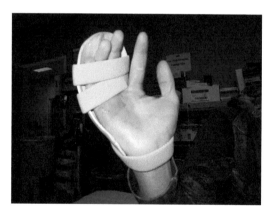

Fig. 19.TT3 Manchester short splint with index finger free for light activity.

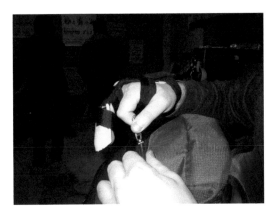

Fig. 19.TT4 Thumb and index free to use zipper.

15–28 DAYS (THIRD AND FOURTH WEEKS POST REPAIR)

- The patient is shown activities that are more in line with typical daily activities but help to achieve active tendon glide. Patients can remove the splint to start trying to bend fingers around cell phone, try to turn a water glass or wine glass on a table surface, try to drag fingers through cream on a table top surface, and try to scrunch tissue or towel and extend fingers.

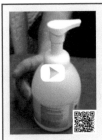

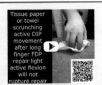

Video 19.TT7
Force free
manipulation
of light objects
encourages distal
interphalangeal
(DIP) flexion after
long finger flexor
tendon repair
(as described by
Gwen van Strien)
(Lalonde, Canada).

Video 19.TT8
Force free
scrunching
manipulation
of light objects
encourages distal
interphalangeal
(DIP) flexion
after flexor
tendon repair
(as described by
Gwen van Strien)
(Higgins, Canada).

29–35 DAYS (FIFTH WEEK POST REPAIR)

- The patient continues to work on full passive composite flexion of all fingers within the orthosis and active extension of each finger in the splint.

- To really work on PIP joint extension, patients are reminded to try and passively block MP joint down into flexion during the active extension exercise.

- The patient continues to work on gentle active tendon glide trying to achieve a full fist position. Again, the patient is taught to avoid forceful jerking movements.

- The patient continues with active synergistic movement of the wrist and fingers with Manchester short splint on.

- The patient continues to use everyday light activities to help achieve active tendon glide and finger dexterity.

- If the DIP joint stops moving, we ultrasound the finger to ensure that there is no rupture and verify if the tendon is just stuck in scar. If that is the case, we start relative motion extension splinting to help get the FDP out of scar. The patient exercises while he or she is living with this orthosis as he or she flexes over 500 times per day. Please see Chapter 54 on Relative Motion Orthosis.[1]

- Relative motion extension orthosis will frequently avoid the need for unnecessary tenolysis which can create more scarring and rupture.

- Relative motion extension orthosis can also be fabricated to help with improving active tendon glide of FDP of the repaired finger. Please see Chapter 54 on Relative Motion Orthosis.

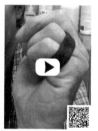

Video 19.TT9
Relative motion extension orthosis to achieve more proximal interphalangeal (PIP) and distal interphalangeal (DIP) joint flexion and avoid tenolysis (Flewelling, Canada).

- Relative motion flexion orthosis can also be fabricated to help with PIP joint flexion contractures. Please see Chapter 54 on Relative Motion Orthosis.

Video 19.TT10 Relative motion flexion splint to achieve more proximal interphalangeal (PIP) joint extension and postoperative feedback. Patient looking at his own ultrasound to help get flexor out of scar (Higgins, Canada).

36–49 DAYS (SIXTH AND SEVENTH WEEKS POST REPAIR)

- Manchester short splint is discontinued at the 6-week mark.
- The patient can continue with full range of motion exercises described above if full movement has not been achieved.
- The patient can start to incorporate the hand into regular activity, still avoiding forceful gripping and heavy-lifting activities.
- Scar massage is started to help soften scar tissue.
- A night extension orthosis is started in patients who have developed PIP joint flexion contractures.

43–70 DAYS MARK (EIGHTH, NINTH, AND TENTH WEEKS POST REPAIR)

- Start grip-strengthening activities for the hand.
- Continue with all exercises if full range of motion has not been achieved.
- Continue with night extension orthosis and/or relative motion flexion/extension programs.
- Start talking about return-to-work programs.

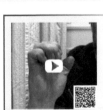

Video 19.TT11 Flexor digitorum profundus (FDP) repair of long finger 7 months post-op (Higgins, Canada).

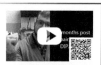

Video 19.TT12
From surgery to 6 months post-op of flexor tendon repair of 5th finger (Higgins, Canada).

Do not lose patience! Sometimes it can take 6 to 8 months for a patient to achieve full hand function status! But it will come! Do not jump in to do tenolysis in a noncompliant patient. You will just add more scar and the patient is not likely to be more compliant.

References

1. Higgins A, Lalonde DH, Bell M, McKee D, Lalonde JF. Avoiding flexor tendon repair rupture with intraoperative total active movement examination. Plast Reconstr Surg 2010;126(3):941–945
2. Lalonde DH, Kozin S. Tendon disorders of the hand. Plast Reconstr Surg 2011;128(1):1e–14e
3. McKee DE, Lalonde DH, Thoma A, Glennie DL, Hayward JE. Optimal time delay between epinephrine injection and incision to minimize bleeding. Plast Reconstr Surg 2013;131(4):811–814
4. Tang JB. Wide-awake primary flexor tendon repair, tenolysis, and tendon transfer. Clin Orthop Surg 2015;7(3):275–281
5. Wong J, McGrouther DA. Minimizing trauma over "no man's land" with flexor tendon retrieval. J Hand Surg Eur Vol 2014;39(9):1004–1006
6. Tang JB, Zhou X, Pan ZJ, Qing J, Gong KT, Chen J. Strong digital flexor tendon repair, extension-flexion test, and early active flexion: experience in 300 tendons. Hand Clin 2017;33(3):455–463
7. Meals C, Lalonde D, Candelier G. Repaired flexor tendon excursion with half a fist of true active movement versus full fist place and hold in the awake patient. Plast Reconstr Surg Glob Open 2019;7(4):e2074
8. Moriya K, Yoshizu T, Tsubokawa N, Narisawa H, Hara K, Maki Y. Clinical results of releasing the entire A2 pulley after flexor tendon repair in zone 2C. J Hand Surg Eur Vol 2016;41(8):822–828
9. Pan ZJ, Pan L, Xu YF, Ma T, Yao LH. Outcomes of 200 digital flexor tendon repairs using updated protocols and 30 repairs using an old protocol: experience over 7 years. J Hand Surg Eur Vol 2020;45(1):56–63
10. Moriya K, Yoshizu T, Tsubokawa N, Narisawa H, Maki Y. Incidence of tenolysis and features of adhesions in the digital flexor tendons after multi-strand repair and early active motion. J Hand Surg Eur Vol 2019;44(4):354–360
11. Al-Dubaiban WI, Al-Abdulkarim AO, Arafah MM, Al-Qattan MM. Flexor tendon-to-volar plate repair: an experimental study and 3 case reports. J Hand Surg Am 2014;39(11):2222–2227
12. Meals C, Lalonde D, Candelier G. Repaired flexor tendon excursion with half a fist of true active movement versus full fist place and hold in the awake patient. Plast Reconstr Surg Glob Open 2019;7(4):e2074
13. Higgins A, Lalonde DH. Flexor tendon repair postoperative rehabilitation: the Saint John Protocol. Plast Reconstr Surg Glob Open 2016;4(11):e1134
14. Lalonde D, Higgins A. Wide awake flexor tendon repair in the finger. Plast Reconstr Surg Glob Open 2016;4(7):e797
15. Khor WS, Langer MF, Wong R, Zhou R, Peck F, Wong JKF. Improving outcomes in tendon repair: a critical look at the evidence for flexor tendon repair and rehabilitation. Plast Reconstr Surg 2016;138(6):1045e–1058e

CHAPTER 20

FLEXOR TENDON REPAIR OF THE HAND, WRIST, AND FOREARM

*Donald H. Lalonde, Chao Chen, Julian Escobar,
Amir Adham Ahmad, and Gökhan Tolga Akbulut*

ADVANTAGES OF WALANT VERSUS SEDATION AND TOURNIQUET IN FLEXOR TENDON REPAIR OF THE HAND, WRIST, AND FOREARM

- All of the general advantages listed in Chapter 2 and Chapter 19 apply to both the surgeon and the patient (no nausea, no tourniquet pain or let-down bleeding, decreased cost without sedation in minor procedure room, safer surgery without sedation, etc.).

- It is often difficult to tell which proximal tendon stumps belong to which distal tendons in a "spaghetti wrist" injury. This can be even more difficult with ragged cuts such as might happen with a table saw accident. The patient will help you identify which proximal tendons belong to which fingers (see ▶ Video 20.1 and Video 20.2).

- You are less likely to have to perform secondary surgery for rupture repair if you test the repairs by having the patient take the fingers through a full range of motion before skin closure.[1] If you see gapping with the stress of full active movement, you can repair the gap, retest the repair to confirm that it is solid, and then close the skin. This is like testing and ensuring blood flow through a microvascular anastomosis before skin closure.

- See Chapter 19 for relevant videos, illustrations, and discussions on finger flexor tendon repairs.

- Many of these injuries happen at night and on weekends—not an ideal time to perform a repair. A major advantage of eliminating sedation for flexor tendon repair is that you do not need to perform the procedure in the main operating room. We do all of our tendon repairs in minor procedure rooms in the clinic outside the main operating room Monday to Friday, 8 AM to 4 PM. We know that we do better surgery at 2 PM than at 2 AM. In addition, our hand therapists can teach patients during the surgery and see the repair (see Chapter 15). This also permits patients to be sober so they can understand their injury and learn how to look after it with intraoperative teaching they can remember.

- You can educate unsedated patients for the 90 or so minutes of the procedure without interruption (see ▶ Video 19.7a). You can tell them that they can move their fingers but not use them, as the therapist will instruct. The patients will remember what you say and be even more motivated to follow hand therapy advice.

- Patients get to see that the repaired tendon works as they watch themselves moving their fingers through a full range of motion before skin closure. They know that their fingers will function well once they get past the postoperative discomfort and stiffness if they put the necessary effort into therapy.

WHERE TO INJECT THE LOCAL ANESTHETIC FOR FLEXOR TENDON REPAIR OF THE HAND

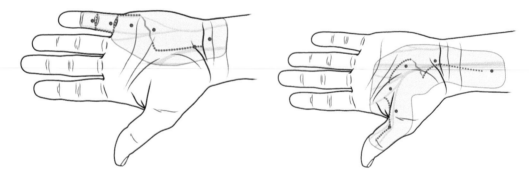

Fig. 20.1 and Fig. 20.2 The orange lines represent the laceration and the dotted red lines are the possible incisions. Red dots are usual injection points. Inject up to 30 mL of buffered 1% lidocaine with 1:100,000 epinephrine starting with 10 mL proximal to the carpal tunnel, then 10 mL in the palm, and 2 mL in the proximal phalanx just under the skin. If the middle phalanx also needs exposure, you can inject another 2 mL there. For the flexor pollicis longus (FPL) laceration in the carpal tunnel **(Fig. 20.2)**, inject up to 40 mL of the same solution starting with 15 mL over FPL on the distal forearm, then 15 mL in the palm and thenar eminence and 2 mL in the thumb proximal phalanx injection point just under the skin. (▶ Video 20.3 shows an FPL repair in the carpal tunnel case.)

SPECIFICS OF MINIMALLY PAINFUL INJECTION OF LOCAL ANESTHETIC IN FLEXOR TENDON REPAIR OF THE HAND

- Local anesthesia injection should barely hurt at all if you follow the simple rules of Chapter 5 for hints to minimize injection pain. The patients will think you are magical.

- We always inject all patients while they are lying down to decrease the risk of their fainting (see Chapter 6).

- Inject local anesthetic into the patient in the waiting area 30 minutes before surgery. This allows the epinephrine to take effect and provides an adequately dry working field.[2]

- You will not cause a palmar compartment syndrome. As soon as you incise the skin, the pressure will come down as the local anesthetic leaks out.

- When performing major nerve blocks such as of the median or ulnar nerves, do not elicit paresthesias. Let the tumescent local anesthetic find and bathe the outside of the nerve so you do not damage it with the sharp needle tip.

- Inject 10 mL under the skin of the thenar eminence. It will bathe the whole thenar pad.

- The goal of the injection is to bathe visible and palpable local anesthetic 2 cm beyond wherever you think you have even a small chance of dissecting in the wrist and hand.

- If you inject 20 mL into the palm, where will it go? Everywhere! Perfect! This is like an extravascular Bier block, but only where you need it.

- The metacarpal phalangeal crease of the thumb has sheath/cutaneous ligaments that are a natural barrier to the diffusion of local anesthetic into the proximal phalanx. Inject into the thenar eminence first to anesthetize the digital nerves of the proximal phalanx so the patient does not feel pain when you insert the needle into the thumb. Inject a further 2 mL into the subcutaneous fat in the proximal phalanx for the epinephrine effect in case the distal end of flexor pollicis longus (FPL) or flexor digitorum profundus (FDP) is there.

WHERE TO INJECT THE LOCAL ANESTHETIC FOR FLEXOR TENDON REPAIR OF THE FOREARM

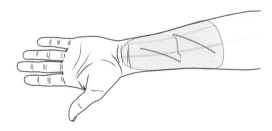

Fig. 20.3 The orange line in the illustration is the laceration and the dotted red lines are the possible incisions. Inject up to 100 mL of 0.5% lidocaine with 1:200,000 epinephrine (buffered with 10 mL of 1% lidocaine with 1:100,000 epinephrine: 1 mL of 8.4% sodium bicarbonate).

SPECIFICS OF MINIMAL PAIN INJECTION OF LOCAL ANESTHETIC IN FLEXOR TENDON REPAIR OF THE FOREARM

- Keep the total dose of infiltration less than 7 mg/kg. If less than 50 mL is required, use premixed 1% lidocaine with 1:100,000 epinephrine. If 50 to 100 mL is required, dilute with saline solution to a concentration of 0.5% lidocaine with 1:200,000 epinephrine. If 100 to 200 mL of solution is required to produce tumescent local anesthesia (see Chapter 4), dilute with saline solution to a concentration of 0.25% lidocaine with 1:400,000 epinephrine.

- Add 10 mL 0.5% bupivacaine with 1:200,000 epinephrine to the injectate if you think the procedure will take more than 3 hours.

- Always inject from proximal to distal to keep the sharp needle tip in anesthetized areas to decrease pain.

- Alternate injecting on the radial side, then the ulnar side, then the radial side, and then the ulnar side. This also decreases pain by letting the distal skin get numb to needle reinsertion.

- You can anesthetize the proximal stumps of the median and ulnar nerves under direct vision after the skin flaps are anesthetized and raised. Use a 30-gauge needle and a 3-mL syringe. Gently lift up the epineurium with small forceps and inject into that loose areolar epineurial tissue so the nerve is bathed all around. Do not inject directly into the nerve fascicles, as you will cause pain and lacerate fascicles and damage axons. After you inject the nerves, repair the tendons so the proximal nerve stumps have time to get numb.

- The goal of the injection is to bathe local anesthetic 2 cm beyond wherever you think you even have a small chance of dissecting in the forearm.

- The more volume that you inject, the greater are the odds that the patient will feel no pain after you begin dissection. Try to avoid "top-ups" of local anesthetic that give patients unnecessary bad memories.

- If you have access to blunt-tipped injection cannulas such as those used to inject dermal fillers, you can inject the local anesthetic painlessly more quickly than with a sharp needle tip[3] (see Chapter 5).

TIPS AND TRICKS FOR PERFORMING FLEXOR TENDON REPAIR OF THE HAND, WRIST, AND FOREARM WITH THE WIDE AWAKE APPROACH

Video 20.1 "Spaghetti wrist." Patient helps identify which proximal tendons belong to which distal tendon ends (Lalonde, Canada).

Video 20.2 Dr Chao Chen of China shows pulling on proximal tendon stumps and having the patient tell you which finger you are pulling on (Chen, China).

- Ask the patient with spaghetti wrist to flex the long finger. You will see the proximal long finger tendon move the most.

- Pull on one of the proximal tendons and ask the patient which "finger" you are pulling on. They will be able to accurately tell you it is the little finger if you are pulling on the little finger FDP tendon.

- You can stimulate unanesthetized proximal nerve fascicles to see which finger they supply. The unsedated patients will tell you which finger is being stimulated because they can feel it.

- Pull the drape down so that patients can see their fingers when you ask them to move. Patients need to look at their fingers to get them to move. They cannot feel their numbed finger move, because they have lost the proprioceptive sense. However, if patients look, they can move the fingers as they wish. Although many patients do not mind looking at the wound, you can cover the wound with a towel as they flex the fingers or thumb while looking at them.

- Do not be afraid to test full flexion and full extension. Your sutures need to be strong enough to take flexion and extension. If they are not, you need to reinforce them.

- See the many added tips and tricks for flexor tendon repair in Chapter 19.

- We do not worry about minor bleeding from cut skin edges, because most little bleeders will stop spontaneously by the time we sew the skin flaps back for exposure. We no longer use cautery but occasionally use a hemostat on larger veins for a few minutes, or we tie them off.

- We use augmented field sterility in our minor procedure rooms for longer cases such as by importing full drapes and gowns from the main operating room (see Chapter 10).

- We wait for at least 30 minutes between local anesthetic injection in the patient waiting area and bringing the patient into the minor procedure room to allow the epinephrine to reach maximal vasoconstriction. We perform a couple of carpal tunnels or see patients for hand consultations from the emergency department while waiting so our time is used productively.

- We ask patients to go to the restroom to relieve themselves after we inject the local anesthetic and just before we start the surgery to avoid unnecessary surgical interruptions and patient discomfort for the longer cases. The patient has no intravenous infusion that would increase the urge to void. If we give preoperative antibiotics, they are administered by mouth.

- When you are trying retrieve or to sew the tendons together, the patient may pull the proximal tendons away from you. If you ask him or her to extend the fingers, the flexor muscles must relax by spinal cord reflex and the patient will stop pulling as much. In addition, you can keep the wrist and fingers passively flexed, which will also help to decrease the tension on the repair.

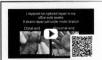

Video 20.3
A repair and subsequently ruptured flexor pollicis longus (FPL) repair under the motor branch in the carpal tunnel (Lalonde, Canada).

Video 20.4
Spaghetti wrist with both nerves and 8-month follow-up (Escobar, Columbia).

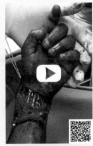

Video 20.5
Spaghetti wrist with both nerves and 8-month follow-up (Ahmad, Malaysia).

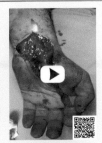

Video 20.6
Spaghetti wrist and hand (Akbulut, Turkey).

References

1. Higgins A, Lalonde DH, Bell M, McKee D, Lalonde JF. Avoiding flexor tendon repair rupture with intraoperative total active movement examination. Plast Reconstr Surg 2010;126(3):941–945
2. McKee DE, Lalonde DH, Thoma A, Glennie DL, Hayward JE. Optimal time delay between epinephrine injection and incision to minimize bleeding. Plast Reconstr Surg 2013;131(4):811–814
3. Lalonde D, Wong A. Local anesthetics: what's new in minimal pain injection and best evidence in pain control. Plast Reconstr Surg 2014; 134(4, Suppl 2):40S–49S

CHAPTER 21

EXTENSOR TENDON REPAIR OF THE FINGER (ZONE 1 MALLET TO ZONE 5 MP JOINT)

Donald H. Lalonde, Egemen Ayhan, Xavier Gueffier, Amanda Higgins, Chris Chun-Yu Chen, Thomas Apard, Paul Sibley, Asif Ilyas, Kamal Rafiqi, and Chye Yew Ng

ADVANTAGES OF WALANT VERSUS SEDATION AND TOURNIQUET IN EXTENSOR TENDON REPAIR OF THE FINGER

- All of the general advantages listed in Chapter 2 apply to both the surgeon and the patient (no nausea, no tourniquet pain or let-down bleeding, decreased cost without sedation in minor procedure room, safer surgery without sedation, etc.).

- Extensor tendon repair is facilitated in children (▶ Video 9.9).

- In zone 5 extensor tendon lacerations over the metacarpophalangeal (MP) joint, you can simulate the relative motion extension splint during WALANT surgery with a sterile tongue depressor or periosteal elevator.[1,2,3,4] This will help you decide whether you need to add a wrist component to the Merritt splint. Wyndell Merritt's relative motion extension splint has revolutionized management of lacerations at the proximal phalanx and dorsal hand levels (see Chapter 22) in the last few years. A relative motion extension splint keeps the affected MP joint more extended than the uninjured MP joints. This lets the repaired tendon move without tension and with less excursion. Patients can return to work with these very functional splints as early as 3 to 5 days after surgery. Don Lalonde has been doing what you see in ▶ Video 21.1 for over 20 years with no ruptures. The ability to educate the unsedated patient during surgery about how to avoid rupture after surgery is important.

- The relative motion extension splint takes the tension off the long extensors, even when fingers are actively flexing.

Video 21.1 Relative motion extension splint decreases excursion in extensor tendon repair in zone 5 and lets people work sooner. See from repair to 8 months post-op with detailed therapy explanation (also see therapy tips below) (Lalonde, Canada).

Video 21.2 Zone 5 relative motion extension splint takes the tension off the extensor tendon repair in the proximal finger (video by Wyndell Merritt).

Video 21.3
Zone 3 Merritt relative motion flexion splinting for boutonniere deformity—how this works, with examples (Lalonde, Canada).

Video 21.4 Merritt relative motion flexion splinting for boutonniere deformity; cadaver demonstration of how it works (Lalonde, Canada).

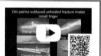

Video 21.5a
WALANT mallet fracture management (Lalonde, Canada).

- You can simulate the relative motion flexion splint (RMFS) during WALANT boutonniere surgery or in clinic consultations with a sterile tongue depressor. The Merritt RMFS has revolutionized acute and chronic boutonniere management in the last few years. Patients can return to work with these very functional splints.

- The RMFS keeps the MP joint of the affected finger more flexed than the MP joints of the adjacent fingers. This increased tension on the long extensors pulls the lateral bands dorsal to the axis of the proximal interphalangeal (PIP) joint while taking the tension off the intrinsic volar pull on the same lateral bands (see ▶ Video 21.3).

- When operating on a boutonniere finger, you can see if the balance of sutures in the lateral bands creates the correct tension to correct the deformity. You can adjust your sutures if the balance is not yet correct after seeing active movement during the surgery.

- WALANT takes away many of the inconveniences of general and motor block anesthesia during the management of fracture mallet injuries.

WHERE TO INJECT THE LOCAL ANESTHETIC FOR EXTENSOR TENDON REPAIR OF THE FINGER

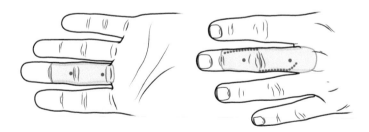

Fig. 21.1(a, b) The orange line in the illustration is the laceration and the dotted red lines are the possible incisions distal to the metacarpophalangeal (MP) joint. Palmar injections: Inject 2 mL of 1% lidocaine with 1:100,000 epinephrine (buffered with 0.2 mL of 8.4% sodium bicarbonate) in the most proximal red injection point in the subcutaneous palmar fat. Perform the most proximal dorsal injection next, and then inject 2 mL in the middle of the subcutaneous fat of the palmar middle phalanx. Dorsal injections: Inject 2 mL of 1% lidocaine with 1:100,000 epinephrine (buffered with 0.2 mL of 8.4% sodium bicarbonate) in the proximal red injection dot in the subcutaneous fat of the dorsal proximal phalanx. Inject the middle phalanx palmar side next and then finally inject 2 mL in the middle of the dorsal middle phalanx subcutaneous fat.

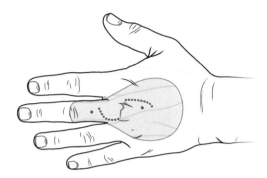

Fig. 21.2 The orange line in the illustration is the laceration at the metacarpophalangeal (MP) joint (zone 5) and the dotted red lines are the possible incisions to expose the tendon. Inject 10 to 15 mL of 1% lidocaine with 1:100,000 epinephrine (buffered with 1.0–1.5 mL of 8.4% sodium bicarbonate) in the proximal red injection dot in the subcutaneous fat of the dorsal hand to be sure the most proximal incision is well bathed with local 2 cm proximal to the incision. Inject 2 to 4 mL in the middle of the dorsal proximal phalanx subcutaneous fat.

- See Chapter 1, Atlas, for more illustrations of the anatomy of diffusion of tumescent local anesthetic in the forearm, wrist, and hand.

SPECIFICS OF MINIMALLY PAINFUL INJECTION OF LOCAL ANESTHETIC IN EXTENSOR TENDON REPAIR OF THE FINGER

- Local anesthesia injection should barely hurt at all if you follow the simple rules of Chapter 5 for hints to minimize injection pain. The patients will think you are magical.

- We always inject all patients while they are lying down to decrease the risk of their fainting (see ▶ Video 6.1).

- Inject the anesthetic solution a minimum of 30 minutes before surgery to allow the epinephrine to take optimal effect and provide an adequately dry working field,[4,5] as outlined in Chapter 4 and Chapter 14.

- With extensor tendon repair, volar local anesthesia injection is not always required.

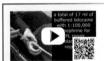

Video 21.5b
Real-time, minimal pain, 4-minute injection for repair of extensor pollicis longus (EPL) (Lalonde, Canada).

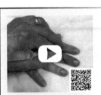

Video 21.5c Real-time, minimal pain, 4-minute injection for repair of zone 2 extensor over long finger (Lalonde, Canada).

TIPS AND TRICKS FOR PERFORMING EXTENSOR TENDON REPAIR OF THE FINGER WITH THE WIDE AWAKE APPROACH

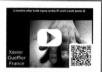

Video 21.6 Conservative management of boutonniere with only relative motion flexion splinting (Gueffier, France).

- Surgery for chronic boutonniere is tricky. In general, conservative serial casting followed by relative motion flexion splinting can solve most problems in cooperative patients. ▶ Video 21.6 shows a patient who had a completely passively extendable PIP joint with the pencil test (see Chapter 54) placing a pencil over the long finger proximal phalanx and under the ring and index proximal phalanges completely extended the long finger PIP joint. Dr Gueffier was able to treat him with only relative motion splinting.

- If you are going to try surgery for chronic boutonniere, almost full passive extension of the PIP joint is a prerequisite. Serial casting may be required to get there before the surgery.

- ▶ Video 21.8 by Egemen Ayhan and Cigdem Ayhan in Turkey shows one possible surgical method for treating chronic boutonniere, with intraoperative pencil test confirming that MP flexion results in complete PIP extension. The patient is then treated with a mandatory RMFS to keep the MP flexed at all times.

Video 21.7 Conservative management of boutonniere with only relative motion flexion splinting (Lalonde, Canada).

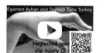

Video 21.8 Surgery and relative motion splint for chronic boutonniere overview (Ayhan, Turkey).

- For postoperative therapy, Egemen Ayhan and his therapist Cigdem Ayhan in Turkey have the patient elevate and immobilize for 3 to 5 days to let swelling come down, let patients get off all pain medicine, and allow pain-guided therapy. They use continuous use relative motion flexion splinting for at least 8 weeks. They also used full-time PIP joint extension splinting for the first 2 to 4 weeks, or until the edema and PIP extensor lag are gone. Coban taping and kinesiotaping also diminish edema during that period. They advise patients to remove the splint (six times, every 2–3 hours) a day for PIP flexion exercises limited to 30 degrees of flexion. They sometimes used flexion block splints to limit these flexion exercises to 30 degrees. Distal interphalangeal (DIP) flexion exercises are done every hour while patients are awake.

Video 21.9
Surgery details for chronic boutonniere (Ayhan, Turkey).

- In ▶ Video 21.10, C.Y. Chen corrected the boutonniere deformity in three steps: (1) arthrotomy was performed to release volar capsule, (2) the central slip was then tightened or repaired, and (3) an elongation of the lateral bands was done by meshing with a scalpel (staged puncture tenotomy). All three steps can be adjusted in the awake patient.

Video 21.10
Boutonniere surgery (Chen, Taiwan).

- Percutaneous extensor tendon repair is useful because the thin finger extensor tendon does not hold a suture very well (▶ Video 21.11). Nylon sutures through both skin and tendon hold the suture better. This is especially true when the skin is frayed, such as from a table saw accident. The ends of the extensor tendon are close enough that the splinting will allow functional healing of the tendon with a gap. You can see that your sutures are tight enough with WALANT, because the finger stays in full extension when you let it go and stop holding it up. Avoiding buried permanent sutures also prevents stitch abscesses later. For the past 10 years, the first author has mostly used monofilament absorbable suture on the extensor side of fingers if he used anything buried at all.

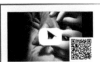

Video 21.11
Transcutaneous extensor tendon repair for the central slip (Lalonde, Canada).

- Take the drape down so the patients can to look at their fingers to get them to extend to test the repair, since they do not feel the numbed fingers. Although most patients do not mind looking at the wound, you can cover the wound with a towel as they watch their appearance when fingers move.

- In contrast to flexor tendon repairs, we do not always make patients test extensor tendon repairs over the proximal phalanx with a full fist of flexion. The sutures may not hold well enough in the thin extensor tendons. Flexor tendon repairs are stronger and withstand full-fist flexion testing easily. In addition, finger extensor repairs can tolerate a gap, as we all witness with most mallet injuries. Flexor tendon lacerations do not tolerate a gap.

Video 21.12
Swan neck rings are great for flexible proximal interphalangeal (PIP) joints (Lalonde, Canada).

- Many patients are interested in looking at the tendon to understand the nature of their problem. Many patients are interested in looking at the tendon to understand the nature of their problem. They can put on a mask and watch the surgery. Many patients love this type of thing. Some patients will tell others it is something they need to put on their bucket list!

- You can perform these operations with field sterility to increase efficiency (see Chapter 10).

Video 21.13 Swan neck repair (Apard, France). Also see ▶ Video 36.7 for another swan neck reconstruction technique.

Video 21.14 Swan neck repair (Ayhan, Turkey). Also see ▶ Video 36.7 for another swan neck reconstruction technique.

Video 21.15 Repair of swan neck with flexor digitorum superficialis (FDS) to bone anchor tenodesis (Lalonde, Canada). Also see ▶ Video 36.7 for another swan neck reconstruction technique.

Video 21.16 Extensor tendon laceration of zones 4 and 5 followed by relative motion extension splint only without wrist splint (Ayhan, Turkey).

Video 21.17 Extensor tendon laceration of extensor pollicis longus (EPL) with nice repair technique for thin flat tendon (Sibley, USA).

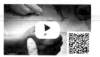

Video 21.18 Sagittal band rupture with nice ultrasound video anatomy and WALANT treatment (Gueffier, France).

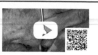

Video 21.19 Sagittal band repair details including relative motion extension splint (Ilyas, USA).

Video 21.20 Sagittal band long finger distally based extensor tendon flap radializes index extensor tendon (Apard, France).

Video 21.21 Rheumatoid synovectomy and repair of radial sagittal bands as well as release ulnar sagittal bands (Rafiqi, Morocco).

Video 21.22 Sagittal band reconstruction of two tendons with nice demonstration of preoperative physical examination (Ng, England).

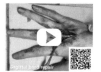

Video 21.23 Extensor tendon sagittal band repair showing nice demonstration of subluxation before and during surgery and correction with simple repair (Chen, Taiwan).

Video 21.24 Extensor tendon sagittal band repair (Ayhan, Turkey).

Video 21.25 Clear ultrasound video diagnosis and treatment of zone 5 extensor laceration (Gueffier, France).

- See ▶ Video 22.TT2 (zone 6) on how to explain to patient how to wean off relative motion extension splint at 4 weeks after injury (Lalonde, Canada).

POSTOPERATIVE THERAPY TIPS FOR ZONES 3–5 EXTENSOR TENDON REPAIRS

ZONE 3 EXTENSOR TENDON INJURY (BOUTONNIERE)

- In boutonniere injuries, the relative motion flexion orthosis (splint) forces the lateral bands dorsally where the torn extensor mechanism can heal like a mallet finger heals while the patient continues to use the finger[2] (see ▶ Video 21.4).

CENTRAL SLIP AND/OR LATERAL BAND INJURIES THAT DO NOT REQUIRE SURGICAL INTERVENTION

- You can use relative motion flexion orthoses to either prevent a possible boutonniere deformity or to treat an existing one.

- Assess the passive motion of the PIP joint. If it can be passively corrected to full extension, then start with a relative motion flexion orthosis.

- If there is a significant flexion contracture of the PIP joint with a soft end feel, then start with serial casting of the PIP joint.

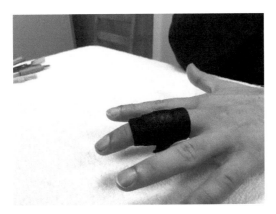

Fig. 21.TT1 Proximal interphalangeal (PIP) joint serial casted in extension; distal interphalangeal (DIP) joint is free to perform passive and active range of motion (ROM) exercises.

- Consider using relative motion flexion serial casting inside an RMFS that will pull up on the lateral bands (see ▶ Fig. 21.TT3 and ▶ Video 21.4).

GUIDELINES TO USING SERIAL CASTING TO CORRECT A PASSIVE SOFT END FEEL PIP EXTENSOR LAG

Video 21.TT1 Proximal interphalangeal (PIP) joint in extension cast and performing active distal interphalangeal (DIP) joint flexion and extension exercises. This can be done while wearing a relative motion flexion splint.

- Use plaster of Paris or other casting material to hold the PIP joint into as much passive extension as possible. Leave the DIP joint free so that the patient can work on passive and active flexion and extension exercises of the DIP joint while the PIP joint is immobilized.

- Use a relative motion flexion orthosis with the cast to help position the MP joint into more flexion than the neighboring MP joints.

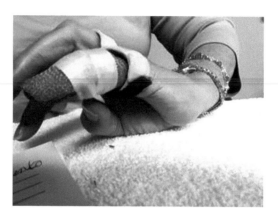

Fig. 21.TT2 A proximal interphalangeal (PIP) joint extension cast with relative motion flexion splint (RMFS) for small finger. The cast allows active distal interphalangeal (DIP) flexion, stretches out the PIP flexion contracture, and the RMFS pulls the lateral bands dorsally by keeping the metacarpophalangeal (MP) joint of the injured finger relatively flexed compared to the others.

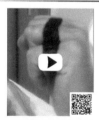

Video 21.TT2 Patient wears only the relative motion flexion splint (RMFS) for the 5th finger for full daytime hours for the last 8 weeks or more of boutonniere daytime management to keep proximal interphalangeal (PIP) joint extension.

- See Chapter 54 on Relative Motion Orthoses for how to make relative motion splints.[6]

- Change the serial cast each week with the goal of achieving more passive extension of the contracted PIP joint. Continue until full passive extension of the PIP joint, or at least a 15 degrees or less persistent flexion contracture of the PIP joint.

- Once you get to less than 15 degrees of PIP joint flexion contracture, continue relative motion flexion splinting to the injured finger for at least 8 more weeks. The patient can feel when the deformity wants to come back without the splint and will guide you in timing for stopping the splint after 8 weeks.

- Patient wears the RMFS full time while performing all activities.

- Patient performs active flexion and extension exercises of all fingers while wearing the relative motion flexion orthosis for the 8 weeks.

- A night extension PIP joint orthosis should be worn with the RMFS while the patient is sleeping for the last 8 weeks of boutonniere management.

- At the 8-week mark, the relative motion flexion orthosis is slowly weaned off over the next month until the patient is no longer wearing the splint and the boutonniere deformity remains corrected.

Video 21.TT3
Patient wearing
relative motion
flexion splint
(RMFS) and
performing flexion
and extension
exercises to the
long finger.

Video 21.TT4
Night extension
splint with relative
motion flexion
splint (RMFS). An
RMFS and a night
extension splint
for sleeping for
the last 2 months
of boutonniere
treatment with
only RMFS in the
daytime.

Video 21.TT5
Summary
of complete
boutonniere
management in
40 seconds.

- Use clinical judgment to either discontinue the night extension splint or the relative motion flexion splinting.

GUIDELINES FOR WHEN SERIAL CASTING IS NOT REQUIRED (FULL PASSIVE PIP EXTENSION IS POSSIBLE IN SPITE OF THE BOUTONNIERE)

- Fabricate a relative motion flexion orthosis for the injured finger for at least 8 weeks.

- Please refer to Chapter 54 on Relative Motion Orthosis for how to fabricate this splint.[6]

- Patient wears the relative motion flexion orthosis full time while performing all activities.

- Patient performs active flexion and extension exercises of all fingers while wearing the relative motion flexion orthosis for 8 weeks.

- Patients are also shown how to hold the PIP joint in extension with the relative motion flexion orthosis and to perform active DIP joint flexion and extension exercises to maintain active lateral band and terminal extensor tendon glide and flexor digitorum profundus (FDP) glide.

- A night extension PIP joint orthosis should be worn with the RMFS while the patient is sleeping.

- At the 8-week mark, the relative motion flexion orthosis is slowly weaned off over the next month until the patient is no longer wearing the splint and the boutonniere deformity remains corrected.

- Use clinical judgment to either discontinue the night extension splint or the relative motion flexion splinting.

CENTRAL SLIP AND/OR LATERAL BAND INJURY THAT REQUIRES SURGICAL INTERVENTION

First 3 to 5 Days Postsurgery

- We place the hand in a resting splint with all interphalangeal joints in full extension and the MP joints and wrist in comfortable slight extension.

- We teach patients during wide awake surgery to keep the hand elevated above the level of the heart all the time either by resting the hand on the opposite shoulder or with the use of pillows.

- We get them to wean off all pain medications by day 5 postoperatively so we can teach them pain-guided hand therapy at 3 to 5 days after surgery.

3 to 5 Days Postsurgery

- See Chapter 22 for videos and discussion on extensor tendon repair of the hand.

- A relative motion flexion orthosis is fabricated for the injured finger. This is the only orthosis worn during the day. This orthosis is worn for 8 weeks.

- Please refer to Chapter 54 on Relative Motion Orthosis for how to fabricate this splint.[6]

- We teach patients to remove the orthosis safely and put bandages over the wound. We show them how to wash the wound safely with mild soap and tap water without putting the hand and wrist in dangerous positions. We show them how to dress the wound with a light layer of Vaseline and Coban dressing.

- Patient wears the relative motion flexion orthosis full time while performing all activities.

- Patient performs active flexion and extension exercises of all fingers while wearing the relative motion flexion orthosis for 8 weeks.

- Patients are also shown how to hold the PIP joint in extension with the relative motion flexion orthosis and to perform active DIP joint flexion and extension exercises to maintain active lateral band and terminal extensor tendon glide and FDP glide.

- A night extension PIP joint extension orthosis should be worn with the relative motion flexion orthosis while the patient is sleeping.

- At the 8-week mark, the relative motion flexion orthosis is slowly weaned off over the next month until the patient is no longer wearing the splint and the boutonniere deformity remains corrected.

- Use clinical judgment to either discontinue the night extension splint or the relative motion flexion splinting.

ZONES 4 (PROXIMAL PHALANX) AND 5 (MP JOINT) EXTENSOR TENDON REPAIR REHABILITATION PROGRAM: THE SAINT JOHN PROTOCOL

- WALANT has allowed us to test the extensor tendon repair and to watch for gaps in the repair that could lead to rupture.[7]

- WALANT provides the opportunity for the hand surgeon and/or hand therapist to determine relative motion orthosis programs that can be used to achieve early active tendon glide (see ▶ Video 21.1 where the surgeon and therapist decide to not use a wrist splint and educate the patient together).

- We have demonstrated with WALANT that there is less tension on the repair site and less excursion when we start early protected movement with a relative motion extension orthosis in zones 5 and 6 (see ▶ Video 21.2).

- In zone 4 extensor tendon repairs, WALANT helps us determine if relative motion flexion or extension splinting works best. We place a sterile tongue blade under and over the injured finger after tendon repair and see the effect of active movement on the supported tendon.

- In zone 5 extensor tendon repairs you do not need to include a wrist orthosis with the program.[1,8,9]

First 3 to 5 Days Postsurgery

- We place the hand in a resting splint with all interphalangeal joints in full extension and the MP joints and wrist in comfortable slight extension.

- We teach patients during wide awake surgery to keep the hand elevated above the level of the heart all the time either by resting the hand on the opposite shoulder or with the use of pillows.

- We get them to wean off all pain medications by day 5 postoperatively so we can teach them pain-guided hand therapy at 3 to 5 days after surgery.

Pain-Guided Therapy Starts Early After a 3 to 5 Days' Pause to Let Bleeding Stop, Swelling Settle, and Patients to Get Off Pain Medication

- It is ideal to start early active tendon glide of a repaired tendon to avoid scar adhesions, which can limit finger range of motion (ROM).

- We wait until 3 to 5 days of immobilization and elevation have passed to permit internal bleeding, clot formation, and swelling to subside.

- This delay also lets patients get off all pain medication so they can start pain-guided therapy and not do what hurts to avoid complications.

3 to 5 Days Postsurgery to the 14-Day Mark (First 2 Weeks)

- The patient is re-taught what positions the hand and wrist they need to avoid to protect the extensor tendon repair.

- See Chapter 22 for more videos and discussion on extensor tendon repair of the hand.

- We teach patients to remove the orthosis safely and put bandages over the wound. We show them how to wash the wound safely with mild soap and tap water without putting the hand and wrist in dangerous positions. We show them how to dress the wound with a light layer of Vaseline and Coban dressing.

Video 21.TT6
Resting hand splint for the first 3 to 5 days following a repair. Keep the hand elevated and quiet to let the bleeding stop, the swelling come down, and the patient to get off all pain medication so they can follow pain-guided therapy and pain-guided healing.

- Coban or compression wrap may be applied to repaired digit to help cover the wound and control edema. We teach patients how to apply this dressing without compromising circulation or the tendon repair.

- A relative motion extension orthosis (with or without a wrist extension orthosis) is fabricated for the hand. This is the orthosis worn during the day.

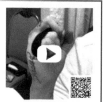

Video 21.TT7
Zone 5 repair: The patient only wore relative motion extension splint and was able to return to work at 2 weeks postsurgery, while wearing splint.

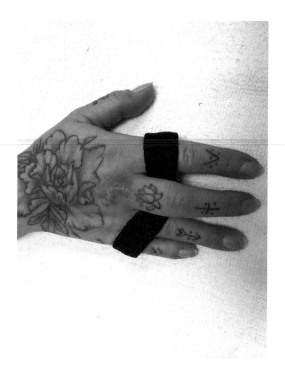

Fig. 21.TT3 Zone 5 repair. The patient has been wearing only this orthosis 4 days postsurgery.

- Please refer to Chapter 53 on Relative Motion Orthosis for how to fabricate this splint.[8]

- A resting hand orthosis with fingers in extension and wrist in comfortable extension is made for nighttime wear for all zones 4, 5, and 6.

- Patients can start to return to work, depending on job demands and employer agreements.

- We **allow** patients to use the hand for activity, as well as perform the recommended ROM exercises with relative motion extension orthosis (+/−) the wrist orthosis[9,10] (see ▶ Video 22.1).

- Patient should avoid heavy lifting, torqueing, and twisting activities with the hand.

- We teach patients to do gentle passive extension ROM exercise, while wearing the relative motion extension orthosis in the injured finger. This is to achieve full extension of the MP joint as well as the interphalangeal (IP) joints of the fingers. The patient may also need to do passive flexion extension exercises to the adjacent fingers that have not been repaired. (This should be done frequently during the day, every waking hour, 10 repetitions, holding for 10 seconds each time.)

- The patient is instructed to perform active tendon glide of all the fingers while wearing the relative motion extension orthosis. The patient should do this without forceful, jerky, or gripping action. Gentle tendon glide is used to make as much of an active fist the relative motion extension orthosis will allow. (This should be done frequently during the day, every waking hour, 10 repetitions, holding for 10 seconds each time.)

15- to 28-Day Mark (Third and Fourth Weeks Post Repair)

- Continue with edema management using Coban or compression wrap if still required. We stop when the edema is gone.
- Continue with full-time wear of the relative motion extension orthosis. At this time the wrist orthosis for zone 4 or 6 may be discontinued. This will depend on patient's activity level and clinical reasoning of the hand therapist.
- Continue with night extension orthosis to help avoid PIP joint flexion contractures from occurring in the fingers.
- The patient continues to do gentle passive extension ROM exercise, while wearing the relative motion extension orthosis as well as passive flexion extension exercises to the adjacent fingers that have not been repaired.
- The patient continues to perform active tendon glide of all the fingers with the relative motion extension orthosis on. The patient should do this without forceful, jerky, or gripping action. Gentle tendon glide is used to make as much of an active fist the relative motion extension orthosis will allow.

29- to 42-Day Mark (Fifth and Sixth Weeks Post Repair)

- Continue with edema management using Coban or compression wrap if still required.
- Continue with full-time wear of the relative motion extension orthosis. At this time the wrist orthosis should be discontinued.
- Change night extension orthosis to a night digit extension orthosis to help avoid PIP joint flexion contractures from occurring in the injured finger.
- The patient continues to do gentle passive extension ROM exercise, **without** the relative motion extension orthosis as well as passive flexion extension exercises to the adjacent fingers that have not been repaired.
- The patient is instructed to perform active flexion and extension tendon glide exercises of all the fingers **without** the relative motion extension orthosis on.
- Patients continue to use their hand for regular activity with the relative motion extension orthosis on.
- Relative motion orthosis is discontinued at week 6.
- Patient should be able to return to work at week 6 if this has not already been initiated earlier in the program.

43- to 56-Day Mark (Seventh and Eighth Weeks Post Repair)

- Night extension orthosis can be discontinued if the patient has full extension of all joints in the repaired digit.

- The patient continues with ROM exercises described above if full movement has not been achieved.

- The patient can start to use hand for all daily activities. Avoid forceful gripping and torqueing activities for another few weeks.

- Scar massage is started to help soften scar tissue.

- Start grip-strengthening activities for the hand.

References

1. Howell JW, Merritt WH, Robinson SJ. Immediate controlled active motion following zone 4-7 extensor tendon repair. J Hand Ther 2005;18(2):182–190

2. Merritt WH. Relative motion splint: active motion after extensor tendon injury and repair. J Hand Surg Am 2014;39(6):1187–1194

3. Burns MC, Derby B, Neumeister MW. Wyndell Merritt immediate controlled active motion (ICAM) protocol following extensor tendon repairs in zone IV-VII: review of literature, orthosis design, and case study—a multimedia article. Hand (N Y) 2013;8(1):17–22

4. Merritt WH, Wong AL, Lalonde DH. Recent developments are changing extensor tendon management. Plast Reconstr Surg 2020;145(3):617e–628e

5. McKee DE, Lalonde DH, Thoma A, Glennie DL, Hayward JE. Optimal time delay between epinephrine injection and incision to minimize bleeding. Plast Reconstr Surg 2013;131(4):811–814

6. Lalonde DH, Flewelling LA. Solving hand/finger pain problems with the pencil test and relative motion splinting. Plast Reconstr Surg Glob Open 2017;5(10):e1537

7. Lalonde D. How the wide awake approach is changing hand surgery and hand therapy: inaugural AAHS sponsored lecture at the ASHT meeting, San Diego, 2012. J Hand Ther 2013;26(2):175–178

8. Hirth MJ, Howell JW, Brown T, O'Brien L. Relative motion extension management of zones V and VI extensor tendon repairs: does international practice align with the current evidence? J Hand Ther 2021;34(1):76–89

9. Hirth MJ, Howell JW, O'Brien L. Relative motion orthoses in the management of various hand conditions: a scoping review. J Hand Ther 2016;29(4):405–432

10. Hirth MJ, Howell JW, O'Brien L. Two case reports—use of relative motion orthoses to manage extensor tendon zones III and IV and sagittal band injuries in adjacent fingers. J Hand Ther 2017;30(4):546–557

CHAPTER 22

EXTENSOR TENDON REPAIR OF THE HAND, WRIST, AND FOREARM (ZONES 6 TO 8)

Donald H. Lalonde, Amanda Higgins, Geoffrey Cook, Amir Adham Ahmad, Thomas Apard, Gökhan Tolga Akbulut, and Julian Escobar

ADVANTAGES OF WALANT VERSUS SEDATION AND TOURNIQUET IN EXTENSOR TENDON REPAIR OF THE HAND, WRIST, AND FOREARM

- All of the general advantages listed in Chapter 2 apply to both the surgeon and the patient (no nausea, no tourniquet pain or let-down bleeding, decreased cost without sedation in minor procedure room, safer surgery without sedation, etc.).

- You can see that your repair is solid enough by watching the patient take the fingers through a full range of motion before you close the skin.

- You can simulate the relative motion extension splint (RMES) during WALANT surgery with a sterile tongue depressor.[1,2,3,4] This will help you decide whether you need to add a wrist component to the Merritt splint. Wyndell Merritt's RMES has revolutionized extensor tendon laceration of the metacarpophalangeal (MP) joint (see ▶ Video 21.1 and ▶ Video 21.2 in Chapter 21) and dorsal hand management in the last few years. Patients can go back to work with these very functional splints as early as a few days after surgery, as shown in ▶ Video 22.1.

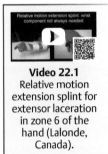

Video 22.1
Relative motion extension splint for extensor laceration in zone 6 of the hand (Lalonde, Canada).

- Patients get to see their finger movement restored during the surgery. They will remember this light at the end of the tunnel when they are working through the pain and stiffness of postoperative healing and therapy.

- You can test the strength of your forearm extensor tendon repairs by asking patients to make a fist and extend their fingers and wrist. If you see gapping, you can strengthen your repairs with more sutures to avoid rupture postoperatively.

- In the forearm, you can easily do primary tendon transfers and test the tension with active movement if you have tendon gaps.

- WALANT is valuable in active extension testing of extensor retinaculum repair.[5]

WHERE TO INJECT THE LOCAL ANESTHETIC FOR EXTENSOR TENDON REPAIR OF THE HAND, WRIST, AND FOREARM

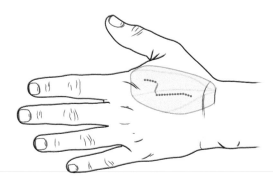

Fig. 22.1 Inject 20 mL of 1% lidocaine with 1:100,000 epinephrine buffered with 2 mL of 8.4% sodium bicarbonate. The orange line in the illustration is the laceration and the dotted red lines are the possible incisions.

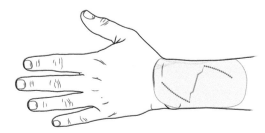

Fig. 22.2 The orange line in the illustration is the laceration and the dotted red lines are the possible incisions. It would take 50 to 60 mL to inflate what is seen in blue. Inject up to 100 mL of 0.5% lidocaine with 1:200,000 epinephrine (buffered with 10 mL of 1% lidocaine with 1:100,000 epinephrine:1 mL of 8.4% sodium bicarbonate).

SPECIFICS OF MINIMALLY PAINFUL INJECTION OF LOCAL ANESTHETIC IN EXTENSOR TENDON REPAIR OF THE HAND

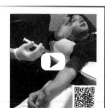

Video 22.2 How to inject local anesthesia in the hand so that it hardly hurts at all (Lalonde, Canada).

- Local anesthesia injection should barely hurt at all if you follow the simple rules of Chapter 5 for hints to minimize injection pain. The patients will think you are magical.

- We always inject all patients while they are lying down to decrease the risk of their fainting (see ▶ Video 6.1).

- The goal of the injection is to get visible and palpable local anesthetic under the skin at least 2 cm outside any area you are likely to dissect.

- Keep the total dose of infiltration less than 7 mg/kg. If less than 50 mL is required, use premixed 1% lidocaine with 1:100,000 epinephrine. If 50 to 100 mL is required, dilute with saline solution to a concentration of 0.5% lidocaine with 1:200,000 epinephrine. If 100 to 200 mL of solution is required to produce tumescent local anesthesia (see Chapter 4), dilute with saline solution to a concentration of 0.25% lidocaine with 1:400,000 epinephrine.

- Add 10 mL 0.5% bupivacaine with 1:200,000 epinephrine to the injectate if you think the procedure will take more than 3 hours.

- Always inject from proximal to distal to keep the sharp needle tip in anesthetized areas to decrease pain.

- Alternate injecting on the radial side, then the ulnar side, then the radial side, and then the ulnar side. This also decreases pain by letting the distal skin get numb to needle reinsertion.

TIPS AND TRICKS FOR PERFORMING EXTENSOR TENDON REPAIR OF THE HAND, WRIST, AND FOREARM WITH THE WIDE AWAKE APPROACH

- To get the extensors to relax, ask the patient to flex the finger. There is a reflex arc in the spinal cord that causes the extensors to relax.

Video 22.3 Extensors reflexively relax when patient is asked to actively flex the finger (Cook, Canada).

- Many of the injuries happen at night and on weekends—not an ideal time to perform a repair. A major advantage of eliminating sedation for flexor tendon repair is that you do not need to perform the procedure in the main operating room. We do all of our tendon repairs in minor procedure rooms in the clinic outside the main operating room, Monday to Friday, 8 AM to 4 PM. We know that we do better surgery at 2 PM than at 2 AM. In addition, our hand therapists can teach patients during the surgery and see the repair (see Chapter 15). This also permits patients to be sober so they can understand their injury and learn how to look after it with intraoperative teaching they can remember.

- ▶ Video 22.4 provides three different extensor tendon repairs of the forearm, including a case of primary tendon graft to extensor pollicis longus (EPL) after rupture from a distal radius fracture.

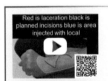

Video 22.4 Three different extensor tendon repairs of the forearm (Lalonde, Canada).

- Do not worry about minor bleeding from cut skin edges because most little bleeders will stop spontaneously by the time you sew the skin flaps back for exposure. We no longer use cautery for most cases but occasionally use a hemostat on bigger vessels for a few minutes or tie them off.

- Patients need to look at their fingers to extend them to test the repair. Patients cannot move numbed fingers well unless they see them. Although most patients do not mind looking at the wound, you can cover the wound with a towel as they watch their fingers move.

- It is worth placing a tongue depressor under the involved finger or fingers to perform the repair and to simulate an RMES intraoperatively. This may allow you to let the patient have early protected movement of the fingers at 3 to 5 days after surgery[3,4] (see Chapter 21).

Video 22.5 Subtotal amputation of thumb with secondary extensor tendon reconstruction (Lalonde, Canada).

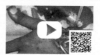

Video 22.6 Extensor pollicis longus (EPL) repair (Ahmad, Malaysia).

Video 22.7 Extensor spaghetti repair (Escobar, Columbia).

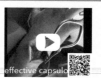

Video 22.8 Extensor carpi ulnaris (ECU) subluxation reconstruction (Apard, France).

Video 22.9 Palmar interosseus reconstruction. Patient could not flex and adduct small finger. Palmar interosseus torn and dorsal to axis of metacarpophalangeal (MP) joint, extending MP and stopping interphalangeal (IP) flexion like boutonniere MP joint (Lalonde, Canada).

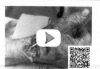

Video 22.10 Spaghetti wrist extensor repair (Akbulut, Turkey).

POSTOPERATIVE THERAPY TIPS FOR ZONES 6–8 EXTENSOR TENDON REPAIRS

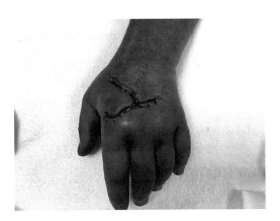

Video 22.TT1
Zone 6 injury with post-operative relative motion and wrist orthoses. Both orthoses are worn together to help protect the repair but let the patient use the hand for functional activity and perform exercises (Higgins, Canada).

Fig. 22.TT1 Zone 6 index and long finger extensor tendon repairs showing zone 6 extensor indicis proprius (EIP) and extensor digitorum communis (EDC) of index and long finger repair.

ZONES 6 (HAND), 7 (EXTENSOR RETINACULUM), AND 8 (FOREARM) EXTENSOR TENDON REPAIR REHABILITATION PROGRAM: THE SAINT JOHN PROTOCOL

- In zone 6 extensor tendon repair, WALANT can help us to determine if a wrist orthosis should be included with the relative motion extension orthosis or if a relative motion extension orthosis on its own is enough protection for the repaired tendon to achieve early glide but avoid rupture.[6]

Video 22.TT2
Zone 6 repair. How to explain to patient how to wean off relative motion extension splint at 4 weeks after injury (Lalonde, Canada).

References

1. Howell JW, Merritt WH, Robinson SJ. Immediate controlled active motion following zone 4-7 extensor tendon repair. J Hand Ther 2005;18(2):182–190
2. Merritt WH. Relative motion splint: active motion after extensor tendon injury and repair. J Hand Surg Am 2014;39(6):1187–1194
3. Merritt WH, Wong AL, Lalonde DH. Recent developments are changing extensor tendon management. Plast Reconstr Surg 2020;145(3):617e–628e
4. Hirth MJ, Howell JW, Brown T, O'Brien L. Relative motion extension management of zones V and VI extensor tendon repairs: does international practice align with the current evidence? J Hand Ther 2021;34(1):76–89
5. Takagi T, Kobayashi Y, Watanabe M. Extensor retinaculum reconstruction using the wide-awake approach. J Hand Surg Am 2017;42(10):844.e1–844.e4
6. Hirth MJ, Howell JW, Feehan LM, Brown T, O'Brien L. Postoperative hand therapy management of zones V and VI extensor tendon repairs of the fingers: an international inquiry of current practice. J Hand Ther 2021;34(1):58–75

CHAPTER 23

TENOLYSIS

Jason Wong, Michael Sauerbier, Peter C. Amadio, Mark Baratz, Xavier Gueffier, Chao Chen, Donald H. Lalonde, and Ian Maxwell

ADVANTAGES OF WALANT VERSUS SEDATION AND TOURNIQUET IN TENOLYSIS

- All of the general advantages listed in Chapter 2 apply to both the surgeon and the patient (no nausea, no tourniquet pain or let-down bleeding, decreased cost without sedation in minor procedure room, safer surgery without sedation, etc.).

- There is no rush when performing tenolysis because there is no tourniquet.[1]

- Your patients can help you, because they are comfortable and cooperative; they can rupture their own adhesions by actively flexing their muscles after you release some of the adhesions.

- Patients can show you where their tendon is stuck with active movement. Sometimes they feel the adhesions rupture in their wrist with active movement when you are thinking they are stuck in their finger as seen in ▶ Video 23.1.

- You know that you have finished the surgery when you see a full range of active finger movement while the patient is on the operating table. This is like testing and ensuring good patency and blood flow through a microvascular anastomosis before you close the skin.

- At the end of the surgery, you can show your patients exercises they can perform. They can do their first exercises on the table in a totally pain-free manner instead of after surgery, when they will be sore. They will remember the exercises and the range of motion they can achieve because they are sedation-free.

- You and the patient will both know how much active movement the finger achieved at the end of the operation. This avoids unrealistic expectations for you and the patient.

Video 23.1 Listen to the patient rupture the adhesions in her wrist when the surgeon thought the tendon was trapped in the finger (Lalonde, Canada).

Video 23.2
Unsedated patient
can remember
the range of
motion obtained
at the end of
surgery (Sauerbier,
Germany).

- In ▶ Video 23.2, Dr Michael Sauerbier performs tenolysis with the wide awake approach. His patient can remember the movement he or she was able to experience on the operating table.

- Patients watch themselves moving the fingers through a full range of motion before the skin is closed. They know that their finger will function well once they get past the postoperative discomfort and stiffness if they put effort into their therapy.

- You are able to talk to unsedated patients for the time that local anesthesia and the tenolysis take to perform. You can educate and warn them about what to do and not do after surgery. We know that the tendon is weaker and has less blood supply after tenolysis. Therefore, to avoid rupture we warn patients to avoid jerk-type movements and heavy lifting for 2 to 3 weeks until the tendon gets stronger.

- The hand therapist can also participate in intraoperative patient evaluation and education if the surgeon allows the therapist into the operating room, as we do (see Chapter 15).

- You can also do this in children. See ▶ Video 9.11 for tenolysis in a 4-year-old by Chao Chen from China.

WHERE TO INJECT THE LOCAL ANESTHETIC FOR TENOLYSIS

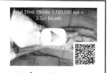

Video 23.3 How
to inject the
local anesthesia
for tenolysis for
the patient seen
in Video 23.5
(Lalonde, Canada).

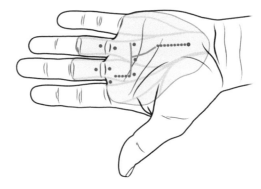

Video 23.4
Real-time,
9-minute lo-
cal anesthesia
injection for
metacarpopha-
langeal (MP) joint
capsulotomy and
metacarpal plate
removal for the pa-
tient seen in Video
23.6 (Lalonde,
Canada).

Fig. 23.1 The orange line represents the patient's original scarring from 60 years before (see Video 23.3 for a tenolysis shown in the drawing). Inject up to 30 mL of 1% lidocaine with 1:100,000 epinephrine and up to 3 mL of 8.4% sodium bicarbonate (1 mL of bicarbonate for each 10 mL of 1% lidocaine with 1:100,000 epinephrine).

- Also see ▶ Video 23.13 for injection of local anesthesia for tenolysis with 3-mL syringe and 30-gauge needle. A small syringe is ideal to push the local anesthetic in scar. A short 0.5-inch needle makes it almost painless for patient.

SPECIFICS OF MINIMALLY PAINFUL INJECTION OF LOCAL ANESTHETIC IN TENOLYSIS

- Local anesthesia injection should barely hurt at all if you follow the simple rules of Chapter 5 for hints to minimize injection pain. The patients will think you are magical.

- As in ▸ Fig. 23.1, inject the first 10 mL into the most proximal red dot injection point, which is the most proximal incision you are likely to use to dissect the proximal tendon. In this case, we actually injected starting at the wrist crease as we opened the carpal tunnel to make certain it would not be too tight after surgery.

- The first few milliliters of local anesthetic go under the skin, and the rest is injected under the superficial palmar fascia.

- After the common digital nerves of the palm are totally numb (30 minutes is ideal), you can make all of the farther distal epinephrine effect injections in a pain-free manner. Alternatively, you can continue injecting slowly in an antegrade fashion so there is always 1 cm of local anesthetic ahead of the needle, as described in Chapter 5 for minimal pain injection.

- Inject the distal palm with 3 mL in each of the red dots just proximal to the preexisting scar.

- Inject another 2 mL in the subcutaneous fat in each of the three most distal red dots in the palm, which are distal to the scar.

- Note that preexisting scar in the hand creates a natural barrier for diffusion of the local anesthetic. You should start proximally, then inject all around a scar, because the local anesthetic will not traverse it easily, and it is hard to inject into scar.

- Inject another 2 mL in the affected proximal phalanges just under the skin.

- Slowly inject (tumesce) until the whole area you will dissect gets a little firm, with visible and palpable local anesthetic swelling. The goal of the injection is to bathe local anesthetic 2 cm beyond wherever you think you even have a small chance of dissecting. You will not cause a palm compartment syndrome. As soon as you incise the skin, the pressure will come down as the local anesthetic leaks out.

- If you inject 20 mL into the palm, where will it go? Everywhere! Perfect! It is like an extravascular Bier block, but only where you need it, and without a tourniquet.

- We keep the total dose of infiltration less than 7 mg/kg. If less than 50 mL is required to produce tumescent local anesthesia (see Chapter 4), we use premixed 1% lidocaine with 1:100,000 epinephrine. If 50 to 100 mL is required, we dilute with saline solution to a concentration of 0.5% lidocaine with 1:200,000 epinephrine.

- Inject patients before they come into the operating room to give the lidocaine and epinephrine at least 30 minutes to work.

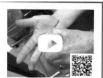

Video 23.5
Tenolysis in a 63-year-old woman who had been unable to flex her long and ring fingers since a tendon repair at age 3 (Lalonde, Canada).

Video 23.6
Metacarpal plate removal and metacarpophalangeal (MP) joint capsulotomy with extensor tenolysis (Lalonde, Canada).

TIPS AND TRICKS FOR PERFORMING TENOLYSIS WITH THE WIDE AWAKE APPROACH

- Patients need to see their hand to move it when it is numb. Take down the barrier drapes so that they can see their fingers move. You can cover the wounds with towels or gauze.

- Keep testing intraoperative active patient flexion until you get a full range of active motion on the operating table before you close the skin.

- Have the patient pull on the tendons (make a fist) from time to time as you dissect. You will see the patient perform mini-ruptures of adhesions. The patient's movement will guide you to where the tendon is still stuck and where you need more dissection to free it.

- We do not like to use sedation because many patients may not be able to cooperate as well to pull and rupture their adhesions. They may also not remember the range of active motion they achieved during surgery.

- Many patients are interested in looking at the tendon to understand the nature of their problem. Satisfying their curiosity can be rewarding.

- It is very helpful to have hand therapists attend the tenolysis. They will be able to witness the achievable range of motion and be able to perform intraoperative teaching of the patient along with the surgeon (see Chapter 15).

Video 23.7 Patient ruptures her own extensor adhesions after wrist fusion for rheumatoid arthritis (Lalonde, Canada).

Video 23.8 Patient ruptures her own adhesions after finger amputation (Wong, England).

Video 23.9 Minimal incision lateral band and adhesion release (Baratz, USA).

Video 23.10 Tenolysis after flexor synovitis (Gueffier, France).

Video 23.11 Clunking caused by old partial flexor digitorum superficialis (FDS) laceration solved with tenolysis (Gueffier, France).

Video 23.12 Extensor tenolysis (Wong, England).

Video 23.13 Injection of local anesthetic for flexor tenolysis after tendon graft (Lalonde and Maxwell, Canada).

POSTOPERATIVE THERAPY TIPS

- We explain to patients during the surgery that we have weakened their tendon by decreasing its blood supply and strength by removing all of the scar adhesions. If they use the hand for heavy lifting early after surgery, they could rupture the weakened tendon. They can apply gradual resistance like after flexor tendon repair. We treat tenolysed flexor tendons as we treat freshly repaired tendons postoperatively, with gentle early protected movement after passive mobilization of the joint to take out the friction (see Chapter 19).

- We teach patients about pain-guided therapy and pain-guided movement starting 3 to 5 days after surgery. Don't do what hurts to avoid rupture and infection.

- We also explain to patients during the surgery that we want them to keep their hand elevated with minimal movement for the first 2 to 4 days to let internal bleeding stop and to allow friction-causing edema to settle. Internal bleeding leads to further internal scarring as the white cells need to "mop up" the old clot. Collagen formation does not start for 3 days. Waiting a few days also allows the avascular tendon to recover from the decrease in blood supply we have caused by cutting adhesions. There is no downside to a rest period, but there are many downsides to immediate forceful movement—especially rupture.

- The patient should start with gentle passive range of motion exercises to the surgical finger. This means using the other hand to gently push the finger toward the palm into a fist position. The patient is encouraged to bend at all three joints, distal interphalangeal (DIP), proximal interphalangeal (PIP), and metacarpophalangeal (MP) joint. The patient should only push the finger for a stretch, it should not cause pain. The patient can then hold this position for a count of 5 seconds. Then the patient uses the other hand to push the surgical finger out straight. Again, emphasizing on trying to achieve extension at all three joints, MCP, PIP and DIP joints. Hold this position for 5 seconds. This is then repeated 10 times. The patient is encouraged to do this exercise as much as possible during the hours awake. This passive exercise helps to warm up tissues and stretch tissues before getting the tendon to glide and pull on bone.

- After passive range of motion, the patient is taught to actively move the finger. This means getting all four fingers to bend and straighten without help. This is trying to achieve tendon glide, through scar formation. The first active exercise is called tuck or a hook. The patient is encouraged to bend the PIP and DIP joints of the four fingers. Hold this position for 5 seconds, then straighten these joints and hold for 5 seconds. This is repeated 10 times, and performed as often as possible when awake. The patient then performs another active exercise that involves all three joints of the finger. The patient tries to make the best fist that he or she can. MP, PIP, and DIP joints are bent together. This is held for 5 seconds.

The patient then straightens the fingers and holds for 5 seconds. This is repeated 10 times as often as possible when awake.

- The patient should notice weekly gains in both passive and active range of motion of the surgical finger.

Reference

1. Tang JB. Wide-awake primary flexor tendon repair, tenolysis, and tendon transfer. Clin Orthop Surg 2015;7(3):275–281

CHAPTER 24

TENDON TRANSFERS

*Donald H. Lalonde, Egemen Ayhan,
Amir Adham Ahmad, Julian Escobar, Xavier Gueffier,
Mark Baratz, Robert E. Van Demark, Jr., Jean Paul Brutus,
Thomas Apard, Geoffrey Cook, Yin Lu, and Paul Sibley*

ADVANTAGES OF WALANT VERSUS SEDATION AND TOURNIQUET IN TENDON TRANSFERS

- All of the general advantages listed in Chapter 2 apply to both the surgeon and the patient (no nausea, no tourniquet pain or let-down bleeding, decreased cost without sedation in minor procedure room for simple transfers like extensor indicis [EI] to extensor pollicis longus [EPL], safer surgery without sedation, etc.).

- When you perform wide awake hand surgery, you do not have to deal with your patient's medical comorbidities, which would only be a problem if you sedate patients. It is safer for your patients to have no sedation. They just get up and go home after surgery, like when they have had a filling at the dentist.

- The biggest advantage of using the wide awake approach for tendon transfer is getting the correct tension on the transfer. It is easy to make a tendon transfer too tight or too loose. You can see that your tendon transfer tension is correct by watching the patient take the thumb or finger through a full range of motion before you close the skin.[1,4,5,6,7,8,10] You can tighten or loosen the transfer and have the comfortable, pain-free patient retest the tension. Both you and your patient know the tension is right before you close the skin.

- Patients are able to see that their transfer is working during surgery. They are motivated to achieve the result they know they will get if they work at it after surgery.

- The surgeon can decide if he or she wants to do a tendon graft versus a tendon transfer based on whether or not he or she sees adequate muscle excursion from the proximal stump of the injured tendon.[9]

Video 24.1
Extensor indicis (EI) to extensor pollicis longus (EPL) transfer: How to get the transfer tension right (Lalonde, Canada).

WHERE TO INJECT THE LOCAL ANESTHETIC FOR EI TO EPL TRANSFER

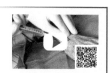

Video 24.2 How to inject local anesthetic for extensor indicis (EI) to extensor pollicis longus (EPL) transfer. Pinch the skin into the needle (Lalonde, Canada).

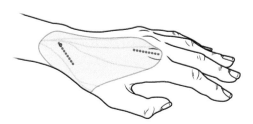

Fig. 24.1 Inject 30 to 40 mL of 1% lidocaine with 1:100,000 epinephrine buffered with 3 to 4 mL of 8.4% bicarbonate (1 mL of sodium bicarbonate for each 10 mL of 1% lidocaine with 1:100,000 epinephrine). The dotted red lines are the possible incisions.

WHERE TO INJECT THE LOCAL ANESTHETIC FOR FLEXOR DIGITORUM SUPERFICIALIS (FDS3 OR FDS4) TO THE FLEXOR POLLICIS LONGUS (FPL) TRANSFER

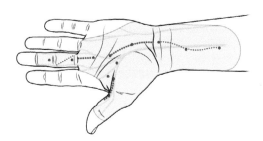

Fig. 24.2 Inject 50 to 100 mL of 0.5% lidocaine with 1:200,000 epinephrine buffered with 10:1 8.4% sodium bicarbonate. The red dots are injection points and the dotted lines are possible incisions.

WHERE TO INJECT THE LOCAL ANESTHESIA FOR RADIAL NERVE PALSY TRIPLE TRANSFER

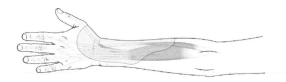

Fig. 24.3 Triple tendon transfer (PT to ECRB, FCR to EDC, and PL to EPL for radial nerve palsy). Blue is the subcutaneous dorsal injection of up to a total of 200 mL of 0.25% lidocaine with 1:400,000 epinephrine.

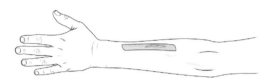

Fig. 24.4 Triple tendon transfer (PT to ECRB, FCR to EDC, and PL to EPL for radial nerve palsy). Pink is the periosteal dorsal injection of up to a total of 200 mL of 0.25% lidocaine with 1:400,000 epinephrine. This is to harvest the periosteal sleeve to lengthen the pronator teres tendon.

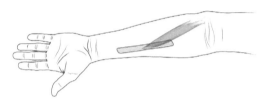

Fig. 24.5 Triple tendon transfer (PT to ECRB, FCR to EDC, and PL to EPL for radial nerve palsy). Pink is the periosteal volar injection of up to a total of 200 mL of 0.25% lidocaine with 1:400,000 epinephrine. This is to harvest the periosteal sleeve to lengthen the pronator teres tendon.

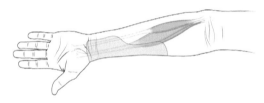

Fig. 24.6 Triple tendon transfer (PT to ECRB, FCR to EDC, and PL to EPL for radial nerve palsy). Blue is the subcutaneous volar injection of up to a total of 200ml of 0.25% lidocaine with 1:400,000 epinephrine.

SPECIFICS OF INJECTING MINIMALLY PAINFUL LOCAL ANESTHETIC FOR TENDON TRANSFERS

- Start by drawing the outline of where you will inject local on the skin with a 2-cm margin beyond wherever you are going to dissect.

- Tumesce (plump up with local anesthetic) the entire area inside the markings.

- If you are going to take muscle insertion (pronator teres with periosteum), you need to inject widely at the periosteal insertion so that you can lift it off the bone painlessly.

- Local anesthesia injection should barely hurt at all if you follow the simple rules of Chapter 5 for hints to minimize injection pain. The patients will think you are magical. How to inject local anesthetic for flexor tendon repair.

- We inject the anesthetic solution a minimum of 30 minutes before surgery to allow the epinephrine to take optimal effect and provide an adequately dry working field.[2,3]

- We inject supine patients on stretchers in a waiting area to decrease the risk of their fainting (see Chapter 6).

Video 24.3 How to inject local anesthetic for pronator teres (PT) to extensor carpi radialis brevis (ECRB), flexor carpi radialis (FCR) to extensor digitorum communis (EDC), and palmaris longus (PL) to extensor pollicis longus (EPL) transfers (Ahmad, Malaysia).[11]

Video 24.4a
Surgery video for pronator teres (PT) to extensor carpi radialis brevis (ECRB), flexor carpi radialis (FCR) to extensor digitorum communis (EDC), and palmaris longus (PL) to extensor pollicis longus (EPL) transfers (Ahmad, Malaysia).

Video 24.4b
Lalonde narrates surgery video for pronator teres (PT) to extensor carpi radialis brevis (ECRB), flexor carpi radialis (FCR) to extensor digitorum communis (EDC), and palmaris longus (PL) to extensor pollicis longus (EPL) transfers (Ahmad, Malaysia).

- To minimize the pain of injection, use a 27-gauge needle (not a 25 gauge) into the most proximal injection point (red dot). This point is marked at least 2 cm proximal to the most proximal place you are likely to dissect.

- You can pinch loose forearm skin and push the skin into the needle to decrease pain.

- Inject the rest of the first 10 mL slowly (over 2 minutes) without moving the needle.

- Continue injecting from proximal to distal, blowing the local anesthetic slowly ahead of the needle so there is always at least 1 cm of visible or palpable local anesthetic ahead of the sharp needle tip that the patient would feel if you advanced it into "live" nerves—"Blow slow before you go."

- Reinsert the needle only into clearly vasoconstricted white skin that has functioning lidocaine and epinephrine so that needle reinsertion is pain-free.

- The goal of the injection is to bathe local anesthetic 2 cm beyond wherever you think you even have a small chance of dissecting.

- We keep the total dose of infiltration to less than 7 mg/kg. If you need less than 50 mL to produce tumescent local anesthesia (see Chapter 4), use buffered 1% lidocaine with 1:100,000 epinephrine. If you want 50 to 100 mL of volume to inject, dilute with saline solution to a concentration of 0.5% lidocaine with 1:200,000 epinephrine. If you need 100 to 200 mL of volume for larger forearm transfers, dilute buffered 50 mL of commercially available 1% lidocaine with 1:100,000 epinephrine with 150 mL of saline solution to produce 200 mL of 0.25% lidocaine with 1:400,000 epinephrine, which is clinically very effective both for local anesthesia and for vasoconstriction.

- You can inject large areas faster with blunt-tipped cannulas but still pain-free. See Chapter 5 for another video clip of cannula injection of tumescent local anesthetic for synovectomy and EI to EPL tendon transfer.

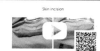

Video 24.4c
Ahmad gives more information on triple tendon transfer for radial nerve palsy (Ahmad, Malaysia).

Video 24.5 How to inject 200 mL painlessly and quickly with a blunt-tipped cannula for a tendon transfer of flexor carpi ulnaris (FCU) to extensor carpi radialis longus (ECRL) (Lalonde, Canada).

Video 24.6 The surgical video of flexor carpi ulnaris (FCU) to extensor carpi radialis longus (ECRL) transfer of the same patient injected with local anesthetic in Video 24.3 (Lalonde, Canada).

TIPS AND TRICKS FOR PERFORMING TENDON TRANSFERS WITH THE WIDE AWAKE APPROACH

- Patients need to look at their fingers or thumb when you ask them to test the transfer, since they may not feel the numbed digits. You need to take sheet barriers down so they can see their numbed fingers or wrist moving. Although most patients do not mind looking at the wound, you can cover the wound with a towel as they watch their fingers and thumb move.

- If you want the thumb EPL to relax, ask the patient to flex the thumb IP joint. The spinal cord reflex will force the EPL to relax. Asking patients to flex will relax extensors. Asking patients to extend will relax flexors.

- Most patients are simply able to move their transfer without thinking about it. The brain can do it automatically in many cases, and they just don't need to "learn" it. However, some are not able to do it right away. For example, you may need to ask them to flex the ring finger to flex the thumb if you have transferred FDS3 to FPL and they can't easily activate it. After a couple of tries, they are usually able to do it almost right away.

- What you see on the table with intraoperative transfer tension testing is what you will get as a result. If the transfer looks too loose, it will be too loose postoperatively. If it looks too tight, it will be too tight postoperatively.

- Use two "temporary" sutures to set your tension where you think it should be. Then have the patient test it to see if you got the tension right. If you only have one suture there, the patient may well rupture it. If the tension looks good, go ahead and do a Pulvertaft or some other weave. If it is too loose, add sutures to make it tighter. If it is too tight, insert sutures where you think they should be, then cut the first sutures that were too tight and test again.

- Do not be afraid to test full flexion and full extension. Your sutures should be strong enough to take it. If they are not, you need to reinforce them.

- We have patients relieve themselves in the restroom after we inject the local anesthetic and just before we start the surgery to avoid unnecessary surgical interruptions for these longer cases. Patients do not receive an intravenous fluid that increases the urge to void. If we give preoperative antibiotics, we give them by mouth.

- For older patients with cardiac comorbidities, you can decrease the concentration of epinephrine and perform the WALANT procedure in the hospital main operating room with monitoring.

- Many patients are interested in looking at the tendon to understand the nature of their problem. You can mask them, show them the tendon, and have them watch it move. It will help greatly that they see the transfer move, because they know that it will work after they overcome the pain and stiffness.

Video 24.7 Local anesthesia extensor indicis proprius (EIP) for thumb opposition via palmaris longus (PL) tendon graft rerouted over ulna (Ayhan, Turkey).

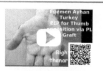

Video 24.8 Thumb opposition transfers including theory, detailed surgery (Camitz procedure), and extensor indicis proprius (EIP) for thumb opposition via palmaris longus (PL) tendon graft rerouted over ulna (Ayhan, Turkey).

Video 24.9 Palmaris longus (PL) to thumb MP joint for thumb opposition (Escobar, Columbia).

Video 24.10a A Flexor digitorum superficialis of the ring finger (FDS4) to flexor pollicis longus (FPL) transfer. The video includes ultrasound location of the tendon ends determined by the surgeon preoperatively (Gueffier, France).

Video 24.10b Longer version transfer of flexor digitorum superficialis (FDS4) to flexor pollicis longus (FPL) with more intraoperative details to get better results (Gueffier, France).

Video 24.11 Flexor digitorum superficialis (FDS4) to flexor pollicis longus (FPL) transfer with early protected movement postoperatively (Ayhan, Turkey).

Video 24.12 Flexor digitorum superficialis (FDS3) to flexor pollicis longus (FPL) transfer, including injection of 70 mL local anesthetic (Lalonde, Canada).

Video 24.13 Flexor digitorum superficialis (FDS3) radius plate removal and FDS4 to flexor pollicis longus (FPL) transfer (Lalonde, Canada).

Video 24.14 Flexor digitorum superficialis (FDS4) two-stage radius plate removal and FDS4 to flexor pollicis longus (FPL) transfer with patient impressions of awake versus asleep (Van Demark, USA).

Video 24.15 Rheumatoid extensor tendon rupture and reconstruction (Brutus, Canada).

Video 24.16 Extensor indicis EI to extensor pollicis longus EPL surgery with intraoperative testing of thumb flexion and extension (Lalonde Canada)

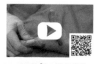

Video 24.17 Extensor indicis (EI) to extensor pollicis longus (EPL) transfer. A patient watching herself extend her thumb and knowing she can get a good result (Baratz, USA).

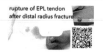

Video 24.18 Extensor indicis (EI) to extensor pollicis longus (EPL) transfer after distal radius fracture (Apard, France).

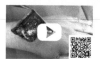

Video 24.19 Side-to-side extensor transfers for rheumatoid hand (Ayhan, Turkey).

Video 24.20 Static correction of claw deformity with bone anchors (Ayhan, Turkey).

Video 24.21 Extensor digiti minimi (EDM) correction of abduction deformity of small finger (Ayhan, Turkey).

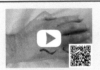

Video 24.22
Local anesthesia for Video 24.21 extensor digiti minimi (EDM) correction of abduction deformity of small finger (Ayhan, Turkey).

Video 24.23
Small-to-ring, side-to-side extensor digitorum communis (EDC) and long flexor digitorum superficialis (FDS) to long and index EDC transfer through interosseus membrane in an 80-year-old with lung problems (Sibley, USA).

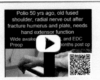

Video 24.24
Polio flexor carpi radialis (FCR) to extensor digitorum communis (EDC) and extensor pollicis longus (EPL) transfer after elective wrist fusion (Cook and Lalonde, Canada).

Video 24.25
Flexor carpi ulnaris (FCU) to extensor digitorum communis (EDC) and palmaris longus (PL) to extensor pollicis longus (EPL) transfers (Lalonde, Canada).

Video 24.26
Extensor indicis (EI) to extensor pollicis longus (EPL) transfer with early controlled movement (Gueffier, France).

Video 24.27
Thumb opposition extensor carpi ulnaris (ECU) to rerouted extensor pollicis brevis (EBP) on abductor pollicis longus (APL) (Yin Lu, China).

References

1. Lalonde DH. Wide-awake extensor indicis proprius to extensor pollicis longus tendon transfer. J Hand Surg Am 2014;39(11):2297–2299
2. Lalonde DH, Wong A. Dosage of local anesthesia in wide awake hand surgery. J Hand Surg Am 2013;38(10):2025–2028
3. McKee DE, Lalonde DH, Thoma A, Glennie DL, Hayward JE. Optimal time delay between epinephrine injection and incision to minimize bleeding. Plast Reconstr Surg 2013;131(4):811–814
4. Bezuhly M, Sparkes GL, Higgins A, Neumeister MW, Lalonde DH. Immediate thumb extension following extensor indicis proprius-to-extensor pollicis longus tendon transfer using the wide-awake approach. Plast Reconstr Surg 2007;119(5):1507–1512
5. Tang JB. Wide-awake primary flexor tendon repair, tenolysis, and tendon transfer. Clin Orthop Surg 2015;7(3):275–281
6. Gao LL, Chang J. Wide awake secondary tendon reconstruction. Hand Clin 2019;35(1):35–41

7. Hong JJ, Kang HJ, Whang JI, et al. Comparison of the wide-awake approach and conventional approach in extensor indicis proprius-to-extensor pollicis longus tendon transfer for chronic extensor pollicis longus rupture. 2020;145(3):723–733

8. Mohammed AK, Lalonde DH. Wide awake tendon transfers in leprosy patients in India. Hand Clin 2019;35(1):67–84

9. Zukawa M, Osada R, Makino H, Kimura T. Wide-awake flexor pollicis longus tendon reconstruction with evaluation of the active voluntary contraction of the ruptured muscle-tendon. Plast Reconstr Surg 2019;143(1):176–180

10. Lalonde D. Discussion: comparison of the wide-awake approach and conventional approach in extensor indicis proprius-to-extensor pollicis longus tendon transfer for chronic extensor pollicis longus rupture. Plast Reconstr Surg 2020;145(3):734–735

11. Abdullah S, Ahmad AA, Lalonde D. Wide awake local anesthesia no tourniquet forearm triple tendon transfer in radial nerve palsy. Plast Reconstr Surg Glob Open 2020;8(8):e3023

CHAPTER 25

TENDON GRAFTS AND PULLEY RECONSTRUCTION

*Donald H. Lalonde, Egemen Ayhan, Alison Wong,
Chao Chen, Nikolas Alan Jagodzinski, Alistair Phillips,
Kamal Rafiqi, Thomas Apard, and Ian Maxwell*

ADVANTAGES OF WALANT VERSUS SEDATION AND TOURNIQUET IN TENDON GRAFTS AND PULLEY RECONSTRUCTION

- All of the general advantages listed in Chapter 2 apply to both the surgeon and the patient (no nausea, no tourniquet pain or let-down bleeding, safer surgery without sedation, etc.).

- The biggest advantage of using the wide awake approach for tendon grafting is getting the correct tension. It is easy to make a tendon graft too tight or too loose. You can see that your tendon reconstruction tension is correct by watching the patient take the thumb or finger through a full range of motion before you close the skin.[1,2,3,4,5,6,7] You can tighten or loosen the transfer and have the comfortable, pain-free patient retest the tension. Both you and your patient know the tension is right before you close the skin.

- You can resect the lumbrical if you are getting a lumbrical plus problem with flexor digitorum profundus (FDP) tendon grafting. You can see this happen at the time of the grafting with active patient movement on the operating table and fix this at the time of grafting.

- Patients are able to see that their transfer is working during surgery. They are motivated to achieve the result they know they will get if they work at it after surgery.

- The surgeon can decide if he or she wants to do a tendon graft versus a tendon transfer based on whether or not he or she sees adequate muscle excursion from the proximal stump of the injured tendon.[8] See ▶ Video 25.3 where flexor pollicis longus (FPL) proximal stump had 2 cm of active excursion so we used it for a tendon graft motor instead of using a tendon transfer and injuring another finger.

WHERE TO INJECT THE LOCAL ANESTHETIC FOR THREE DIFFERENT TENDON TRANSFERS

In the case shown in ▶ Video 25.1, inject 110 mL of 0.25% lidocaine with 1:400,000 epinephrine buffered with 10:1 8.4% sodium bicarbonate.

Video 25.1 How to inject local anesthesia for flexor tendon grafting using flexor digitorum superficialis (FDS) as grafts for flexor digitorum profundus (FDP) reconstruction (Lalonde, Canada).

Video 25.2 How to inject local anesthesia for palmaris longus (PL) graft to reconstruct flexor digitorum profundus (FDP5) with FDP4 motor (Gueffier, France).

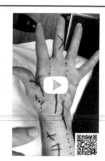

Video 25.3 How to inject local anesthesia with cannula for graft or transfer, and find two ends of flexor pollicis longus (FPL) ruptured on distal radius fracture plate with ultrasound for tendon grafting with palmaris longus (PL) and half flexor carpi radialis (FCR) (Lalonde, Canada).

- ▶ Video 25.5 demonstrates FPL reconstruction with tendon grafting after a distal radius fracture plate induces tendon rupture. The patient is prepared for either tendon transfer or tendon graft based on how much active movement there remains in the proximal FPL motor 2 months after rupture. The FPL proximal stump has 2 cm of active movement so we decided to graft instead of damaging another finger with transfer.[8]

SPECIFICS OF INJECTING MINIMALLY PAINFUL LOCAL ANESTHETIC FOR TENDON GRAFTS AND PULLEY RECONSTRUCTION

- Start by drawing the outline of where you will inject local anesthetic on the skin with a 2-cm margin beyond wherever you are going to dissect.

- Tumesce (plump up with local anesthetic) the entire area inside the markings.

- Local anesthesia injection should barely hurt at all if you follow the simple rules of Chapter 5 for hints to minimize injection pain. The patients will think you are magical.

- We inject the anesthetic solution a minimum of 30 minutes before surgery to allow the epinephrine to take optimal effect and provide an adequately dry working field.[9,10]

- We inject supine patients on stretchers in a waiting area to decrease the risk of their fainting (see Chapter 6).

- To minimize the pain of injection, use a 27-gauge needle (not a 25 gauge) into the most proximal injection point (red dot). This point is marked at least 2 cm proximal to the most proximal place you are likely to dissect.

- You can pinch loose forearm skin and push the skin into the needle to decrease pain.

- Inject the rest of the first 10 mL slowly (over 2 minutes) without moving the needle.

- Continue injecting from proximal to distal, blowing the local anesthetic slowly ahead of the needle so there is always at least 1 cm of visible or palpable local anesthetic ahead of the sharp needle tip that the patient would feel if you advanced it into "live" nerves—"Blow slow before you go."

- Reinsert the needle only into clearly vasoconstricted white skin that has functioning lidocaine and epinephrine so needle reinsertion is pain-free.

- The goal of the injection is to bathe local anesthetic 2 cm beyond wherever you think you even have a small chance of dissecting.

- We keep the total dose of infiltration less than 7 mg/kg. If you need less than 50 mL to produce tumescent local anesthesia (see Chapter 4), use buffered 1% lidocaine with 1:100,000 epinephrine. If you want 50 to 100 mL of volume to inject, dilute with saline solution to a concentration of 0.5% lidocaine with 1:200,000 epinephrine. If you need 100 to 200 mL of volume for larger forearm transfers, dilute buffered 50 mL of commercially available 1% lidocaine with 1:100,000 epinephrine with 150 mL of saline solution to produce 200 mL of 0.25% lidocaine with 1:400,000 epinephrine, which is clinically very effective both for local anesthesia and for vasoconstriction.

- To inject local anesthesia for finger pulley reconstruction, the process is the same as in Chapter 19.

- You can inject large areas faster with blunt-tipped cannulas but still pain-free. See ▸ Video 24.5 for a video clip of cannula injection of tumescent local anesthetic for a tendon transfer of flexor carpi ulnaris (FCU) to extensor carpi radialis longus (ECRL). Cannula injection of local anesthetic was also used in ▸ Video 25.3.

TIPS AND TRICKS FOR PERFORMING TENDON GRAFTS AND PULLEY RECONSTRUCTION WITH WIDE AWAKE APPROACH

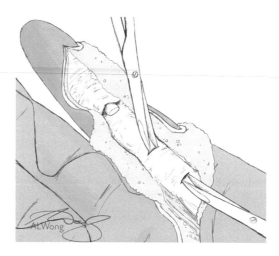

Fig. 25.1 Instead of two-stage Hunter implant (rod) tendon graft reconstruction, dig out the A2 pulley from the scar. Get on the bone and under where the A2 pulley still exists in the scar cocoon and with small spreads of fine blunt-tipped scissors (Steven's tenotomy scissors). You can dig out the tunnel that will easily accommodate the flexor digitorum superficialis (FDS) tendon graft as was done in Video 25.1 and Video 25.4.

Video 25.4
Original A2 pulley use for tendon graft 10 months after injury (amputation and replantation). Flexor digitorum superficialis (FDS) of long became the motor of flexor digitorum profundus (FDP) index via tendon graft (Chen, China).

- Dig the A2 pulley out of scar for primary tendon grafting instead of two-stage Hunter implant (rod) reconstruction as in ▸ Fig. 25.1 and ▸ Video 25.1 and ▸ Video 25.4.

- Patients need to look at their fingers or thumb when you ask them to test the transfer, since they cannot feel the numbed digits. You need to take sheet barriers down so they can see their numbed fingers or wrist moving. Although most patients do not mind looking at the wound, you can cover the wound with a towel as they watch their fingers and thumb move.

- If you want the thumb extensor pollicis longus (EPL) to relax, ask the patient to flex the thumb interphalangeal (IP) joint. The spinal cord reflex will force the EPL to relax. Asking patients to flex will relax extensors. Asking patients to extend will relax flexors.

- Most patients are simply able to move their tendon grafts without thinking about it. The brain can do it automatically in many cases, and they just don't need to "learn" it. However, some are not able to do it right away. For example, you may need to ask them to flex the ring finger to flex the thumb if you have transferred FDS3 to FPL and they can't easily activate it. After a couple of tries, they are usually able to do it almost right away.

- What you see on the table with intraoperative tendon graft tension testing is what you will get as a result. If the graft looks too loose, it will be too loose postoperatively. If it looks too tight, it will be too tight postoperatively.

- Use two "temporary" sutures to set your tension where you think it should be. Then have the patient test it to see if you got the tension right. If you only have one suture there, the patient may well rupture it. If the tension looks good, go ahead and do a Pulvertaft or some other weave. If it is too loose, add sutures to make it tighter. If it is too tight, insert sutures where you think they should be, then cut the first sutures that were too tight and test again.

- Do not be afraid to test full flexion and full extension. Your sutures should be strong enough to take it. If they are not, you need to reinforce them.

- We have patients relieve themselves in the restroom after we inject the local anesthetic and just before we start the surgery to avoid unnecessary surgical interruptions for these longer cases. Patients do not receive an intravenous fluid that increases the urge to void. If we give preoperative antibiotics, we give them by mouth.

- For older patients with cardiac comorbidities, you can decrease the concentration of epinephrine and perform the WALANT procedure in the hospital main operating room with monitoring.

- Many patients are interested in looking at the tendon to understand the nature of their problem. You can mask them, show them the tendon, and have them watch it move. It will help greatly that they see the transfer move, because they know that it will work after they overcome the pain and stiffness.

- In ▶ Video 25.5, we reconstructed the extensor retinacular pulley only to find that it downgraded finger extension so the pulley was abandoned and the patient ended up with better movement with a little bowstringing. This procedure was performed while Dr Alistair Phillips and Dr Nikolas Alan Jagodzinski were visiting Dr Lalonde in Canada.

Video 25.5
Extensor tendon graft reconstruction with attempted and abandoned retinacular pulley reconstruction (Lalonde, Canada).

Video 25.6
Lacerated extensor tendon defect measured with active movement with suture spanning gap replaced with primary palmaris longus (PL) tendon graft over metacarpophalangeal (MP) joint (Chen, China).

- In ▶ Video 25.6, Chao Chen from China has a gap of extensor tendon. He places a temporary suture to bridge the gap while watching a full range of active movement. He now has measured this gap and replaces that with a palmaris longus tendon graft.

- In ▶ Video 19.9 Egemen Ayhan from Turkey demonstrates pulley reconstruction at the time of flexor tendon repair.

Video 25.7 Extensor tendon reconstruction with palmaris longus (PL) tendon graft anchored to sagittal band so it can become effective with active intraoperative movement (Lalonde, Canada).

Video 25.8 A2 pulley reconstruction with extensor retinaculum in a mountain climber (Apard, France).

Video 25.9 Pulley reconstruction (Rafiqi, Morocco).

Video 25.10 Tendon graft and subsequent tenolysis with demonstration of local anesthesia with patient on chronic oxygen (Maxwell and Lalonde, Canada).

THERAPY TIPS AFTER TENDON GRAFTING AND PULLEY RECONSTRUCTION

- Like in flexor tendon repair, eliminating any gap and seeing stability of pulley reconstruction with full-fist flexion and extension testing during the surgery gives us the confidence to move away from full-fist place and hold to true active movement as advocated by Tang,[11] Higgins,[12] and Lalonde[13] (see Chapter 19).

Video 25.TT1
Early protected movement after tendon graft (Ayhan, Turkey).

References

1. Lalonde DH. Wide-awake extensor indicis proprius to extensor pollicis longus tendon transfer. J Hand Surg Am 2014;39(11):2297–2299
2. Bezuhly M, Sparkes GL, Higgins A, Neumeister MW, Lalonde DH. Immediate thumb extension following extensor indicis proprius-to-extensor pollicis longus tendon transfer using the wide-awake approach. Plast Reconstr Surg 2007;119(5):1507–1512
3. Tang JB. Wide-awake primary flexor tendon repair, tenolysis, and tendon transfer. Clin Orthop Surg 2015;7(3):275–281
4. Gao LL, Chang J. Wide awake secondary tendon reconstruction. Hand Clin 2019;35(1):35–41
5. Hong JJ, Kang HJ, Whang JI, et al. Comparison of the wide-awake approach and conventional approach in extensor indicis proprius-to-extensor pollicis longus tendon transfer for chronic extensor pollicis longus rupture. Plast Reconstr Surg 2020;145(3):723–733
6. Mohammed AK, Lalonde DH. Wide awake tendon transfers in leprosy patients in India. Hand Clin 2019;35(1):67–84
7. Lalonde D. Discussion: comparison of the wide-awake approach and conventional approach in extensor indicis proprius-to-extensor pollicis longus tendon transfer for chronic extensor pollicis longus rupture. Plast Reconstr Surg 2020;145(3):734–735
8. Zukawa M, Osada R, Makino H, Kimura T. Wide-awake flexor pollicis longus tendon reconstruction with evaluation of the active voluntary contraction of the ruptured muscle-tendon. Plast Reconstr Surg 2019;143(1):176–180
9. Lalonde DH, Wong A. Dosage of local anesthesia in wide awake hand surgery. J Hand Surg Am 2013;38(10):2025–2028
10. McKee DE, Lalonde DH, Thoma A, Glennie DL, Hayward JE. Optimal time delay between epinephrine injection and incision to minimize bleeding. Plast Reconstr Surg 2013;131(4):811–814
11. Tang JB, Zhou X, Pan ZJ, Qing J, Gong KT, Chen J. Strong digital flexor tendon repair, extension-flexion test, and early active flexion: experience in 300 tendons. Hand Clin 2017;33(3):455–463
12. Higgins A, Lalonde DH. Flexor tendon repair postoperative rehabilitation: the Saint John Protocol. Plast Reconstr Surg Glob Open 2016;4(11):e1134
13. Meals C, Lalonde D, Candelier G. Repaired flexor tendon excursion with half a fist of true active movement versus full fist place and hold in the awake patient. Plast Reconstr Surg Glob Open 2019;7(4):e2074

CHAPTER 26

CARPAL TUNNEL DECOMPRESSION OF THE MEDIAN NERVE

Donald H. Lalonde, Andrew W. Gurman, Xavier Gueffier, Shu Guo Xing, Jin Bo Tang, Amir Adham Ahmad, and Thomas Apard

ADVANTAGES OF WALANT VERSUS SEDATION AND TOURNIQUET IN CARPAL TUNNEL DECOMPRESSION

- All of the general advantages listed in Chapter 2 apply to both the surgeon and the patient (no nausea, no tourniquet pain or let-down bleeding, decreased cost without sedation in minor procedure room, safer surgery without sedation, etc.). The world is shifting to pure local anesthesia for carpal tunnel surgery.[18,21,22,23,24]

- Patients who have had bilateral carpal tunnel surgery overwhelmingly prefer their WALANT hand compared with their intravenous (IV) regional anesthesia hand.[11] Patients love the simplicity of WALANT carpal tunnel release for many reasons (▶ Video 2.3).

- When you perform wide awake hand surgery, you do not have to deal with your patient's medical comorbidities, which would only be a problem if you sedate patients. It is safer for your patients to have no sedation. They just get up and go home after surgery, like when they have had a filling at the dentist.

- A major advantage of ending sedation for carpal tunnel surgery is that you do not need to perform the procedures in the main operating room. You can do all of your carpal tunnel surgeries in minor treatment rooms in the clinic outside the main operating room with evidence-based field sterility (see Chapter 10).

- You can easily perform 15 or more carpal tunnel releases in 1 day with only one nurse using field sterility in the office or clinic. You can also see consultation and recheck patients between operations (see Chapter 14).

- You avoid tourniquet let-down bleeding and other tourniquet complications. A 2020 systematic review and meta-analysis[15] and prospective randomized controlled trial[16] and other studies[20] have shown more pain but no significant clinical benefit with using a tourniquet compared to WALANT. Adding epinephrine does decrease surgical time if no tourniquet is used.[17]

- You do not need to use a cautery, particularly if you inject the epinephrine 30 minutes before the first incision. We have not opened a cautery for over 25 years for carpal tunnel release. Hematoma has not been a problem, even in patients on anticoagulants.

- Your patient remains pain-free with the median and ulnar nerve block for up to 5 hours using the technique described below.[1] Most do not need narcotics, especially after good perioperative teaching on how to take pain medicine.[10]

Video 26.1
Patient's impressions of carpal tunnel surgery at the end of the operation
(also see ▶ Video 2.3) (Lalonde, Canada).

- Although patients can "tolerate" 7 minutes of tourniquet control, they hate it. (see surgeon's impression of having a tourniquet on his own arm in ▶ Video 2.4). They will not experience any tourniquet pain at all if you simply use epinephrine with the lidocaine. There is high-level published evidence that the tourniquet hurts twice as much as the injection of a local anesthetic in carpal tunnel surgery.[2,3] Patients appreciate the tourniquet-free experience.

- Patients may be able to drive themselves home after WALANT carpal tunnel release.[12]

- WALANT carpal tunnel surgery is much less expensive than traditional tourniquet surgery with sedation and therefore actually available in developing countries.[13,14,19]

- You can educate your patient during pain-free injection of local anesthesia to decrease the risks of postoperative complications and narcotic use (see ▶ Video 14.1 and ▶ Video 14.2).

- Clearly these advantages are evident to most surgeons now because in a recent survey of the American Society for Surgery of the Hand members published in *Journal of Hand Surgery Global Online* in June 2020, only 14% of 869 members who responded to the survey did not offer WALANT to their carpal tunnel patients.[18]

WHERE TO INJECT THE LOCAL ANESTHETIC FOR AN OPEN CARPAL TUNNEL RELEASE

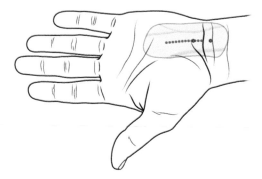

Fig. 26.1 For carpal tunnel release, 20 mL of 1% lidocaine with 1:100,000 epinephrine (buffered with 10 mL lido/epi:1 mL of 8.4% sodium bicarbonate) is injected.

SPECIFICS OF MINIMALLY PAINFUL INJECTION OF LOCAL ANESTHETIC IN OPEN CARPAL TUNNEL RELEASE

- Local anesthesia injection should barely hurt at all if you follow the simple rules of Chapter 5 for hints to minimize injection pain. The patients will think you are magical.

- Also see ▶ Video 14.1 and ▶ Video 4.2 for patient education during local anesthesia injection during carpal tunnel surgery.

- We inject the anesthetic solution a minimum of 30 minutes before surgery to allow the epinephrine to take optimal effect and provide an adequately dry working field.[4]

- We inject supine patients lying down on stretchers in a waiting area to decrease the risk of their fainting (see ▶ Video 6.1).

- To minimize the pain of injection, use a fine 27-gauge needle (not a 25 gauge) into the most proximal red dot injection point.

- Ask the patient to look away. Press with a fingertip very firmly just proximal to the injection site before you put in the needle to add the sensory "noise" of touch and pressure to decrease the pain. Ask them to take a deep breath and do not move as you insert the needle.

- Insert the first needle perpendicularly into the subcutaneous fat. Stabilize the syringe with two hands and have your thumb ready on the plunger to avoid the pain from needle wobble until the skin needle site is numb. Inject the first visible 0.5-mL bleb and then pause. Ask the patient to tell you when the needle pain is all gone. After he or she tells you the pain is gone, inject the rest of the first 10 mL slowly (over 2 minutes) without moving the needle.

- Ask the patient to tell you if he or she feels further episodes of pain during the injection so you can score your injection technique, as outlined in Chapter 5. If the patient feels pain twice, you score an eagle, three times a birdie, four times a bogie, and so on. It takes 5 minutes to perform the injection for a carpal tunnel release and consistently get a hole-in-one, where the patient feels only the stick of the first 27-gauge needle in the injection process.[5,6,7]

- Inject 10 mL of buffered 1% lidocaine with 1:100,000 epinephrine just ulnar to palmaris longus at the proximal injection point, as shown in the Fig. 26.1. This should be near the median nerve, but *never in the nerve*. Do not elicit paresthesias (electric shock feeling).

- The first 2 mL is injected just subcutaneous in the fat. Notice the location of small subcutaneous veins and avoid them.

- Advance slowly and more deeply to get under superficial fascia of the forearm to inject the remaining 8 mL for the median nerve block. This will also numb the ulnar nerve. If you are not under the forearm fascia, you may not block the nerve.

- After the initial 10 mL, come back to the subcutaneous plane with the needle tip and slowly infiltrate the second 10 mL from proximal to distal in an antegrade direction down the palm between the skin and the

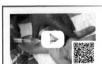

Video 26.2 Hole-in-one injection of local anesthesia for carpal tunnel surgery while teaching patients about postoperative management (Lalonde, Canada).

Video 26.3 Eagle score with injection because he did not reinsert in an area clearly numbed. Score yourself each time you inject (see Chapter 5) (Lalonde, Canada).

Video 26.4 Injecting the local anesthetic or operating with the hand above the head is sometimes more comfortable. Always ask patients how their shoulder/elbow position feels to make them comfortable. You can also inject local anesthetic and operate with patient on their side (Lalonde, Canada).

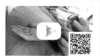

Video 26.5 Blunt-tipped cannula injection of local anesthetic for carpal tunnel surgery (Lalonde, Canada).

superficial palmar fascia. Blow the local anesthetic slowly ahead of the needle so there is always at least 1 cm of visible or palpable local anesthetic ahead of the sharp needle tip that the patient would feel if you advanced it into "live" nerves. Follow the rule of "Blow slow before you go." (See Chapter 5 for further tips on how to inject local anesthetic with minimal pain.)

- When reinserting the needle, do so into skin that is within 1 cm of clearly vasoconstricted white skin that has functioning lidocaine and epinephrine so the needle reinsertion is pain-free.

- To avoid all pain in suturing the wound, be sure to have visible or palpable local anesthetic at least 1 cm on either side and 1 cm past the distal end of the palmar incision.

- Some surgeons think that 10 mL is an unnecessarily large volume for the median nerve block. Dalhousie New Brunswick medical students had bilateral median nerve blocks with 5 mL on one side and 10 mL on the other side. There were clearly more median nerve block failures in the 5-mL group than the 10-mL group.[8]

- In some patients, the forearm fascia acts as a barrier to local anesthesia diffusion. If you only inject subcutaneously in the wrist, and do not have the needle under the forearm fascia, you may not get a median nerve block as the local anesthetic may not penetrate the forearm fascia.

- Some people only inject under the skin with no intention of getting a median nerve block, and routinely successfully do carpal tunnel surgery under local anesthetic this way. This works well. However, a possible disadvantage of this approach is that patients with "live" median nerves sometimes feel "electric jolts" when the nerve is touched during the surgery.

- When you perform wide awake carpal and cubital tunnel at the same time, or carpal tunnel with lacertus tunnel (see Chapter 28) releases at the same time, simply decrease the concentration of the local anesthetic to 0.5% lidocaine with 1:200,000 epinephrine. See Chapter 30 for doing multiple nerves at the same time.

- You can also inject with a blunt-tipped cannula to increase the speed of painless injection compared with sharp needle tip injection (also see Chapter 5). The blunt needle tip can push quickly with no pain past "live" unanesthetized nerves by gliding in the fat. Sharp needle tips will pierce nerves and cause pain if the local anesthetic is not bathing the nerve well ahead of the needle tip and if the operator is not moving slowly enough to let the local anesthetic work before the needle tip reaches the nerves.

- A blunt-tipped, 37-mm-long, 27-gauge cannula into a needle hole created in numbed skin with a 25-gauge needle works well in the subcutaneous fat over the carpal tunnel.

WHERE TO INJECT THE LOCAL ANESTHETIC FOR AN ENDOSCOPIC CARPAL TUNNEL RELEASE

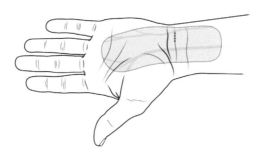

Fig. 26.2 For an endoscopic carpal tunnel release procedure, inject 20 to 25 mL of 1% lidocaine with 1:100,000 epinephrine (buffered with 10 mL lido/epi:1 mL of 8.4% sodium bicarbonate).

SPECIFICS OF MINIMALLY PAINFUL INJECTION OF LOCAL ANESTHETIC IN ENDOSCOPIC CARPAL TUNNEL RELEASE

- Gurman's technique: The anesthesia is the same as for open techniques, i.e., two 10-mL syringes of 1% lidocaine with epinephrine (1:100,000) and sodium bicarbonate.

- Inject 5 mL infiltrated subcutaneously in the distal forearm, extending proximally from the wrist crease.

- The second 5 mL goes under the forearm fascia in the distal forearm, near the median nerve. NEVER elicit paresthesias of the median nerve because you may damage the nerve with the sharp tip of the needle. You can inject near it but not in it.

- Inject the last 10 mL into the palm. Wait at least for 30 minutes.

- Dr Gurman feels that the tenosynovium is less juicy this way than when he uses general anesthesia and a tourniquet, and that his visualization is better.

- Use cotton-tipped applicators to soak up any blood or excess fluid from the local.

- You could apply a regular arm tourniquet for your first case or two, but do not inflate it. You won't need it, but you may be more relaxed knowing that it is there.

- Dr Gurman has more tips. The occasional patient will have pain as he passes the trocar under the transverse carpal ligament or when he makes the incision for the distal portal. The distal portal is easy; you

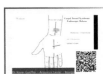

Video 26.6 How to inject local anesthesia and perform endoscopic carpal tunnel release (Gueffier, France).

Video 26.7 How to inject local anesthesia for endoscopic carpal tunnel release (Gurman, USA).

just inject a little more local in the skin. For the deep pain, it is also rather easy. He stops as soon as the patient complains of pain, and he withdraws the trocar, leaving the cannula in place. He then injects about 3 to 4 mL of local using an IV catheter attached to the end of a syringe. He then withdraws the cannula, leaving the catheter in the palm. You are already in the deep palmar space, at the point of pain, and the anesthetic will flow freely. There is no risk to the nerve or tendons from a needle since the angiocath is a blunt, flexible plastic tube. You can reinsert in a couple of minutes, and the patient will be fine.

- Always inject from proximal to distal so that it hurts less as described in Chapter 5.

- The injection takes longer than the procedure, but the patients are amazed at how little pain they feel when you do it this way.

TIPS AND TRICKS FOR PERFORMING OPEN CARPAL TUNNEL PROCEDURES WITH THE WIDE AWAKE APPROACH

Video 26.8 Typical patient education advice during surgery or bandage application to decrease complications (Lalonde, Canada).

- Managing patient expectations of WALANT carpal tunnel surgery begins with a calm, matter-of-fact approach about WALANT during the consultation as in ▶ Video 7.1. Make it sound as simple as going to the dentist for a filling, but easier because no one is working in their mouth.

- Educating the patient on postoperative activities during the injection (▶ Video 26.2), the surgery, and the bandage application (▶ Video 26.7) will greatly decrease the risk zof complications. These 10 to 15 minutes of time invested in the patient is a much more effective use of the surgeon's time than talking to the nurses about the weather (see Chapter 8).

Video 26.9 Buried simple interrupted absorbable Monocryl sutures you do not need to remove are much more comfortable and convenient for patients and surgeons (Lalonde, Canada).

- One of the best things that Dr Lalonde did in carpal tunnel surgery was to abandon transcutaneous nylon sutures about 20 years ago. He only uses simple interrupted buried dermal Monocryl absorbable 5-0 sutures as demonstrated in ▶ Video 26.9. Transcutaneous nylon has been shown to cause more infections in palmar closure than buried Monocryl.[9]

- Inject two to four patients with local anesthetic outside the operating room before operating on the first one. This will give at least half an hour for the local anesthetic to work on these waiting patients, both for lidocaine numbing and for epinephrine vasoconstriction. It takes 26 minutes to achieve peak vasoconstriction in humans after 1:100,000 epinephrine injection (level I evidence).[4]

- After you inject the first patient, he or she will usually feel well enough to go sit in the waiting area with the injected hand raised until the surgery. You can then inject the second patient, then the third one. Then you can perform the surgery on the first one. While the nurse turns over the room and brings in the second patient after the first procedure, you are injecting the fourth patient. No surgeon time is lost in turnover. One surgeon and one nurse can comfortably perform 15 carpal tunnels with field sterility in an 8-hour working day (see Chapter 14).

- In Canada, almost all carpal tunnel procedures are performed with field sterility in the manner shown in ▶ Video 26.12. The cost is much less with much less garbage production. The patient's convenience and satisfaction are much higher with field sterility outside the main operating room than with full sterility in the main operating room (see Chapter 10).

- Field sterility permits one hand surgeon and one nurse to perform 15 or more carpal tunnel procedures per day at a very leisurely pace (see Chapter 14).

- Get your assistant to pull very firmly on the Senn retractors to decrease the little bleeding that sometimes occurs, especially if the patient is hypertensive or receiving anticoagulants.

- There is no need to stop anticoagulation for carpal tunnel surgery with WALANT.

- *Never cut or suture where the skin is not white.* If there are no epinephrine molecules there causing vasoconstriction, there will likely not be any lidocaine molecules there either.

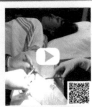

Video 26.10
Surgery from start to finish including intraoperative advice (Lalonde, Canada).

Video 26.11
Narrated description of open carpal tunnel surgery technique (Lalonde, Canada).

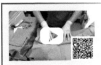

Video 26.12 Sterile setup for typical Canadian carpal tunnel release in minor procedure room outside the main operating room (Lalonde, Canada).

Video 26.13
Intraoperative advice on how to take pain medicine and follow pain-guided healing. Advising the patient after injection of local anesthetic for carpal tunnel release (Lalonde, Canada).

Video 26.14
See the median nerve gliding with active movement. Advising the patient after injection of local anesthetic for carpal tunnel release (Ahmad, Malaysia).

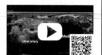

Video 26.15
Ultrasound-guided carpal tunnel release (Apard, France).

- Offer patients a guided tour of their carpal tunnel surgery. Many will accept and be delighted that they were given the opportunity to experience seeing the inside of their hand.

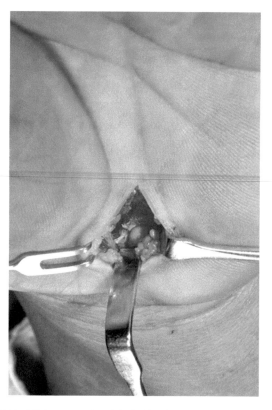

Fig. 26.3 With WALANT, visibility is good with little bleeding, even with a 2 to 3 cm incision (Shu Guo Xing and Jin Bo Tang).

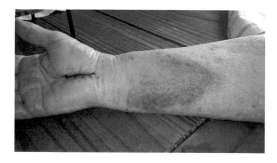

Fig. 26.4 Early bruising seen the day after surgery with 10 mL of local anesthetic injected in the wrist which can appear red and may make patients think they have an infection. This is not an infection. There is no heat or fever. It resolves in time and without treatment.

- For more in-depth learning about ultrasound in hand surgery and carpal tunnel release, see Chapter 49 and Chapter 50.

TIPS AND TRICKS FOR PERFORMING ENDOSCOPIC CARPAL TUNNEL SURGERY WITH THE WIDE AWAKE APPROACH

- To see Xavier Gueffier's surgery video of endoscopic carpal tunnel, see ▶ Video 26.6.

- Waiting at least 30 minutes between injection and surgery is even more important in endoscopic surgery. This is important to minimize bleeding into the endoscopic field.

- You can clear vision-obstructing fluid from the endoscopy port with a cotton-tipped swab if necessary.

- The greatest bleeding problems come from the incision site if you cut a superficial vein, which can then ooze into the wound and even into the endoscope device when you introduce it. Being cautious to avoid those superficial bleeders is extremely helpful to obviate that problem. The transverse carpal ligament itself is very avascular, and there will not be many problems with bleeding from the ligament itself.

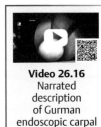

Video 26.16
Narrated description of Gurman endoscopic carpal tunnel surgery.

References

1. Chandran GJ, Chung B, Lalonde J, Lalonde DH. The hyperthermic effect of a distal volar forearm nerve block: a possible treatment of acute digital frostbite injuries? Plast Reconstr Surg 2010;126(3):946–950

2. Braithwaite BD, Robinson GJ, Burge PD. Haemostasis during carpal tunnel release under local anaesthesia: a controlled comparison of a tourniquet and adrenaline infiltration. J Hand Surg [Br] 1993;18(2):184–186

3. Ralte P, Selvan D, Morapudi S, Kumar G, Waseem M. Haemostasis in open carpal tunnel release: tourniquet vs local anaesthetic and adrenaline. Open Orthop J 2010;4:234–236

4. McKee DE, Lalonde DH, Thoma A, Glennie DL, Hayward JE. Optimal time delay between epinephrine injection and incision to minimize bleeding. Plast Reconstr Surg 2013;131(4):811–814

5. Lalonde D, Wong A. Local anesthetics: what's new in minimal pain injection and best evidence in pain control. Plast Reconstr Surg 2014; 134(4, Suppl 2):40S–49S

6. Lalonde DH. "Hole-in-one" local anesthesia for wide-awake carpal tunnel surgery. Plast Reconstr Surg 2010;126(5):1642–1644

7. Farhangkhoee H, Lalonde J, Lalonde DH. Teaching medical students and residents how to inject local anesthesia almost painlessly. Can J Plast Surg 2012;20(3):169–172

8. Lovely LM, Chishti YZ, Woodland JL, Lalonde DH. How much volume of local anesthesia and how long should you wait after injection for an effective wrist median nerve block? Hand (N Y) 2018;13(3):281–284

9. Rochlin DH, Sheckter CC, Curtin CM. Which stitch? Replacing anecdote with evidence in minor hand surgery. Plast Reconstr Surg Glob Open 2019;7(4):e2189

10. Alter TH, Ilyas AM. A prospective randomized study analyzing preoperative opioid counseling in pain management after carpal tunnel release surgery. J Hand Surg Am 2017;42(10):810–815

11. Ayhan E, Akaslan F. Patients' perspective on carpal tunnel release with WALANT or intravenous regional anesthesia. Plast Reconstr Surg 2020;145(5):1197–1203

12. Thompson Orfield NJ, Badger AE, Tegge AN, Davoodi M, Perez MA, Apel PJ. Modeled wide-awake, local-anesthetic, no-tourniquet surgical procedures do not impair driving fitness: an experimental on-road noninferiority study. J Bone Joint Surg Am 2020;102(18):1616–1622

13. Alter TH, Warrender WJ, Liss FE, Ilyas AM. A cost analysis of carpal tunnel release surgery performed wide awake versus under sedation. Plast Reconstr Surg 2018;142(6):1532–1538

14. Gabrielli AS, Lesiak AC, Fowler JR. The direct and indirect costs to society of carpal tunnel release. Hand (N Y) 2020;15(2):NP1–NP5

15. Olaiya OR, Alagabi AM, Mbuagbaw L, McRae MH. Carpal tunnel release without a tourniquet: a systematic review and meta-analysis. Plast Reconstr Surg 2020;145(3):737–744

16. Iqbal HJ, Doorgakant A, Rehmatullah NNT, Ramavath AL, Pidikiti P, Lipscombe S. Pain and outcomes of carpal tunnel release under local anaesthetic with or without a tourniquet: a randomized controlled trial. J Hand Surg Eur Vol 2018;43(8):808–812

17. Sraj S. Carpal tunnel release with wide awake local anesthesia and no tourniquet: with versus without epinephrine. Hand (N Y) 2019;1558944719890038. [published online ahead of print, December 7, 2019] doi: 10.1177/1558944719890038

18. Grandizio LC, Graham J, Klena JC, Current trends in WALANT surgery: a survey of American Society for Surgery of the Hand members. Journal of Hand Surgery Global Online 2020;2(4):186–190

19. Castro Magtoto IJ, Alagar DL. Wide awake local anesthesia no tourniquet: a pilot study for carpal tunnel release in the Philippine orthopedic center. J Hand Surg Asian Pac Vol 2019;24(4):389–391

20. Kang SW, Park HM, Park JK, et al. Open cubital and carpal tunnel release using wide-awake technique: reduction of postoperative pain. J Pain Res 2019;12:2725–2731

21. Munns JJ, Awan HM. Trends in carpal tunnel surgery: an online survey of members of the American Society for Surgery of the Hand. J Hand Surg Am 2015;40(4):767–71.e2

22. Peters B, Giuffre JL. Canadian trends in carpal tunnel surgery. J Hand Surg Am 2018;43(11):1035.e1–1035.e8

23. Gunasagaran J, Sean ES, Shivdas S, Amir S, Ahmad TS. Perceived comfort during minor hnd surgeries with wide awake local anaesthesia no tourniquet (WALANT) versus local anaesthesia (LA)/tourniquet. J Orthop Surg (Hong Kong) 2017;25(3):2309499017739499

24. Far-Riera AM, Pérez-Uribarri C, Sánchez Jiménez M, Esteras Serrano MJ, Rapariz González JM, Ruiz Hernández IM. Estudio prospectivo sobre la aplicación de un circuito WALANT para la cirugía del síndrome del túnel carpiano y dedo en resorte [Prospective study on the application of a WALANT circuit for surgery of tunnel carpal syndrome and trigger finger]. Rev Esp Cir Ortop Traumatol 2019;63(6):400–407

CHAPTER 27

CUBITAL TUNNEL DECOMPRESSION OF THE ULNAR NERVE

*Donald H. Lalonde, Alistair Phillips,
Thomas Apard, and Amir Adham Ahmad*

ADVANTAGES OF WALANT VERSUS SEDATION AND TOURNIQUET IN CUBITAL TUNNEL DECOMPRESSION SURGERY

- All of the general advantages listed in Chapter 2 apply to both the surgeon and the patient (no nausea, no tourniquet pain or let-down bleeding, decreased cost without sedation in minor procedure room, safer surgery without sedation, etc.).

- Positioning patients with their elbow above their head is much easier for your access as the surgeon. The anesthesiologist and his or her equipment will not be occupying your valuable surgical access space.

- Patients can position themselves comfortably, so the elbow and the shoulder are not sore during the surgery. They can have the surgery by easily lying on their side (▶ Fig. 27.3) or on their abdomen for prone surgery with their arm on an arm board (▶ Video 27.1) or at their side (▶ Video 30.4). This is simple and can be much more comfortable in the awake patients. They do not wake up from general anesthesia with shoulder pain that we caused by putting their shoulder in a position it does not like.

- There is no tourniquet, so you have much easier access to the proximal incision.

- You can see whether the ulnar nerve subluxates with active movement by watching patients actively flex and extend the elbow through a full range of motion before you close the skin. If the nerve subluxates, you can transpose it if required.

- You and your patient may see return of M5 power in ring and small finger flexor digitorum profundus (FDP) during the surgery after cubital tunnel release if you examine for it (see ▶ Video 27.5).

Video 27.1 Prone position can be much more comfortable for patients (Apard, France).

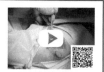

Video 27.2 Checking active movement to verify that subluxation is stopped after transposition and 5-0 Vicryl suspension of epineurium for chronic painful subluxation (Lalonde, Canada).

- There is some evidence that there is less pain in patients who have had cubital tunnel release with WALANT as opposed to sedative anesthesia with a tourniquet.[1]

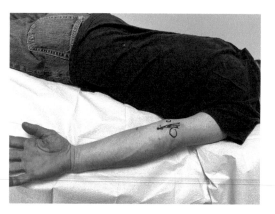

Fig. 27.1 Prone position for cubital tunnel release can be very comfortable for patients who like to sleep on their abdomen, and is very simple in the unsedated patient.

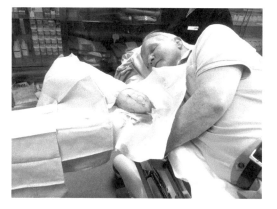

Fig. 27.2 This patient with a stiff elbow and a sore shoulder has been placed in a comfortable position for a cubital tunnel release with field sterility. We negotiated different positions until he found this one worked best to accommodate his stiff elbow and sore shoulder from old injuries.

- You can decrease costs and garbage from unnecessary full operating room sterility by performing cubital tunnel decompression with field sterility or augmented field sterility in minor procedure rooms or in the office (see Chapter 10 and ▶ Fig. 27.3).

WHERE TO INJECT THE LOCAL ANESTHETIC FOR CUBITAL TUNNEL DECOMPRESSION

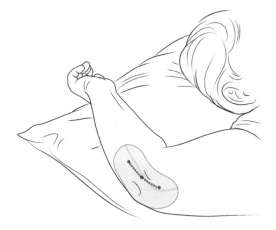

Fig. 27.3 Inject 60 mL of 0.5% lidocaine with 1:200,000 epinephrine buffered with 3 mL of 8.4% sodium bicarbonate for a ratio of 10 mL lido/epi:1 mL of 8.4% sodium bicarbonate.

SPECIFICS OF MINIMALLY PAINFUL INJECTION OF LOCAL ANESTHETIC FOR CUBITAL TUNNEL DECOMPRESSION

- Local anesthesia injection should barely hurt at all if you follow the simple rules of Chapter 5 for hints to minimize injection pain. The patients will think you are magical.

- Mix 30 mL of 1% lidocaine with 3 mL of 8.4% bicarbonate into a 50-mL bag of saline solution that contains only 30 mL. (You remove 20 mL from the 50-mL bag before adding the lidocaine.) This gives you 63 mL of 0.5% lidocaine with 1:200,000 epinephrine buffered 10:1 with 8.4% sodium bicarbonate.

- Inject 20 mL subcutaneously in the most proximal part of the incision, followed by 20 mL in the middle of the incision, and then 20 mL at the end of the incision.

- You can start with a 10-mL syringe and a 27-gauge needle to decrease pain. You can then switch to a 20-mL syringe with a short 25-gauge needle for the next injections for a little more speed, being careful to not inject too fast.

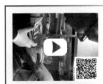

Video 27.3 How to inject local anesthesia for cubital tunnel release (Lalonde, Canada).

- You don't need to move the needle much and will likely hurt less if you just inject subcutaneously with the needle in one place letting the local anesthesia find its way.

- Do not try to get into the cubital tunnel with the needle tip. You may injure the nerve and it is not necessary to go there.

- The nerve may not be anesthetized but if you are gentle and do not manipulate the nerve, there will be no pain. Just decompressing the nerve is all you have to do.

- Inject the anesthetic solution a minimum of 30 minutes before surgery to allow the epinephrine to take optimal effect and provide an adequately dry working field.

- We inject supine patients on stretchers in a waiting area to decrease the risk of their fainting.

- If you want to perform endoscopic cubital tunnel decompression that goes farther distally in the forearm, you can inject another 20 mL or more distally in the forearm so that you have at least 2 cm of palpable or visible local anesthetic beyond your area of dissection.

- For those who prefer anterior transposition, the soft tissue in the new nerve path will need to be more extensively flooded with another 20 mL of local anesthetic.

- We have not worked out the technique for submuscular transposition at this time, since we do not do that operation. You would likely need to inject beneath the deep forearm fascia to accomplish that operation as a wide awake procedure.

TIPS AND TRICKS FOR PERFORMING CUBITAL TUNNEL DECOMPRESSION WITH THE WIDE AWAKE APPROACH

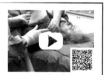

Video 27.4 Cubital tunnel surgery in a patient with a sore elbow.

Video 27.5 Testing for flexor digitorum profundus (FDP5) power return during surgery after release of the cubital tunnel (Ahmad, Malaysia).

- Ask the patients about which position is most comfortable for them to show you their cubital tunnel. Inject the local anesthetic in that position. If they are comfortable during the 5- to 10-minute injection process, they will likely be comfortable in that position for the duration of the surgery. When the patients cannot abduct the shoulder comfortably, we have done the operation easily with the patients on their back, abdomen, or side with the arm either by their side, on an arm board, or above on the head.

- The position of the arm as seen in ▶ Fig. 27.3 is a good position to see the cubital tunnel clearly during the surgery. It is Dr Lalonde's favorite position. Also see ▶ Video 30.4 for Lalonde's cubital and carpal tunnel releases in prone position in the main operating room with field sterility.

- When the elbow is flexed, the nerve is tight in the canal, and there is less space to get your scissors in to open the roof of the canal. Ask the patient to extend the elbow until that maneuver is easy, then return the arm to elbow flexion. The awake cooperative patient makes this easy.

- Whether you use four towels with field sterility or half sheets for enhanced field sterility or full sterility, apply the drapes loosely enough to allow active full elbow flexion and extension.

- We do not routinely need cautery for cubital tunnel release, because we wait at least half an hour for the epinephrine to work. An hour is even better.

- Close the skin with buried intradermal simple interrupted 5-0 Monocryl sutures as shown in detail for carpal tunnel closure in ► Video 26.9. Buried simple interrupted sutures of absorbable monofilament Monocryl mean that there are no sutures to remove.

- After cubital tunnel release, get the patient to actively flex and extend the elbow to see if the nerve is subluxating. If you feel that a subluxating nerve will be a problem for the patient, you can tack it anteriorly on the forearm fascia as in anterior transposition.

- We let them take off the outside bandage the next day and get in the shower and get wounds wet. The skin tapes airdry after the shower. They remove the skin tapes like Band-Aid at 10 days. They reapply the outside bandage for 4 to 5 days to remind them to do pain-guided healing.

- We instruct the patients to keep the hand up and quiet for the first couple of days until they are off all acetaminophen or ibuprofen, which is all they need for pain if they elevate and immobilize their hand. Once they are off all painkillers and they know what hurts, they can start to lower the hand and use it providing they do not do what hurts. This is pain-guided healing or common sense.

- Test for weakness of FDP ring and small fingers before surgery, and again during surgery after cubital tunnel release. You and your patient may see return of M5 power in ring and small finger FDP during the surgery after cubital tunnel release if you examine for it (see ► Video 27.5).

Reference

1. Kang SW, Park HM, Park JK, et al. Open cubital and carpal tunnel release using wide-awake technique: reduction of postoperative pain. J Pain Res 2019;12:2725–2731

CHAPTER 28

LACERTUS SYNDROME: MEDIAN NERVE RELEASE AT THE ELBOW

*Elisabet Hagert, Donald H. Lalonde, Egemen Ayhan,
Jean Paul Brutus, Amir Adham Ahmad, and Daniel McKee*

Lacertus syndrome is proximal compression of the median nerve at the elbow under the lacertus fibrosus (bicipital aponeurosis). You can easily release this with good results in the right patients, as described in ▶ Video 28.1. It is a simple procedure, similar to carpal tunnel release with WALANT. For many surgeons, this has replaced the more complex traditional operation of pronator syndrome surgery.

You make the diagnosis of lacertus syndrome on a clinical examination triad consisting of:

- Weakness in the flexor carpi radialis (FCR), flexor pollicis longus (FPL), and flexor digitorum profundus muscles of the index finger (FDP2)

- Pain over the median nerve at the medial edge of the lacertus fibrosus[1]

- Positive scratch collapse test over the median nerve at the elbow

▶ Video 28.2 demonstrates clinical examination of lacertus syndrome showing weakness of FCR, FDP2, FPL, tenderness under lacertus fibrosis, and positive scratch collapse test.

Video 28.1 How Don Lalonde learned about lacertus syndrome from Elisabet Hagert (Lalonde, Canada).

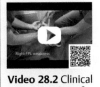

Video 28.2 Clinical examination of lacertus syndrome (Hagert, Sweden).

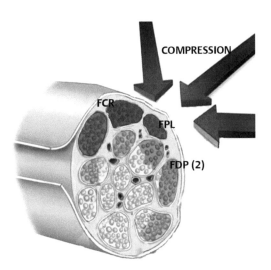

Fig. 28.1 Nerves most compressed by lacertus at the elbow. FCR, flexor carpi radialis; FDP2, digitorum profundus muscles of the index finger; FPL, flexor pollicis longus.

241

- Although less prominent than motor signs, sensory symptoms in the median nerve distribution are present in some patients, especially in the palmar cutaneous branch distribution which branches off the median nerve proximal to the wrist crease.

- Consider this diagnosis if patients complain of weakness or numbness in the palmar cutaneous distribution, or after failed carpal tunnel release.

- You will not make this diagnosis with nerve conduction studies. You make the diagnosis of lacertus syndrome through a history and a thorough physical motor examination.[2]

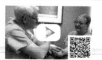

Video 28.3
Recognizing lacertus syndrome in a carpal tunnel consultation (Lalonde, Canada).

Video 28.4
Demonstrating tenderness under lacertus in the physical examination and explaining lacertus compression to carpal tunnel consultation patient from Video 28.3 (Lalonde, Canada).

Video 28.5 Explaining WALANT concurrent carpal and lacertus releases procedure to patient in Video 28.3 and Video 28.4 in the preoperative consultation (Lalonde, Canada).

ADVANTAGES OF WALANT VERSUS SEDATION AND TOURNIQUET IN MEDIAN NERVE RELEASE AT THE ELBOW

- All of the general advantages listed in Chapter 2 apply to both the surgeon and the patient (no nausea, no tourniquet pain or let-down bleeding, decreased cost without sedation in minor procedure room for simple transfers like extensor indicis [EI] to extensor pollicis longus [EPL], safer surgery without sedation, etc.).

- You can see that you have solved your patient's problem by watching him or her get the power back to his or her FPL, FDP2, and FCR on the operating table before you close the skin, as shown in ▶ Video 28.1 in this chapter.

- Your patient can see that you have solved the problem when he or she watches power return to the FPL, FDP2, and FCR on the operating table (see Video 28.14 for possible explanation).

- Your fingertip can feel the superficialis sling actively flex over the median nerve inside the wound. You ask the patient to flex the long and ring fingers and feel the effect on the superficialis sling. You can choose to divide it through a separate incision if you feel it is a problem.

WHERE TO INJECT THE LOCAL ANESTHETIC FOR LACERTUS TUNNEL RELEASE AT THE ELBOW

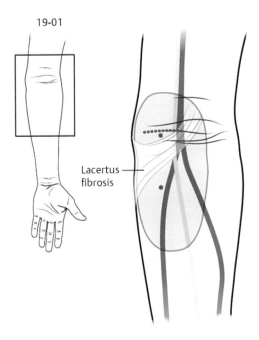

19-01

Lacertus fibrosis

Fig. 28.2 Inject at least 30 mL of 1% lidocaine with epinephrine 1:100,000 with 3 mL 8.4% sodium bicarbonate solution above and below Scarpa's superficial fascia, but superficial to the deep muscular fascia. You are not anesthetizing the median nerve. In large patients, Lalonde will inject 60 mL or more 0.5% lidocaine with 1:200,000 epinephrine.

SPECIFICS OF MINIMAL PAIN INJECTION OF LOCAL ANESTHETIC IN LACERTUS TUNNEL RELEASE AT THE ELBOW

- Local anesthesia injection should barely hurt at all if you follow the simple rules of Chapter 5 for hints to minimize injection pain. The patients will think you are magical.

- We inject the anesthetic solution a minimum of 30 minutes before surgery to allow the epinephrine to take optimal effect and provide an adequately dry working field.[2,3]

- We inject supine patients on stretchers in a waiting area to decrease the risk of their fainting (see Chapter 6).

- Inject in the fat just under the skin and under the superficial fascia from proximal to distal. There is no need to inject under the deep forearm muscle fascia. The goal is to leave the median nerve motor branches unanesthetized so you can test muscle power after you divide the lacertus.

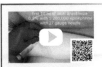

Video 28.6
Injecting the local anesthesia for lacertus syndrome (Lalonde, Canada).

- To minimize pain of injection, start with a fine 27-gauge needle (not a 25 gauge) into the most proximal injection point (red dot). Inject the first 10 mL slowly without moving the needle.

- Reinsert the needle farther distally into skin that is within 1 cm of clearly white and vasoconstricted tissue. If the epinephrine is working, so is the lidocaine. Needle reinsertion should not hurt.

- The more volume you inject, the greater the odds that no additional anesthetic will be required after you start to dissect. Try to avoid the need to "top-up" the anesthetic. The usual culprit is insufficient volume of tumescent local anesthetic.

- The anesthesia should cover the area between the medial epicondyle and biceps tendon, as well as distally past the lacertus fibrosus and the superficialis sling.

- In large patients, Lalonde will inject 60 mL or more 0.5% lidocaine with 1:200,000 epinephrine.

- Also see Chapter 30 for more videos on lacertus local anesthesia release.

TIPS AND TRICKS FOR PERFORMING LACERTUS TUNNEL RELEASE AT THE ELBOW WITH THE WIDE AWAKE APPROACH

Video 28.7
Surgical release of lacertus fibrosus (Hagert, Sweden).

- Resisted active elbow flexion during the surgery helps identify the biceps and lacertus fibrosus with your fingertip in the wound.

- In this condition, the brachial artery is frequently not palpable with a finger in the wound before you cut the thickened lacertus. After lacertus release, the brachial artery should be easily palpable from above the elbow to past the superficialis sling.

- Lift up on the skin flap with your retractor; do not push down on the muscular fascia as this can cause pain.

- Dr Lalonde likes to get down to the muscle fascia in one big spread with curved mayo scissors and do the rest of the suprafascial dissection with an army navy retractor.

- When manipulating the lacertus, warn the patient that he or she may feel pressure.

- Be careful not to manipulate the median nerve because the patient may feel unnecessary paresthesias. However, it may be helpful to warn the patient that he or she may feel a temporary pain akin to an "electrical current" out into the forearm and/or hand and that this is not dangerous. It just means that you are releasing the nerve.

- Once you have divided the lacertus fibrosus and released the median nerve, carefully let your finger slide distally and proximally over the nerve to rule out other compression points. If there is doubt as to possible entrapment of the median nerve at the superficialis sling, ask the patient to flex the ring and then the long fingers while you palpate at the level of the superficialis arcade. If you feel a constriction, consider releasing the superficialis arcade through a separate small transverse skin incision. You have already numbed this area.

• When you have adequately released the nerve, test the strength of the FPL and FDP2 to check for immediate improvement (see ▶ Video 28.6 and Video 28.7). Ask patients to look at their hand as you test the strength, so they can see the action in the thumb and index finger. You can cover the wound with a towel if they do not want to see it. Patients will be pleased to see the power of their thumb and index finger return.

• If your patient had a remote carpal tunnel release and still has numbness, test the return of sensation during the surgery as soon as you have released the lacertus. It may come back instantly during the surgery as happened to the patient in ▶ Video 28.9.

• Close the skin with buried intradermal simple interrupted 5-0 Monocryl sutures as shown in detail for carpal tunnel closure in ▶ Video 26.9. Buried simple interrupted sutures of absorbable monofilament Monocryl mean that there are no sutures to remove.

• As with all these operations, we let the patients take off the bandages and get in the shower the next day with just skin tapes on the wound. The skin tapes air dry after the shower and come off at about 10 days like a Band-Aid. They reapply the outside bandage for 4 to 5 days until they are used to pain-guided healing.

Video 28.8 A webinar lecture in 2020 providing more information on lacertus syndrome (Hagert, Sweden).

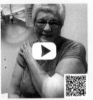

Video 28.9 Patient with remote carpal tunnel release and persistent numbness enjoyed immediate return of full sensation during the surgery as soon as we released the lacertus (Lalonde, Canada).

Video 28.10 Patient who was only able to half flex long and index fingers regained full flexion during surgery right after lacertus release (Lalonde, Canada).

Video 28.11 Patient with previous carpal tunnel release and persistent numbness and weakness experiences full return of sensation and power right after lacertus release (Lalonde, Canada).

Video 28.12 Bilateral lacertus release with power return during the surgery on both sides (Ahmad, Malaysia).

Video 28.13 Examination, surgery, and return of power (Ayhan, Turkey).

Immediate postoperative result after ... lea... elbow an... d... pic... tunnel release under V...

Video 28.14 Immediate postoperative examination showing unoperated hand weakness (Brutus, Canada).

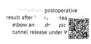

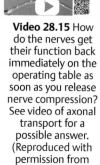

Video 28.15 How do the nerves get their function back immediately on the operating table as soon as you release nerve compression? See video of axonal transport for a possible answer. (Reproduced with permission from Dr Goshima.[4])

References

1. Hagert E. Clinical diagnosis and wide-awake surgical treatment of proximal median nerve entrapment at the elbow: a prospective study. Hand (N Y) 2013;8(1):41–46
2. Hagert CG, Hagert E. Manual muscle testing—a clinical examination technique for diagnosing focal neuropathies in the upper extremity. In: Slutsky DJ, ed. Upper Extremity Nerve Repair: Tips and Techniques. A Master Skills Publication. Rosemont, IL: American Society for Surgery of the Hand; 2008
3. McKee DE, Lalonde DH, Thoma A, Glennie DL, Hayward JE. Optimal time delay between epinephrine injection and incision to minimize bleeding. Plast Reconstr Surg 2013;131(4):811–814
4. Goshima Y, Usui H, Shiozawa T, et al. Computational analysis of the effects of antineoplastic agents on axonal transport. J Pharmacol Sci 2010;114(2):168–179

CHAPTER 29

RADIAL AND PERONEAL NERVE DECOMPRESSION

Elisabet Hagert and Donald H. Lalonde

ADVANTAGES OF WALANT VERSUS SEDATION AND TOURNIQUET IN RADIAL TUNNEL RELEASE IN THE FOREARM

- All of the general advantages listed in Chapter 2 apply to both the surgeon and the patient (no nausea, no tourniquet pain or let-down bleeding, decreased cost without sedation in minor procedure room, safer surgery without sedation, etc.).

- The greatest advantages with WALANT in radial tunnel syndrome are the ability to perform intraoperative clinical examination to check for immediate return of strength in the extensor carpi ulnaris (ECU) and the ability to have complete control over possible bleeding (▶ Video 29.4).

CLINICAL DIAGNOSIS OF RADIAL TUNNEL COMPRESSION IN THE FOREARM

- The radial tunnel syndrome is an entrapment of the posterior interosseous nerve (PIN) at the level of the proximal supinator edge, the "arcade of Frohse."

- The diagnosis is based on a clinical triad ▶ Video 29.1 which consists of:
  - Weakness in the ECU.
  - Positive scratch collapse test over the PIN at the level of the arcade of Frohse.
  - Pain over the PIN at the point of entrance under the proximal supinator edge (arcade of Frohse), located about three fingers distal to the lateral epicondyle.[1]

- Most instances of radial tunnel syndrome will not be revealed on electromyography (EMG)/neurography, but only through a thorough physical examination.[2]

- Elisabet Hagert presents a very useful lecture describing the anatomy, diagnosis, and treatment of radial tunnel syndrome in a 2020 7-minute lecture shown in ▶ Video 29.2.

Video 29.1 Clinical diagnosis of radial tunnel syndrome (Hagert, Sweden).

Video 29.2 What you should know about radial tunnel syndrome (Hagert, Sweden).

WHERE TO INJECT THE LOCAL ANESTHETIC FOR RELEASE OF THE POSTERIOR INTEROSSEOUS NERVE AT THE ARCADE OF FROHSE

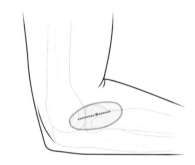

Fig 29.1 Dorsal injection for radial tunnel release.

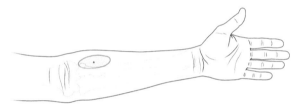

Fig. 29.2 Volar injection for radial tunnel release.

- Inject 20 to 30 mL 1% lidocaine with 1:100,000 (North America) or 1:200,000 epinephrine (Europe) with 2 to 3 mL 8.4% sodium bicarbonate over the dorsal aspect of the arcade of Frohse. The arcade of Frohse (the maximum point of tenderness on physical examination) is marked before starting anesthesia, usually about three fingerbreadths distal to the lateral epicondyle (LE). The anesthesia should cover the area from just distal to the LE and obliquely about 4 to 5 cm in a distal direction.

- Inject 10 mL buffered 1% lidocaine with 1:100,000 epinephrine over the volar aspect of the arcade of Frohse, situated just underneath the volar edge of the brachioradialis muscle in the proximal forearm.

Video 29.3
Local anesthesia injection for radial nerve release in the forearm (Hagert, Sweden).

SPECIFICS OF MINIMAL PAIN INJECTION OF RADIAL TUNNEL RELEASE IN THE FOREARM

- Local anesthesia injection should barely hurt at all if you follow the simple rules of Chapter 5 for hints to minimize injection pain. The patients will think you are magical.

- An additional 10 mL of 1% lidocaine with 1:100,000 (North America) or 1:200,000 epinephrine (Europe) should be available during surgery to add intraoperatively as the dissection is brought to the depth of the forearm and over the supinator edge (arcade of Frohse) (see ▶ Video 29.3).

- Use a total of 20 + 10 mL of lidocaine-epinephrine for a smaller arm, 30 + 10 mL in patients with more subcutaneous tissue or larger arm.

- We inject the anesthetic solution a minimum of 30 minutes before surgery to allow the epinephrine to take optimal effect and provide an adequately dry working field, as outlined in Chapter 4.

- We inject supine patients lying down on stretchers in a waiting area to decrease the risk of fainting (see Chapter 6).

TIPS AND TRICKS FOR PERFORMING RADIAL TUNNEL RELEASE IN THE FOREARM WITH THE WIDE AWAKE APPROACH

- The dissection should be carried between the extensor carpi radialis brevis and longus. This is best done using gentle finger dissection, as this will carry the approach softly to the proximal supinator edge and the arcade of Frohse. Using scissors at this stage may cause unnecessary dissection into muscle fibers, rendering the dissection more difficult.

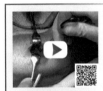

Video 29.4
Surgical release of the posterior interosseus nerve in the forearm (Hagert, Sweden).

- Always have an additional 10 mL of lidocaine-epinephrine available for direct infiltration during surgery. Once the dissection is carried beneath the extensors and to the proximal edge of the supinator, most patients will feel a deep pain that needs to be further anesthetized.

- When the PIN has been adequately released, test the strength of the ECU to check for immediate improvement (▶ Video 29.3).

- Close the skin with buried intradermal simple interrupted 5-0 Monocryl sutures as shown in detail for carpal tunnel closure in ▶ Video 26.9. Buried simple interrupted sutures of absorbable monofilament Monocryl mean that there are no sutures to remove.

SPECIFICS OF MINIMAL PAIN INJECTION OF SUPERFICIAL RADIAL RELEASE IN THE FOREARM

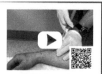

Video 29.5 Local injection for surgical release of the superficial radial nerve in the forearm for Wartenberg's syndrome (Lalonde, Canada).

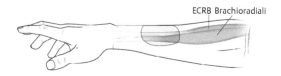

Fig. 29.3 Superficial radial nerve release injection. ECRB, extensor carpi radialis brevis.

- Inject 15 to 25 mL local anesthesia for superficial radial nerve in the forearm for Wartenberg's syndrome in the blue area.
- Inject 10 mL of 1% lidocaine (10 mg/mL) with epinephrine with 1 mL of 8.4% sodium bicarbonate over the volar aspect of the arcade of Frohse, situated just underneath the volar edge of the brachioradialis muscle in the proximal forearm.

Video 29.6 Surgical release of the superficial radial nerve in the forearm for Wartenberg's syndrome (Lalonde, Canada).

SPECIFICS OF MINIMAL PAIN INJECTION OF PERONEAL NERVE IN THE LEG

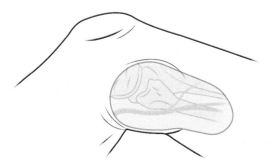

Fig. 29.4 Peroneal nerve release injection.

- Inject 60 to 80 mL of 0.5% lidocaine with 1:200,000 epinephrine in the blue area of dissection.

- Prepare 100 mL of 0.5% lidocaine with 1:200,000 epinephrine and inject 60 to 80 mL over the area of dissection as shown in ▶ Video 29.7.

- ▶ Video 29.8 shows the incision and the final exposure of the peroneal nerve. For a much more detailed video on how to perform this operation, please see Dr Susan Mackinnon's video on common peroneal nerve decompression available at https://www.youtube.com/watch?v=GDC0wDHtdy0.[3]

Video 29.7 Local injection for surgical release of the peroneal nerve in the leg (Lalonde, Canada).

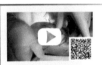

Video 29.8 WALANT surgical release of the peroneal nerve in the leg (Lalonde, Canada).

References

1. Hagert E, Hagert CG. Upper extremity nerve entrapments: the axillary and radial nerves—clinical diagnosis and surgical treatment. Plast Reconstr Surg 2014;134(1):71–80
2. Hagert E, Lalonde D. Nerve entrapment syndromes. In: Chang J, Neligan PC, eds. Nelligan's Plastic Surgery. Elsevier; 2017:525–548
3. Common peroneal nerve release at the fibular head—standard (Feat. Dr. Mackinnon). https://www.youtube.com/watch?v=GDC0wDHtdy0. Uploaded on September 10, 2018. Accessed August 29, 2020

Chapter 30

Simultaneous Release of Carpal Tunnel with Cubital Tunnel or Lacertus

Donald H. Lalonde

ADVANTAGES OF WALANT VERSUS SEDATION AND TOURNIQUET IN COMBINED SURGERIES

- All of the general advantages listed in Chapter 2 apply to both the surgeon and the patient (no nausea, no tourniquet pain or let-down bleeding, decreased cost without sedation in minor procedure room, safer surgery without sedation, etc.).

- Performing either a cubital tunnel, a lacertus release, or a carpal tunnel with WALANT is much less of an "event" than with sedation and a tourniquet. If you are going to ask patients to immobilize and elevate their hand for a carpal tunnel for a couple of days till they are off all pain killers and follow pain-guided healing, it is more efficient for patients to do both elbow and hand surgeries at the same time as they only have to recover once for two operations.

SPECIFICS OF MINIMALLY PAINFUL INJECTION OF LOCAL ANESTHETIC AND SURGERY FOR COMBINED CUBITAL AND CARPAL TUNNEL DECOMPRESSION

- See Chapter 26 and Chapter 27 for specifics and drawings on how much and where to inject for carpal tunnel and cubital tunnel, respectively.

- Inject 60 mL of buffered 0.5% lidocaine with 1:200,000 epinephrine for the elbow and 20 mL of the same solution for the hand.

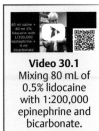

Video 30.1
Mixing 80 mL of
0.5% lidocaine
with 1:200,000
epinephrine and
bicarbonate.

- For combined carpal tunnel and cubital tunnel releases at the same time, we start injecting the cubital tunnel with local anesthetic first and operate on it after the carpal tunnel release. This gives the epinephrine longer time to work at the cubital tunnel, where hemostasis is more important. We usually don't need a cautery to do this combination of surgeries.

Video 30.2 Injecting for both cubital tunnel and carpal tunnel releases in the same operation (Lalonde, Canada).

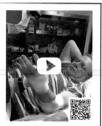

Video 30.3 Intraoperative patient advice on postoperative showering and pain-guided healing after cubital and carpal tunnel surgery (Lalonde, Canada).

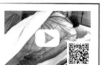

Video 30.4 Prone position field sterility for cubital and carpal tunnel surgery with arm at side (not on arm board).

Video 30.5 Patient's impressions 1 minute after cubital and carpal tunnel releases, and 1 minute before he went home (Lalonde, Canada).

- As with all combined surgeries, alternate injections from the elbow to the hand each time you need to reinsert a needle, so the patient is less likely to feel reinsertion pain because the local anesthetic has more time to work before the sharp needle tip is reinserted.

- We use buried 5-0 Monocryl sutures that don't need to be removed (see ▶ Video 26.9) and cover the wounds with skin tape for the elbow operations to keep the clothing off the wound. We use no skin tapes on the carpal tunnels, just temporary bandages for a few days in between showers.

- We let them take off the outside bandage the next day and get in the shower and get wounds wet. The skin tapes air-dry after the shower. They reapply the outside bandage to remind them to do pain-guided healing.

- We instruct the patients to keep the hand up and quiet for the first couple of days until they are off all acetaminophen or ibuprofen, which is all they need for pain even for combined operations if they elevate and immobilize their hand. Once they are off all painkillers and they know what hurts, they can start to lower and hand and use it providing they do not do what hurts. This is pain-guided healing or common sense (see ▶ Video 30.3).

SPECIFICS OF LOCAL ANESTHESIA INJECTION AND SURGERY FOR LACERTUS AND CARPAL TUNNEL RELEASES IN THE SAME OPERATION

- See Chapter 26 and Chapter 28 for specifics and drawings on how much and where to inject for carpal tunnel and lacertus releases, respectively.

- Inject 60 mL of buffered 0.5% lidocaine with 1:200,000 epinephrine for the lacertus and 20 mL of the same solution for the hand.

- For combined carpal tunnel and lacertus releases at the same time, we start injecting the lacertus with local anesthetic first so the local anesthesia has more time to work. I operate on the lacertus first so the patient can see the power come back to the thumb and index finger before I operate on the carpal tunnel release. This gives the epinephrine longer time to work at the cubital tunnel, where hemostasis is more important. We usually don't need a cautery to do this combination of surgeries.

- As with all combined surgeries, alternate injections from the elbow to the hand each time you need to reinsert a needle, so the patient is less likely to feel reinsertion pain because the local anesthetic has more time to work before the sharp needle tip is reinserted.

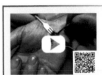

Video 30.6
Lacertus and carpal tunnel examination, injection, releases, and return of power (Lalonde, Canada).

SPECIFICS OF LOCAL ANESTHESIA INJECTION AND SURGERY FOR LACERTUS AND CUBITAL TUNNEL RELEASES IN THE SAME OPERATION

- See Chapter 27 and Chapter 28 for specifics and drawings on how much and where to inject for cubital tunnel and lacertus releases, respectively.

- Inject 50 to 70 mL of buffered 0.33% lidocaine with 1:300,000 epinephrine for the lacertus and 60 mL of the same solution for the cubital tunnel.

- For combined carpal tunnel and lacertus releases at the same time, we start injecting the lacertus with local anesthetic first so the local anesthesia has more time to work. I operate on the lacertus first so the patient can see the power come back to the thumb and index finger before I operate on the cubital tunnel release. This also gives the epinephrine longer time to work at the cubital tunnel, where hemostasis is more important. We usually don't need a cautery to do this combination of surgeries.

- As with all combined surgeries, alternate injections from the lacertus to the cubital tunnel each time you need to reinsert a needle, so the patient is less likely to feel reinsertion pain because the local anesthetic has more time to work before the sharp needle tip is reinserted.

- As in all the other operations, we let the patients take off the bandages and get in the shower the next day with just skin tapes on the wound. The skin tapes air-dry after the shower and come off at about 10 days like a Band-Aid.

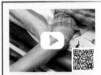

Video 30.7
Lacertus and cubital tunnel local injection (Lalonde, Canada).

SPECIFICS OF LOCAL ANESTHESIA INJECTION AND SURGERY FOR ALL THREE LACERTUS, CUBITAL TUNNEL, AND CARPAL TUNNEL RELEASES IN THE SAME OPERATION

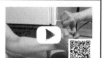

Video 30.8 Clinical examination of lacertus, cubital tunnel, and carpal tunnel patient in Video 30.9 and Video 30.10.

Video 30.9 Injection of local anesthesia for lacertus, cubital tunnel, and carpal tunnel of the patient in Video 30.8 and Video 30.10.

Video 30.10 The patient in Video 30.8 and Video 30.9 offers her 6 months' impressions of simultaneous release of lacertus, cubital tunnel, and carpal tunnel in one sitting.

- See Chapter 26, Chapter 27, and Chapter 28 for specifics and drawings on how much and where to inject for carpal tunnel, cubital tunnel, and lacertus releases, respectively.

- Inject 60 mL of buffered 0.25% lidocaine with 1:400,000 epinephrine for the lacertus, 60 mL for the cubital tunnel, and 20 mL for the carpal tunnel.

- As in all the other combined surgeries, alternate injections from the lacertus to the cubital tunnel to the palm each time you need to reinsert a needle, so the patient is less likely to feel reinsertion pain because the local anesthetic has more time to work before the sharp needle tip is reinserted.

- Always reinsert a needle within 1 to 2 cm of clearly vasoconstricted tumesced skin so the patient does not feel needle reinsertion pain.

- I operate on the lacertus first so the patient can see the power come back to the thumb and index finger before I operate on the cubital tunnel, where I can sometimes see the return of flexor digitorum profundus of the 5th finger (FDP5) power.

- After I inject the local anesthetic, I ask the patients to go to the restroom before the surgery so they are comfortable during the procedure.

- I usually don't need a cautery to do this combination of surgeries.

- As in all the other operations, we let the patients take off the bandages and get in the shower the next day with just skin tapes on the wound. The skin tapes air-dry after the shower and come off at about 10 days like a Band-Aid.

CHAPTER 31

LACERATED NERVES

*Donald H. Lalonde, Steven Koehler, Chao Chen,
and Julian Escobar*

ADVANTAGES OF WALANT VERSUS SEDATION AND TOURNIQUET IN REPAIR OF LACERATED NERVES

- All of the general advantages listed in Chapter 2 apply to both the surgeon and the patient (no nausea, no tourniquet pain or let-down bleeding, decreased cost without sedation in minor procedure room, safer surgery without sedation, etc.).

- You are able to see how much tension there is on your nerve repair with the patient's active movement before you close the skin. You may decide to let the patient go back to work 3 to 7 days postoperatively with a relative motion flexion splint (see the relative motion flexion splint in ▶ Video 31.1 and other videos in Chapter 21, Chapter 22, and Chapter 54).

- During surgery you will have the unhurried time to explain to the patient all of the problems of a nerve laceration including neuroma, time of recovery, etc. You can explain in simple terms what to expect over the next few months, including his or her ability to return to work and the best way to take pain medications after surgery. Your patient can remember and absorb all of this in a pain-free, unsedated state.

Video 31.1
Relative motion flexion splint allows early protected movement after digital nerve repair (Lalonde, Canada).

WHERE TO INJECT THE LOCAL ANESTHETIC FOR REPAIR OF DIGITAL NERVE LACERATIONS

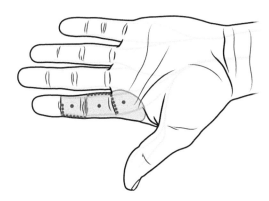

Fig. 31.1 The orange line in the illustration is the laceration and the dotted red lines are the possible incisions. Inject 8 mL of 1% lidocaine with 1:100,000 epinephrine (buffered with 10 mL lido/epi: 1 mL of 8.4% sodium bicarbonate).

SPECIFICS OF MINIMALLY PAINFUL INJECTION OF LOCAL ANESTHETIC FOR REPAIR OF LACERATED NERVES

- Local anesthesia injection should barely hurt at all if you follow the simple rules of Chapter 5 for hints to minimize injection pain. The patients will think you are magical.

- Inject the anesthetic solution a minimum of 30 minutes before surgery to allow the lidocaine and epinephrine to take optimal effect and provide an adequately dry working field, and for the digital nerves to be completely numb.

- Inject the patient in the waiting area outside the procedure room so no time is wasted.

- We inject supine patients lying down on stretchers to decrease the risk of their fainting (Chapter 6).

- To minimize the pain of injection, perform a digital nerve block as outlined in Chapter 1 and ▶ Video 1.1.

WHERE TO INJECT THE LOCAL ANESTHETIC FOR REPAIR OF A MEDIAN NERVE LACERATION IN THE FOREARM

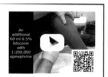

Video 31.2
Local anesthesia injection and surgery for sural nerve grafting to a median nerve defect (Koehler, USA).

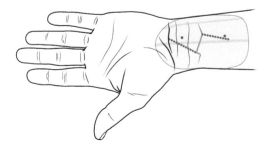

Fig. 31.2 Inject 30 to 50 mL of 1% lidocaine with 1:100,000 epinephrine (buffered with 10 mL lido/epi:1 mL of 8.4% sodium bicarbonate).

SPECIFICS OF INJECTING THE LOCAL ANESTHETIC FOR REPAIR OF A MEDIAN NERVE LACERATION IN THE FOREARM

- Local anesthesia injection should barely hurt at all if you follow the simple rules of Chapter 5 for hints to minimize injection pain. The patients will think you are magical.

- When performing major nerve blocks such as of the median or ulnar nerves, do not elicit paresthesias. Let the tumescent local anesthetic find and bathe the outside of the nerve so you do not damage it with the sharp needle tip.

- Inject the anesthetic solution a minimum of 60 minutes before surgery to allow the lidocaine and epinephrine to take optimal effect in large nerves like the median or ulnar nerves. It takes a very long time (100 minutes) for nonultrasound-guided nerve blocks to COMPLETELY numb large nerves like the median nerve in the distal forearm.[1]

- It takes a long time for the local anesthesia to diffuse into large nerves and the proximal nerve stump may still be sensitive even though you are cutting skin and dissecting soft tissue painlessly all around the nerve.

- You can anesthetize the proximal stumps of the median and ulnar nerves under direct vision after the skin flaps are anesthetized and raised. Use a 30-gauge needle and a 3-mL syringe. Gently lift up the epineurium with small forceps and inject into that loose areolar epineurial tissue. This will balloon the outside covering of the nerve to accelerate fascicle infiltration by the lidocaine. Do not inject directly into the nerve fascicles, as you will cause pain and lacerate fascicles and damage axons.

- Inject the patient in the waiting area outside the procedure room so no time is wasted.

- We inject supine patients lying down on stretchers to decrease the risk of their fainting (Chapter 6).

- Always start by injecting well proximal to the laceration where the nerve is "live" to start anesthetizing the big median or ulnar nerve.

- Inject 25 mL of 1% lidocaine with 1:100,000 epinephrine buffered 10:1 with 8.4% sodium bicarbonate 2 to 3 cm proximal to the laceration.

- The first 15 mL is injected just under the skin and the remaining 10 mL is placed subfascially.

- Gradually advance the needle as you inject the 25 mL, as described in Chapter 5, for minimal pain injection. The fascia is 3 to 5 mm under the skin, depending on the patient's size.

- It is best to have extra local anesthetic at hand, because some of it may well come out through the laceration.

- We keep the total dose of infiltration less than 7 mg/kg. If less than 50 mL is required to produce tumescent local anesthesia (see Chapter 4), we use premixed 1% lidocaine with 1:100,000 epinephrine. If 50 to 100 mL is required, we dilute with saline solution to a concentration of 0.5% lidocaine with 1:200,000 epinephrine.

- It is wise to have at least 5 cm of visible palpable local anesthetic proximal to the laceration along the path of the nerve in case the proximal stump has migrated proximally.

TIPS AND TRICKS FOR REPAIRING LACERATED NERVES WITH THE WIDE AWAKE APPROACH

- For digital nerve injuries, you can simulate relative motion flexion splinting for early protected movement to begin 3 to 5 days after surgery. Repair the nerve and insert a tongue depressor to simulate the splint, as in ▶ Video 31.1. If the nerve stays together with no tension

Video 31.3
Stimulation of
proximal stump
to determine if
group fascicles are
sensory or motor
(Chen, China).

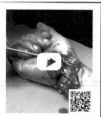

Video 31.4
Checking nerve
movement with
full-fist flexion
and extension
after ulnar nerve
repair (Escobar,
Columbia).

with active flexion and extension, you can prescribe a relative motion flexion splint to be worn postoperatively. If the nerve comes apart with tongue depressor simulation, then clearly you would treat this patient with standard immobilization after surgery.

- We perform these nerve repairs in the minor procedure room outside the operating room with field sterility (see Chapter 10) and loupe magnification. We have access to a microscope there, but loupes have been as effective and more efficient.

- After nerve repairs in the wrist and forearm, examine your nerve gliding and make sure there is no gapping with active movement of the wrist and fingers. Protect your nerve postoperatively accordingly.

- You can stimulate the unanesthetized proximal stump to determine which group fascicles are motor and which are sensory by having the patient tell you what he or she is feeling as in ▶ Video 31.3.

Reference

1. Lovely LM, Chishti YZ, Woodland JL, Lalonde DH. How much volume of local anesthesia and how long should you wait after injection for an effective wrist median nerve block? Hand (N Y) 2018;13(3):281–284

CHAPTER 32

DUPUYTREN'S CONTRACTURE

*Donald H. Lalonde, Xavier Gueffier, Thomas Apard,
Duncan McGrouther, Jason Wong, and Kamal Rafiqi*

ADVANTAGES OF WALANT VERSUS SEDATION AND TOURNIQUET IN DUPUYTREN'S CONTRACTURE

- All of the general advantages listed in Chapter 2 apply to both the surgeon and the patient (no nausea, no tourniquet pain or let-down bleeding, decreased cost without sedation in minor procedure room, safer surgery without sedation, etc.).

- With the wide awake approach, you can see how much active extension the patient can really achieve after cord resection and before the skin is closed. In the case in ▶ Video 32.1, after complete cord resection, posterior interphalangeal (PIP) extension was still very limited because of metacarpophalangeal (MP) hyperextension. We showed the relative motion flexion splint concept to the patient during surgery so that he would understand why it was important to wear his relative motion flexion splint after surgery. It helped him to get a much better result than we would have obtained without relative motion flexion splinting.

- You and the patient both find out during surgery whether or not the patient is likely to regain full active extension, thus avoiding the patient's having unrealistic expectations after surgery.

- Many of these patients are older and could have severe problems with general anesthesia and sedation because of medical comorbidities. With WALANT, they will just get up and go home as they do after they have a dental procedure (see ▶ Video 2.2 and ▶ Video 32.3).

- Patients get to see that the cord and nodule are gone as they watch themselves moving their fingers through a full range of motion before we close the skin. They realize that their fingers can work well once they get past the postoperative discomfort and stiffness.[1,2]

- Procedures requiring correction of multiple digits and revisions are not time-limited by the use of a tourniquet.

Video 32.1
Relative motion flexion splinting is a priceless new treatment of Dupuytren posterior interphalangeal (PIP) extensor lag. See local injection for this patient in ▶ Video 32.4 (Lalonde, Canada).

Video 32.2
Passive versus active extension after Dupuytren cord resection and pencil test to determine value of relative motion flexion splinting to correct posterior interphalangeal (PIP) extensor lag (Gueffier, France).

Video 32.3 Patient with Dupuytren's surgery in two fingers needs oxygen tank to sleep sitting up and night (Lalonde, Canada).

- When a patient is being treated for recurrent Dupuytren's contracture, his or her mindset may be quite different from a primary surgery for the condition. The patient may feel that during the initial repair there was minimal follow-up and perhaps not enough discussion about the fact that the disease would likely recur in the future. The wide awake procedure allows you to have a prolonged consultation with the patient during the surgery to discuss the recurrent nature of this condition and postoperative rehabilitation options.

WHERE TO INJECT THE LOCAL ANESTHETIC FOR DUPUYTREN'S CONTRACTURE

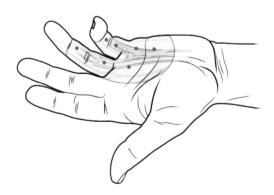

Fig. 32.1 Inject 10 mL of 1% lidocaine with 1:100,000 epinephrine (buffered with 10 mL lido/epi:1 mL of 8.4% sodium bicarbonate) in the most proximal red dot under the skin. Follow this with 2 mL in each of the six remaining red dots, alternating from the ring to the small finger, always injecting proximal first and distal last.

SPECIFICS OF MINIMALLY PAINFUL INJECTION OF LOCAL ANESTHETIC IN DUPUYTREN'S CONTRACTURE

Video 32.4 Injecting local anesthetic for Dupuytren's surgery. Inject up to 25 mL of 1% lidocaine with 1:100,000 epinephrine (buffered with 10 mL lido/epi:1 mL of 8.4% sodium bicarbonate) (Lalonde, Canada).

- Local anesthesia injection should barely hurt at all if you follow the simple rules of Chapter 5 for hints to minimize injection pain. The patients will think you are magical.
- Inject the anesthetic solution a minimum of 30 minutes before surgery to allow the lidocaine and epinephrine to take optimal effect and provide an adequately dry working field, and for the digital nerves to be completely numb.
- Inject supine patients lying down on stretchers before they come into the operating room.
- To minimize the pain of injection, start with a 30-gauge needle and a 3-mL syringe in the most proximal injection point.
- Inject another 10 to 20 mL in the distal palm, always reinserting the needles in areas that are clearly 1 cm inside the blanched border of vasoconstricted skin.

- The cords can act as a barrier to the diffusion of local anesthetic. That is why you may need to inject on both sides of a cord. You should be able to see and palpate the local anesthetic under the skin anywhere you will make an incision and dissect.

- Inject another each 2 mL in the middle of proximal and middle phalanx wherever you are going to dissect. If you are going to dissect into the distal phalanx, you will only need 1 mL in the middle of the subcutaneous fat there.

- If you are going to be doing forceful joint manipulation or joint dissection, you may well need another 4 mL proximal to the dorsal MP joint as well as on the ulnar side of the small finger to make sure all dorsal joint branches are blocked.

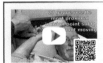

Video 32.5
Injecting local anesthetic for Dupuytren's surgery into another patient with palmar and finger cords with 7-month follow-up (Lalonde, Canada).

TIPS AND TRICKS FOR PERFORMING DUPUYTREN'S CONTRACTURE SURGERY WITH THE WIDE AWAKE APPROACH

- Your first WALANT case should not be a Dupuytren's procedure because WALANT surgery is not bloodless surgery. This operation can be difficult for novice surgeons and trainees and can increase the risk of nerve damage. Dupuytren's procedure, especially recurrent Dupuytren's, is the least dry operation in wide awake surgery. This is because the cords frequently wrap around the digital arteries, which are still pumping blood when bathed with 1:100,000 epinephrine. Their little branches bleed when avulsed by cord dissection. We recommend that you not perform Dupuytren's procedure with WALANT until you are comfortable with this procedure as well as using WALANT for other procedures.

- One concern with performing WALANT Dupuytren's fasciectomy is that the blood in the field of view can obscure the disease. It is possible that you can leave more resectable disease behind that you might have removed under a bloodless field approach.

- Injection of 100 mg of tranexamic acid with each 10 mL of local anesthesia can be helpful to promote stability of clots (Dr Lalonde thanks Dr John B. Moore IV of USA for this idea).

- Consider performing this operation standing instead of sitting so you can easily walk around the table to get a better look at the cord and digital nerves from both sides. Parts of the dissection are easier from the other side.

- You can apply a loose, uninflated tourniquet to the upper arm as a safety net.

- After the resection, patients need to look at the fingers to get them to move, since they cannot feel the numbed fingers. Although most patients do not mind looking at the wound, you can cover the wound with a towel as they flex all fingers together while looking at them.

- For dermofasciectomy, our preferred full-thickness skin graft donor site is the inner upper arm, 5 cm above the medial epicondyle and below the tourniquet (if you apply one). Clearly, this area will require further local anesthesia.

Video 32.6
With good intraoperative education, most patients only need ibuprofen and/or acetaminophen after WALANT Dupuytren's surgery (same patient as ▶ Video 32.5) (Lalonde, Canada).

Video 32.7
Amputation of middle phalanx with K-wiring of distal phalanx on proximal phalanx with WALANT (Apard, France).

Video 32.8
Injection of
local anesthetic,
surgery, and
relative motion
flexion splinting
postoperative
rehabilitation
(Gueffier, France).

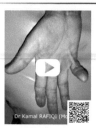

Video 32.9
Dupuytren 5th
finger cord (Rafiqi,
Morocco).

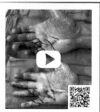

Video 32.10
Malingue flaps
(Apard, France).

- Also for dermofasciectomy, we restrict the resection to the proximal segment of the digit, whereas Logan's group[3] has generally recommended extending farther proximally. We remove a short segment of longitudinal cord at the distal palmar crease to release a contracted MP joint. However, we leave Dupuytren's tissues proximal and distal to the grafted area because they regress as tension is relieved.

References

1. Denkler K. Dupuytren's fasciectomies in 60 consecutive digits using lidocaine with epinephrine and no tourniquet. Plast Reconstr Surg 2005;115(3):802–810
2. Nelson R, Higgins A, Conrad J, Bell M, Lalonde D. The wide-awake approach to Dupuytren's disease: fasciectomy under local anesthetic with epinephrine. [published correction appears in Hand (N Y). 2010 Jun;5(2):213] Hand (N Y) 2010;5(2):117–124
3. Armstrong JR, Hurren JS, Logan AM. Dermofasciectomy in the management of Dupuytren's disease. J Bone Joint Surg Br 2000;82(1):90–94

CHAPTER 33

GANGLIONS AND OTHER SMALL SOFT TISSUE OPERATIONS

Lei Zhu, Donald H. Lalonde, Jason Wong, Shu Guo Xing, Jin Bo Tang, Jean Paul Brutus, and Xavier Gueffier

ADVANTAGES OF WALANT VERSUS SEDATION AND TOURNIQUET IN GANGLION, LIPOMA, SKIN CANCER, AND OTHER SOFT TISSUE MASS EXCISION

- All of the general advantages listed in Chapter 2 apply to both the surgeon and the patient (no nausea, no tourniquet pain or let-down bleeding, decreased cost without sedation in minor procedure room, safer surgery without sedation, etc.).

TIPS AND TRICKS FOR PERFORMING SKIN CANCER EXCISION ON THE HAND WITH WALANT

- During skin cancer excision, the large volume of tumescent local anesthetic used in this technique actually hydrodissects the tumor off the tendon paratenon for you. This promotes the take of a skin graft and creates a nice tissue plane, permitting you to get under the cancer for complete excision of the tumor.

- Many skin cancer patients are older and may have problems with general anesthesia and sedation because of medical comorbidities. With WALANT, they will simply get up and go home after the procedure, just like after they have a dental procedure.

- When applying skin grafts to the hand after cancer excision, you can educate patients during surgery about how important it is that they keep their hand elevated and "on strike," doing absolutely nothing with it for the next week while the skin graft takes after cancer excision. At the end of the procedure, patients can sit up and elevate their hand with total understanding of what to do. If patients are sedated or undergo general anesthesia, they may not understand what to do and may be too groggy during postoperative recovery to grasp the teaching. They may well keep their hand dependent and may even have problems with vomiting, which could lead to further hematoma under the graft. If they are sedated, they may require hospital admission for the procedure to get safe general anesthesia and monitoring.

Video 33.1
Squamous cell
skin cancer in two
80-year-olds on
anticoagulants
(Lalonde, Canada).

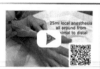

Video 33.2
Local anesthetic
injection for
squamous cell
cancer in hand
(Lalonde, Canada).

- See ▶ Video 8.1 for giving advice to a wide-awake patient while excising skin cancer from the hand.

- Local anesthesia injection should barely hurt at all if you follow the simple rules of Chapter 5 for hints to minimize injection pain. The patients will think you are magical.

- In the first hand cancer case, in ▶ Video 33.1, we injected at least 20 mL of buffered 1% lidocaine with 1:100,000 epinephrine (buffered with 10 mL lido/epi:1 mL of 8.4% sodium bicarbonate). We injected from proximal to distal all around and under the tumor edge. We let the tumescent local anesthetic lift the tumor away from the tendons. After we removed the tumor, we injected an additional 20 mL in his medial arm where we harvested a skin graft an hour later. For a full hour, the hand with cancer was elevated and compressed with a saline gauze so it stopped bleeding as the patient was on anticoagulants. During that hour, we performed other surgery such as carpal tunnel release. We then covered the wound with the skin graft as seen in the video.

- Do not insert the needle in the tumor itself. Blow all around it first, from proximal to distal. You will elevate the tumor off the tendons with the large volume of tumescent local anesthetic as shown in ▶ Video 33.2.

- The more volume that you inject, the wider will be the amount of loose areolar tissue between the epitenon and the cancer. This will facilitate preservation of live epitenon over the tendon with complete cancer excision.

- In ▶ Video 33.1, we performed both wide awake skin cancer excisions in men in their eighties in a minor procedure room outside of the main operating room with field sterility.

- We marked the incision line before injecting the local anesthetic. The skin is healthy where it is soft and folds as you push it into the rigid cancer with your finger. The healthy skin becomes tumescent and no longer folds readily after you have injected the local anesthetic.

- We harvested thick split-thickness skin graft with a number 10 blade on the loose skin of the arm in both cases. We then excised the exposed dermis of the donor site and closed the wound primarily with buried dermal sutures. No suture removal was required. It healed nicely as a line scar much more quickly than it would have healed as a split-thickness donor site.

- We immobilized the hands with a volar splint for a week and reminded the patient that he should keep his hand "on strike," elevated without movement during the week. We got a healed wound and a complete excision of the cancer.

TIPS AND TRICKS FOR PERFORMING GANGLION EXCISION WITH THE WIDE AWAKE APPROACH

- Local anesthesia injection should barely hurt at all if you follow the simple rules of Chapter 5 for hints to minimize injection pain. The patients will think you are magical.

- We usually use about 15 to 20 mL of 1% lidocaine with 1:100,000 epinephrine (buffered with 10 mL lidocaine with 1:100,000 epinephrine: 1 mL of 8.4% sodium bicarbonate). Slowly infiltrate at least 15 mL of tumescent injection to the dorsal aspect of the wrist which will block the sensory branches of the radial, ulnar, and posterior interosseous nerves.

- Inject around the ganglion to avoid piercing it (Fig. 33.1).

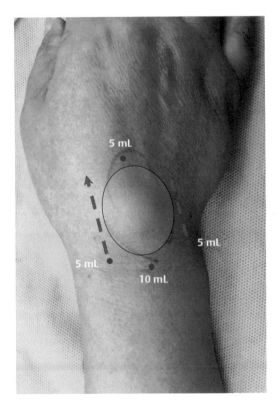

Fig. 33.1 The injection method for the excision of ganglion cyst. Vertical injection is performed in the proximal and distal points.

- We often encounter the bigger vessels need to excise wrist ganglions. We no longer use cautery for most cases but occasionally use a hemostat on bigger vessels for a few minutes or tie them off.

- The pedicle of the ganglion cyst is often located inside the wrist joint. It is important to block the nerve branches innervating the dorsal wrist capsule so that you can have pain-free access. We occasionally need to add the injection to the capsule around the pedicle of the ganglion cyst during the operation.

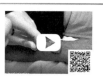 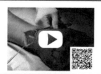

Video 33.3 Dorsal wrist ganglion local anesthesia injection (Lalonde, Canada).

Video 33.4 Dorsal wrist ganglion excision surgery (Xing, China).

Video 33.5 Volar triggering wrist ganglion excision surgery (Brutus, Canada).

TIPS AND TRICKS FOR PERFORMING LIPOMA EXCISION WITH THE WIDE AWAKE APPROACH

Video 33.6 Excision of lipoma in the forearm (Xing, China).

- Local anesthesia injection should barely hurt at all if you follow the simple rules of Chapter 5 for hints to minimize injection pain. The patients will think you are magical.

- Bathe 2 cm of soft tissue surrounding the lipoma generously and wait for at least 30 minutes while doing other procedures or local injection.

- If less than 50 mL is required, we use premixed 1% lidocaine with 1:100,000 epinephrine. If 50 to 100 mL is required, we dilute with saline solution to a concentration of 0.5% lidocaine with 1:200,000 epinephrine. If 100 to 200 mL is required, we dilute with saline solution to a concentration of 0.25% lidocaine with 1:400,000 epinephrine (all solutions buffered with 10 mL of 1% lido/1:100,000 epi:1 mL of 8.4% sodium bicarbonate).

TIPS AND TRICKS FOR EXCISION OF OTHER BENIGN LESIONS

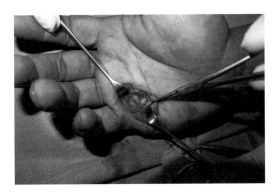

Fig. 33.2 Giant cell tumor (Zhu, China). A large volume of local anesthesia (15 mL) helps to hydrodissect the capsule of the tumor from the loose surrounding tissue. Magnification is helpful to preserve the capsule and completely excise the lesion. Waiting at least 30 minutes for vasoconstriction is helpful; 45 to 60 minutes is even better.

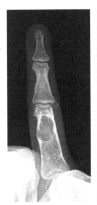
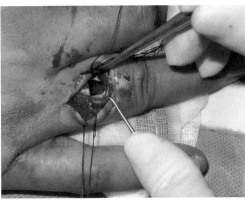

Fig. 33.3 Enchondroma (Zhu, China). Inject local anesthesia 2 mL volar and 2 to 3 mL dorsal till tissues are tumesced (plump and pale with vasoconstriction). Chisel hole in cortex, curette lesion, rinse with saline and then 95% alcohol, and then pack with artificial bone.

Video 33.7
Minimally painful local anesthesia injection for palmar pyogenic granuloma (Lalonde, Canada).

Video 33.8
Ultrasound video showing preoperative appearance and excision of giant cell tumor wrapped around flexor tendon (video by Elise Gueffier) (Gueffier, France).

Video 33.9
Ultrasound video showing preoperative appearance and removal of wood splinter foreign body (Lalonde, Canada).

CHAPTER 34

FLAP HARVEST AND TRANSFER IN THE HAND

Shu Guo Xing, Jin Bo Tang, Chung-Chen Hsu, Jason Wong, Egemen Ayhan, and Xavier Gueffier

ADVANTAGES OF WALANT VERSUS SEDATION AND TOURNIQUET IN FLAP HARVEST AND TRANSFER IN THE HAND

- All of the general advantages listed in Chapter 2 apply to both the surgeon and the patient (no nausea, no tourniquet pain or let-down bleeding, decreased cost without sedation in minor procedure room, safer surgery without sedation, etc.).

- Most patients needing soft tissue reconstruction are traumatic and need repair primarily or in delayed primary stage. With WALANT, we can perform the operation immediately when they arrive at the hospital without waiting to get into the main operating room with general anesthesia.

- You do not need to deal with your patient's medical comorbidities, which would be a problem if you perform the operation under general anesthesia and sedation. With WALANT, they will simply get up and go home after the procedure.[1,2]

- You do not need to perform the operation in the main operating room. You can do it in minor treatment rooms in the clinic outside the main operating room with evidence-based field sterility (see Chapter 10).[1,2,3,4]

- Your patient remains pain-free with WALANT for up to 4 to 5 hours. They do not need narcotics after good perioperative teaching on how to take pain medicine.

- See Chapter 8 for videos on giving advice to patients on postoperative activities during the surgery.

WHERE TO INJECT THE LOCAL ANESTHETIC FOR FLAP HARVEST AND TRANSFER IN THE HAND

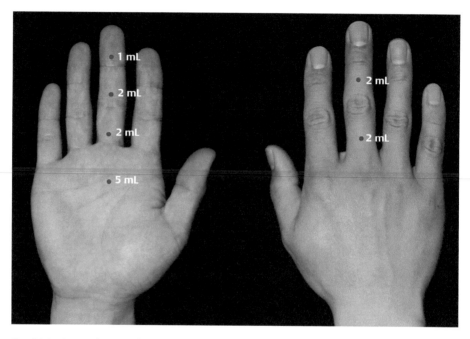

Fig. 34.1 Injection location for extended Segmuller flap and homodigital reverse digital artery flap: *Left*: Sites of injection on palmar aspect of the finger. *Right*: Sites of injection on dorsal aspect of the finger. The most proximal injection can be only 4 to 5 mL instead of 10 mL.

- Local anesthesia injection should barely hurt at all if you follow the simple rules of Chapter 5 for hints to minimize injection pain. The patients will think you are magical.

- Inject 1% lidocaine with 1:100,000 epinephrine buffered with 8.4% sodium bicarbonate in a 10:1 ratio (1 mL of 8.4% bicarbonate for each 10 mL of 1% lidocaine with 1:100,000 epinephrine).

- The local anesthetic is less than 15 to 20 mL per digital ray for harvesting the extended Segmuller flap or for a flap from dorsum of the hand (► Fig. 34.1, ► Fig. 34.2, and ► Fig. 34.3).

- Inject 10 mL in the most proximal injection point (volar to the level of metacarpophalangeal [MP] joint). The first few milliliters go under the skin, and the rest is injected under the superficial palmar fascia without moving the needle. This injection at the base of the finger acts as a temporary sympathetic block in the finger distal to the injection that may help prevent vasospasm. Hyperemia in the finger distal to the white epinephrine at the digit base makes this clear.

- The anesthesia of this injection also helps the authors remove the wound dressings without pain.

- To decrease the pain of distal injections, you can wait for the local anesthesia to numb the common digital nerves after the most proximal injection, and then inject another 2, 2, and 1 mL under volar finger skin in the fat between the two digital nerves at the level of the MP, proximal interphalangeal (PIP), and distal interphalangeal (DIP) joint creases, respectively.

- Finally, inject 2 mL each in the dorsal central aspects of the proximal and middle phalanges.

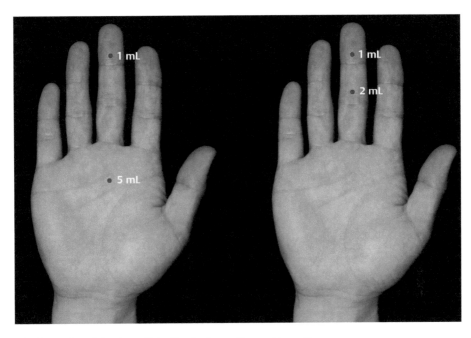

Fig. 34.2 Location of the sites of injection for harvesting an Atasoy flap.

- The proximal injection may be less than 10 mL. We sometimes only inject 4 to 5 mL, or do not inject to this proximal point at all. Instead, we inject 2 to 3 mL at the PIP joint level, which also produces satisfactory anesthesia.

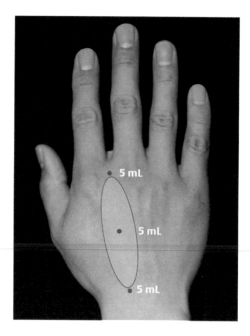

Fig. 34.3 Location of the injection for dorsal metacarpal artery perforator flap.

- Inject about 20 mL to harvest this flap.

- First, inject about 5 to 10 mL proximal to the designed flap. After waiting for 5 minutes, inject 5 mL each to the central and metacarpal head parts of the flap.

- We are careful to inject beside the likely location of the flap perforator, not right in the perforator. We do not want to damage the perforator with the needle.

- Then inject up to 10 mL in the area between the defect and the flap.

SPECIFICS OF MINIMALLY PAINFUL INJECTION OF LOCAL ANESTHETIC IN FLAP HARVEST AND TRANSFER IN THE HAND

- Local anesthesia injection should barely hurt at all if you follow the simple rules of Chapter 5 for hints to minimize injection pain. The patients will think you are magical.

- In Nantong, we inject the anesthetic solution about 5 to 15 minutes (or sometimes less than 5 minutes) before surgery to allow the epinephrine to take effect. We do not typically wait for more than 15 minutes, as we think it is fine to have some blood in the field in our patients.[5]

- We always inject all patients while they are lying down to decrease the risk of their fainting (see Chapter 6).

- To minimize the pain of injection, use a fine 27-gauge needle into the most proximal injection point. This point is marked at least 1 cm proximal to the most proximal place you are likely to dissect.

- Only reinsert the needle into clearly numb areas to avoid pain after the first injection.

- You may inject an additional 2 mL each in the dorsal central aspects of the proximal and middle phalanges.

TIPS AND TRICKS FOR PERFORMING FLAP HARVEST AND TRANSFER IN THE HAND WITH THE WIDE AWAKE APPROACH

- Flap surgery is not a contraindication for WALANT. The safety and possibility of the local anesthetic with epinephrine in the hand in microvascular dissection and flap harvest have been proven. Based on the transient vasoconstrictive effects of epinephrine on the vasculature of only capillaries (▶ Fig. 34.4), soft tissue flaps will not suffer avascular necrosis in 4 to 5 hours because we can routinely successfully perform digital replantation after 6 to 8 hours of ischemia.[6,7,8,9,10]

- Dr Prasetyono routinely decreases his concentration of epinephrine to 1:1,000,000 for safe flap harvest and good anesthesia.[11]

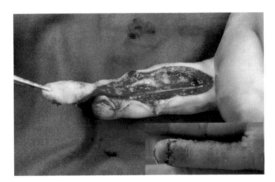

Fig. 34.4 The homodigital reverse digital artery flap surgery under WALANT. We can clearly see digital arteries pulsate, though they were bathed with 1:100,000 epinephrine during the operation. The bottom right inserted picture is a postoperative view during follow-up.

- We do not apply this method to patients with unilateral or bilateral digital bundle injuries (recent or previous), a history of a peripheral vascular disorder, or considerable procedural anxiety who prefer intravenous sedation or brachial plexus block anesthesia.

- After local anesthetic injection, we typically wait only 10 to 15 minutes to start flap dissection. We have found that there is no need to wait for 20 to 30 minutes to begin surgery in these patents.[5] During these 10 to 15 minutes, we perform preoperative preparation by cleansing the skin and draping the area.

- We do not use digital or other tourniquets to aid in the identification and dissection of structures. At the time of the skin incisions, there is some bleeding, but, as we reach the deep tissues, the bleeding decreases, and the field is clear enough to allow the procedure. All the cases had adequate bleeding control (▶ Fig 34.4 and ▶ Fig. 34.5). The authors could clearly see digital arteries pulsate even though they were bathed with 1:100,000 epinephrine.

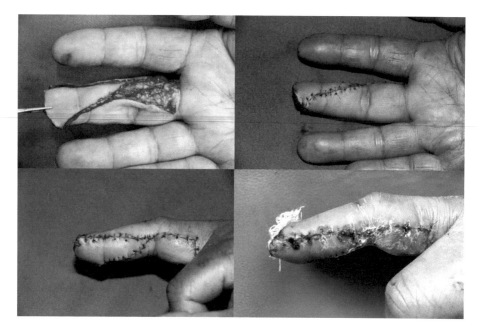

Fig. 34.5 The Segmuller flap surgery under WALANT. The patient had adequate bleeding control and was pain-free.

- The Nantong group has used this anesthesia method in more than 100 fingers for harvest of pedicled flaps and transfer after traumatic defects of fingertips as well as dorsal and central finger wounds. No patients required termination of the procedure because of pain. All flaps survived without overt venous congestion or flap failure because of the vasoconstrictive effects of epinephrine after the operation.

- It is difficult to assess flap perfusion with capillary refill or skin color because of the vasoconstrictive action of epinephrine under WALANT. If you want to verify the blood supply of the flaps during the operation, you can inject phentolamine (1 mg diluted in 1–10 mL saline) to reverse the vasoconstrictive effects of epinephrine. The flap will pink up nicely and quickly after the injection. For pedicle or advancement flaps, digital artery-based pedicled flaps, Atasoy flaps, and Moberg flaps (▶ Fig. 34.6) are safe to use with epinephrine and lidocaine, so such phentolamine injections are not necessary.

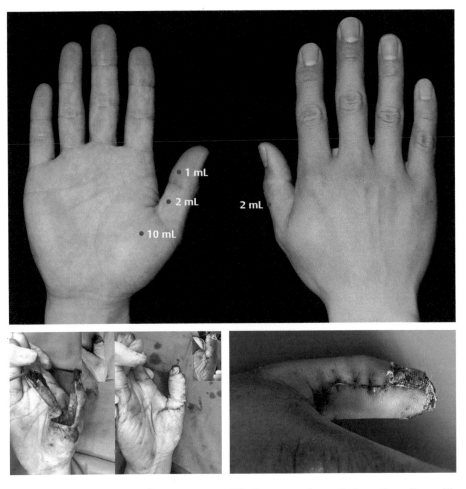

Fig. 34.6 Moberg flap surgery under WALANT. It is difficult to assess flap perfusion with capillary refill or skin color after the surgery, but the phentolamine was not used because observation and monitoring were not critically necessary for this kind of traditional flap. Inserted pictures are intraoperative dorsal views.

- After the surgery, monitoring of the pedicle flaps and advancement flaps is not necessary. If you want to monitor blood perfusion of the skin or are worried about the effect of epinephrine, you could inject phentolamine immediately after surgery as a routine in all patients who have this anesthesia though we have not done so in a single case.

- We also consider it proper to use epinephrine in the finger or thumb when the tip needs artificial dermal templates. However, we suggest avoiding epinephrine when amputation is treated with a composite graft without anastomosis of the vessels.

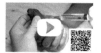

Video 34.1 Moberg
flap local anesthesia
and flap elevation
(Xing, China).

Video 34.2
Metacarpal artery
island local injection
and flap harvest
(Quaba flap) (Wong,
England).

Video 34.3
Homodigital island
flap (Hsu, Taiwan).

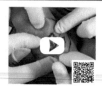

Video 34.4
Dufourmentel flap
(Gueffier, France).

Video 34.5
Innervated digital
artery perforator
flap and bone
graft fingertip
reconstruction
(Ayhan, Turkey).

References

1. Lalonde DH. Reconstruction of the hand with wide awake surgery. Clin Plast Surg 2011;38(4):761–769
2. Lalonde DH. Conceptual origins, current practice, and views of wide awake hand surgery. J Hand Surg Eur Vol 2017;42(9):886–895
3. Tang JB, Gong KT, Zhu L, Pan ZJ, Xing SG. Performing hand surgery under local anesthesia without a tourniquet in China. Hand Clin 2017;33(3):415–424
4. Gong KT, Xing SG. How to establish and standardize wide-awake hand surgery: experience from China. J Hand Surg Eur Vol 2017;42(8):868–870
5. Xing SG, Mao T. Purposeful waiting after injection of anaesthetics with epinephrine is mostly unnecessary for wide-awake surgery. J Hand Surg Eur Vol 2019;44(9):990–991
6. Tang JB, Landín L, Cavadas PC, et al. Unique techniques or approaches in microvascular and microlymphatic surgery. Clin Plast Surg 2017;44(2):403–414
7. Tang JB, Elliot D, Adani R, Saint-Cyr M, Stang F. Repair and reconstruction of thumb and finger tip injuries: a global view. Clin Plast Surg 2014;41(3):325–359
8. Xing SG, Mao T. The use of local anaesthesia with epinephrine in the harvest and transfer of an extended Segmuller flap in the fingers. J Hand Surg Eur Vol 2018;43(7):783–784
9. Xing SG, Tang JB. Extending applications of local anesthesia without tourniquet to flap harvest and transfer in the hand. Hand Clin 2019;35(1):97–102
10. Wong J, Lin CH, Chang NJ, Chen HC, Lin YT, Hsu CC. Digital revascularization and replantation using the wide-awake hand surgery technique. J Hand Surg Eur Vol 2017;42(6):621–625
11. Prasetyono TOH, Nindita E. The safety of one-per-mil tumescent infiltration into tissue that has survived ischemia. Arch Plast Surg 2019;46(2):108–113

CHAPTER 35

INFECTION SURGERY, COMPARTMENT SYNDROME RELEASE, AND TIBIAL HEMATOMA DRAINAGE

Donald H. Lalonde and Gökhan Tolga Akbulut

ADVANTAGES OF WALANT VERSUS SEDATION AND TOURNIQUET FOR INFECTION SURGERY SUCH AS FIGHT BITE DEBRIDEMENT AND FLEXOR SYNOVITIS

- All of the general advantages listed in Chapter 2 apply to both the surgeon and the patient (no nausea, no tourniquet pain or let-down bleeding, decreased cost without sedation in minor procedure room, safer surgery without sedation, etc.).

- Patients with lesions like fight bite infections have traditionally gone to the main operating room for debridement and irrigation because of the need for general anesthesia. Now that we know how to numb these patients with minimally painful local anesthesia injection, the debridement and irrigation can safely and easily be performed in the emergency department.[1]

- Patients can be admitted for intravenous antibiotics directly to the emergency department and bypass the main operating room altogether (▶ Video 35.1 and ▶ Video 35.3).

- Unsedated patients can remember surgeon's education during the injection of the local anesthesia and during the whole debridement process. Patients will recover much faster and are much less likely to have postoperative complications when they understand: (1) why it is so important to keep the hand elevated and immobilized for the first days until they are off all pain killers and (2) how to take pain medicine properly, get off it as quickly as possible, and follow pain-guided healing. See ▶ Video 35.4b to hear Dr Lalonde explain pain-guided healing to a patient with early infective flexor synovitis that responded to immobilization, elevation, pain-guided healing, and antibiotics without requiring surgery. Many patients with early flexor synovitis do not require surgery.

- In the clinic or emergency department in countries that regulate water cleanliness, you can wash a numbed infected draining hand with large volumes of clean tap water to wash out the pus from the wound in a sink. This also avoids contaminating clean main operating room theaters with pus.

WHERE TO INJECT THE LOCAL ANESTHETIC FOR FIGHT BITE DEBRIDEMENT

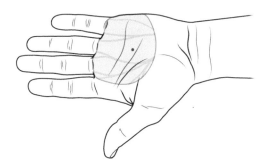

Fig. 35.1 Inject 10 to 15 mL of 1% lidocaine with 1:100,000 epinephrine buffered with 1 mL of 8.4% bicarbonate in the palm volar and 1 cm proximal to the fight bite. You do not need to move the needle. Just inject under the skin.

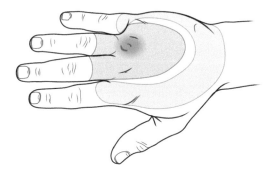

Fig. 35.2 Inject 40 mL of local anesthesia (*blue*) containing 1% lidocaine with 1:100,000 epinephrine buffered with 4 mL of 8.4% bicarbonate in the dorsum outside of the red zone of cellulitis. Always inject from proximal to distal. Inject the radial side, then the ulnar side, then back to the radial side, then back to the ulnar side until the cellulitis is surrounded by a ring of tumescent local anesthesia.

SPECIFICS OF MINIMALLY PAINFUL INJECTION OF LOCAL ANESTHETIC FOR INFECTION SURGERY LIKE A FIGHT BITE

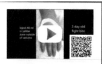

Video 35.1 How to inject local anesthesia for fight bite debridement and washout in the emergency department (Lalonde, Canada).

- Local anesthesia injection should barely hurt at all if you follow the simple rules of Chapter 5 for hints to minimize injection pain. The patients will think you are magical.

- In infected hands, injecting directly into inflamed tissues does not work very well because of three reasons: (1) It is painful, (2) the swollen tissues do not easily accept the extra local anesthetic volume, and (3) the hyperemia washes out lidocaine quickly, even with epinephrine.

- Instead of injecting into the infected area, inject tumescent local anesthetic proximally outside the zone of cellulitis.

- First inject 10 to 15 mL in the palm as shown in ▶ Fig. 35.1. Center the injection between the nerve branches going to the most affected fingers. Do not move the 27-gauge needle after starting the injection in the fat. The palm under the skin of the dorsal cellulitis should be tumesced enough that you can see and feel the local anesthetic in the palm under the entire affected area.

- Then inject the dorsal central area proximal to the cellulitis as shown in ▶ Fig. 35.2. Inject the first 10 mL without moving the 27-gauge needle. Inject the second 10 mL either on the radial or ulnar side of the first injection, but always reinsert needles within 1 cm of an area clearly inflated with local anesthesia so that subsequent needle pokes do not hurt.

- Alternate radial and ulnar injections until the entire dorsal skin proximal to the cellulitis is tumesced with a ring around the zone of cellulitis.

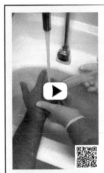

Video 35.2 How to educate patients about infection management and debride the fight bite in the emergency department (Lalonde, Canada).

WHERE TO INJECT THE LOCAL ANESTHETIC FOR SUPPURATIVE FLEXOR SYNOVITIS DRAINAGE AND IRRIGATION

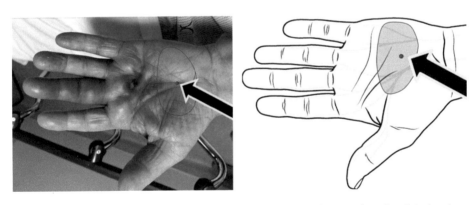

Fig. 35.3 Inject 20 mL of buffered 1% lidocaine with 1:100,000 epinephrine in the palm of the hand just distal to the transverse carpal ligament where the nerve trunks divide into common digital nerves. The smaller the nerve, the faster and more completely it numbs. This is much more effective and works much faster than a median nerve block proximal to the wrist crease. Nonultrasound-guided median nerve blocks at the wrist take an average of 100 minutes to be effective.[3]

Video 35.3
Local anesthesia injection for flexor synovitis (Lalonde, Canada).

Video 35.4a
Drainage and irrigation of flexor synovitis in the emergency department in an 81-year-old man with multiple medical comorbidities (Lalonde, Canada).

Video 35.4b Many cases of early flexor synovitis can be treated nonsurgically with antibiotics, elevation, immobilization, and pain-guided healing (Lalonde, Canada).[2]

TIPS AND TRICKS FOR PERFORMING INFECTION SURGERY WITH THE WIDE AWAKE APPROACH IN THE EMERGENCY DEPARTMENT

- One of the first things Dr Lalonde does after he meets the patient is to inject the palmar and then the dorsal with anesthesia as in ▶ Video 35.1. This gives the local anesthesia at least 30 minutes to work while he gets the rest of the history, does the paperwork, teaches the patient, and builds an immobilization splint.

- Teach the patient about the importance of immobilization and elevation. He tells them, "We did not spend 2 billion years evolving pain because it is bad for us. It is your body's only way to say to you: 'Don't move and don't let the hand down by your side! You are helping the germs when you do that!'" He tells them to try to get off all pain medicine as soon as possible so they can hear their body tell them when it is safe to put the hand down and to move with pain-guided healing.

- We can wash very dirty hand injuries in the emergency department with tap water in the sink after numbing the hand. There is level I evidence that this is as effective as sterile saline.[4]

- Many cases of hand osteomyelitis can be managed with oral antibiotics instead of intravenous antibiotics.[5]

ADVANTAGES OF WALANT VERSUS SEDATION AND TOURNIQUET FOR COMPARTMENT SYNDROME RELEASE

- Compartment syndrome release in the emergency department avoids the transfer time to the main operating room, as well as induction of general anesthesia time.

- Patients with other medical or surgical comorbidities are spared the need for general anesthesia.

SPECIFICS OF MINIMALLY PAINFUL INJECTION OF LOCAL ANESTHETIC FOR COMPARTMENT SYNDROME RELEASE

- Local anesthesia injection should barely hurt at all if you follow the simple rules of Chapter 5 for hints to minimize injection pain. The patients will think you are magical.

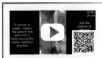

Video 35.5 How to inject local anesthesia for compartment syndrome release of the forearm (Lalonde, Canada).

- We inject the anesthetic solution a minimum of 30 minutes before surgery to allow the epinephrine to take optimal effect and provide an adequately dry working field.

- We inject supine patients on stretchers in a waiting area to decrease the risk of their fainting (see Chapter 6).

- Prepare 400 mL of 0.25% lidocaine with 1:400,000 epinephrine with 50 mL of 1% lidocaine with 1:100,000 epinephrine and 5 mL of 8.4% bicarbonate as described in Chapter 4.

- Start with 10-mL syringes on each of the volar and then dorsal compartment release incisions proximally.

- Always inject proximal to distal.

- Then use 20-mL syringes with 25-gauge, 1.5-inch needles. *Blow slow before you go…* (as in Chapter 5 for minimal pain injection). Alternate between volar and dorsal back to volar back to dorsal to give the local anesthesia time to numb the needle reinsertion sites.

Video 35.6 Compartment syndrome releases of the forearm in minor procedure room (Lalonde, Canada).

Video 35.7 Compartment syndrome releases of the forearm (Akbulut, Turkey).

Video 35.8 Local anesthetic injection and surgery for acute compartment syndrome release in coronary care unit after stenting of axillary artery thrombosis after cardiac arrest and no blood flow to upper extremity for 4 hours (Lalonde, Canada).

HOW AND WHERE TO INJECT THE LOCAL ANESTHETIC FOR TIBIAL HEMATOMA DRAINAGE

Video 35.9
Tibial hematoma anesthesia and drainage with 80 mL of 0.5% lidocaine with 1:200,000 epinephrine (Lalonde, Canada).

- Local anesthesia injection should barely hurt at all if you follow the simple rules of Chapter 5 for hints to minimize injection pain. The patients will think you are magical. Always inject proximal to distal.

- Start with 20 mL at the upper border of the hematoma just under the skin.

- Only reinsert needles in areas clearly inside 1 cm of the white vasoconstricted border of skin.

- Inject another 20 mL on the medial side of the hematoma subcutaneously.

- Inject another 20 mL on the lateral side of the hematoma subcutaneously.

- Keep alternating medial and lateral injection until you have firm palpable local anesthesia solution all around the hematoma.

- Finally inject the last 20 mL inside the hematoma at the level of the tibia.

- Give the local anesthesia 30 minutes to work and then evacuate the hematoma.

- We either put a vacuum-assisted closure (VAC) device on it or treat it with daily shower, Vaseline on a gauze, and Coban wrap until it is healed, in the same way Dr Lalonde treats fingertip amputations and other wounds with secondary healing, daily shower, Vaseline, and Coban tape dressing.[6,7]

References

1. Harper CM, Dowlatshahi AS, Rozental TD. Challenging dogma: optimal treatment of the "fight bite". Hand (N Y) 2020;15(5):647–650
2. DiPasquale AM, Krauss EM, Simpson A, Mckee DE, Lalonde DH. Cases of early infectious flexor tenosynovitis treated non-surgically with antibiotics, immobilization, and elevation. Plast Surg (Oakv) 2017;25(4):272–274
3. Lovely LM, Chishti YZ, Woodland JL, Lalonde DH. How much volume of local anesthesia and how long should you wait after injection for an effective wrist median nerve block? Hand (N Y) 2018;13(3):281–284
4. Moscati RM, Mayrose J, Reardon RF, Janicke DM, Jehle DV. A multicenter comparison of tap water versus sterile saline for wound irrigation. Acad Emerg Med 2007;14(5):404–409
5. Kargel JS, Sammer DM, Pezeshk RA, Cheng J. Oral antibiotics are effective for the treatment of hand osteomyelitis in children. Hand (N Y) 2020;15(2):220–223
6. Krauss EM, Lalonde DH. Secondary healing of fingertip amputations: a review. Hand (N Y) 2014;9(3):282–288
7. Janis JE, Kwon RK, Lalonde DH. A practical guide to wound healing. Plast Reconstr Surg 2010;125(6):230e–244e

CHAPTER 36

FINGER JOINT ARTHROPLASTY, FUSION, AND LIGAMENT REPAIR

Donald H. Lalonde, Amanda Higgins, Jason Wong, Chye Yew Ng, Xavier Gueffier, Thomas Apard, and Asif Ilyas

ADVANTAGES OF WALANT VERSUS SEDATION AND TOURNIQUET IN ARTHROPLASTY AND FUSION OF THE PROXIMAL INTERPHALANGEAL (PIP) JOINT

- All of the general advantages listed in Chapter 2 apply to both the surgeon and the patient (no nausea, no tourniquet pain or let-down bleeding, decreased cost without sedation in minor procedure room, safer surgery without sedation, etc.).[1]

- If you choose a dorsal approach in arthroplasty, you can see that you have repaired the extensor mechanism properly to get the best possible active extension without rupture of the repair. You watch the patient take the finger through a comfortable pain-free range of motion before skin closure. Sometimes the closing sutures in the extensor tendon will burst with intraoperative testing of full flexion and extension of the PIP joint. It is better to know and fix it before you close the skin so that a boutonniere deformity does not develop later.

- In fusion, the patient gets to help choose the final angle after seeing the joint move with temporary K-wire fixation.

- With intraoperative teaching and the nonsedated patients' ability to observe and remember the intraoperative movement, they will have a realistic expectation of the best possible outcome of range of movement when they leave the operating room.

- You are sure that the active movement motion is optimal by adjusting the extensor mechanism and PIP joint before closing the wound.

WHERE TO INJECT THE LOCAL ANESTHETIC FOR PIP JOINT ARTHROPLASTY AND FUSION

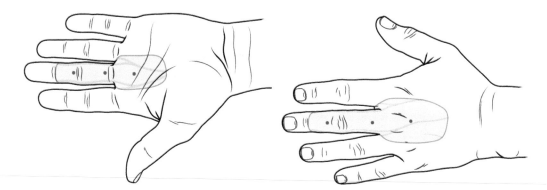

Fig. 36.1 (a) Palmar injections: Inject 5 to 10 mL of 1% lidocaine with 1:100,000 epinephrine (buffered with 0.5–1.0 mL of 8.4% sodium bicarbonate) in the most proximal red injection point on the palmar side. Do the most proximal dorsal injection next, and then inject 2 mL in the middle of each of the palmar proximal and middle phalanges in the subcutaneous fat. **(b)** Dorsal injections: Inject 4 to 5 mL of 1% lidocaine with 1:100,000 epinephrine (buffered with 0.4–0.5 mL of 8.4% sodium bicarbonate) in the proximal red injection dot on the dorsal hand. Do the two palmar injections next, and then inject 2 mL in the middle of each of the dorsal proximal and middle phalanges in the subcutaneous fat.

SPECIFICS OF MINIMALLY PAINFUL INJECTION OF LOCAL ANESTHETIC IN PIP JOINT ARTHROPLASTY

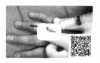

Video 36.1
Proximal interphalangeal (PIP) arthroplasty and fusion injection of local anesthesia (Lalonde, Canada).

- Local anesthesia injection should barely hurt at all if you follow the simple rules of Chapter 5 for hints to minimize injection pain. The patients will think you are magical.

- Inject just under the skin. There is no need to inject into the sheath. It would only add unnecessary pain. The local anesthetic will diffuse into the sheath.

- Inject the anesthetic solution a minimum of 30 minutes before surgery to allow the epinephrine to take optimal effect and provide an adequately dry working field as outlined in Chapter 4 and Chapter 14.

- We inject supine patients lying down on stretchers to decrease the risk of their fainting (see Chapter 6).

- To minimize the pain of injection, start with a fine 27- or 30-gauge needle (not a 25 gauge).

- In this operation, inject 4 mL in the most proximal red dot injection point of the palm first, and then inject 4 mL in the most proximal red dot injection point of the dorsal hand after that. This will give at least a little time for the distal injection points to numb up before you inject them.

- The distal injections are for the epinephrine vasoconstriction effect, since the skin is already numb from the proximal nerve blocks.

INJECTION OF LOCAL ANESTHETIC IN DISTAL INTERPHALANGEAL (DIP) FUSION

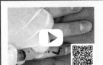

Video 36.2 Distal interphalangeal (DIP) fusion injection of local anesthesia (Lalonde, Canada).

TIPS AND TRICKS FOR PERFORMING INTERPHALANGEAL JOINT ARTHROPLASTY AND FUSION WITH THE WIDE AWAKE APPROACH

- Consider performing all hand surgery operations standing so you can easily walk around the table and ensure that the reconstructed finger looks good when flexing and extending from all positions.

- After implant placement or fusion, get the patient to take the fingers through a full range of motion. You may want to adjust the bone to improve the movement you see before you repair the soft tissues.

- After tendon closure, ask the patient to take the fingers through a full range of motion. You may want to adjust the extensor tendon closure to improve the movement you see before you let the patient leave the operating room.

- If you have patients take part in selecting the final angle of fusion, they may be more likely to be satisfied with the result. You can ask for their opinion after inserting temporary K-wires and having them see their resulting movement.

- If you use K-wires for fusion, you can educate the patient about pain-guided healing and movement after surgery to decrease the risk of infections around the K-wires.

- Patients need to look at the fingers to get them to move, because they cannot feel the numbed finger. You need to take down drapes so they can see their fingers. Although most patients do not mind looking at the wound, you can cover the wound with a towel as the patient flexes all fingers together while looking at them.

- Many patients are interested in looking at the opened finger to understand the nature of their problem. You can put a mask on the patients and show them the tendons and joint. Have them watch their finger move. They will remember how well it works, and this will motivate them to achieve the same movement with therapy.

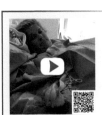

Video 36.3 Proximal interphalangeal (PIP) arthroplasty surgery (Lalonde, Canada).

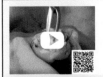

Video 36.4 Distal interphalangeal (DIP) fusion surgery (Lalonde, Canada).

Video 36.5 Patient chooses final angle of distal interphalangeal (DIP) fusion during the surgery (Lalonde, Canada).

- Close the skin with buried intradermal simple interrupted 5-0 Monocryl sutures as shown in detail for carpal tunnel closure in ▶ Video 26.9. Buried simple interrupted sutures of absorbable monofilament Monocryl mean that there are no sutures to remove.

- Surgeon's intraoperative patient education about postoperative care to avoid complications is ideal in all WALANT operations.

Video 36.6
Intraoperative
education
to decrease
complications
after distal
interphalangeal
(DIP) fusion
surgery (Lalonde,
Canada).

Video 36.7
Volar plate
reconstruction
to correct swan
neck deformity
(Ng, England).
Also see Videos
21.13–21.15 for
more swan neck
reconstruction
options.

Video 36.8
Volar plate
reconstruction
(Wong, England).

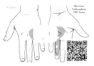

Video 36.9
Proximal
interphalangeal
(PIP) arthroplasty
revision (Gueffier,
France).

Video 36.10
Proximal
interphalangeal
(PIP) prosthesis
arthroplasty
(Apard, France).

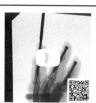

Video 36.11 Distal
interphalangeal
(DIP) fusion (Ilyas,
USA).

THERAPY TIPS FOR INTERPHALANGEAL JOINT ARTHROPLASTY

- We get our patients to elevate and immobilize their hand for 3 to 5 days after surgery. This decreases the risk of bleeding in the wound after surgery as blood clots generate more scar. It also allows the swelling to come down to facilitate movement. It permits patients to get off all pain medication to allow pain-guided therapy after surgery. This movement delay does not significantly add to scar formation because collagen formation does not start until day 3.

- We start relative motion flexion splinting for our dorsal approach PIP joint arthroplasty patients at 3 to 5 days after surgery with pain-guided therapy if they are off all pain medication. They carry this on for a month or two after the surgery to let the extensor mechanism heal while the tissues are gliding.

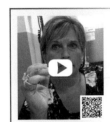

Video 36.TT1
Postoperative proximal interphalangeal (PIP) arthroplasty therapy (Lalonde, Canada).

Reference

1. Gunasagaran J, Sean ES, Shivdas S, Amir S, Ahmad TS. Perceived comfort during minor hand surgeries with wide awake local anaesthesia no tourniquet (WALANT) versus local anaesthesia (LA)/tourniquet. J Orthop Surg (Hong Kong) 2017;25(3):2309499017739499

CHAPTER 37

THUMB METACARPOPHALANGEAL JOINT FUSION AND ULNAR COLLATERAL LIGAMENT REPAIR

Donald H. Lalonde, Elisabet Hagert, Jean Paul Brutus, Paul Sibley, Amir Adham Ahmad, Xavier Gueffier, and Thomas Apard

ADVANTAGES OF WALANT VERSUS SEDATION AND TOURNIQUET IN THUMB METACARPOPHALANGEAL JOINT FUSION

- All of the general advantages listed in Chapter 2 apply to both the surgeon and the patient (no nausea, no tourniquet pain or let-down bleeding, decreased cost without sedation, safer surgery without sedation, etc.).[1]

- You can walk around the operating table and assess how the thumb looks with patient's active movement after you fix the metacarpophalangeal (MP) joint with temporary K-wires. You and the patient can compare the active movement of the K-wired thumb to the normal thumb on the other hand.

- Patients can participate in choosing the final angle of fixation, because you can reposition the K-wires if you choose to do so.

- Both you and the patient leave the operating room with realistic expectations of final possible thumb active movement.

- You get to assess the stability of your fixation with active movement to feel better about not inserting a trans-MP articular K-wire with ulnar collateral ligament (UCL) repair.

- Patients get to see that the thumb will be able to move before the skin is closed. They know that all can work well once they get past the postoperative discomfort and stiffness. They will be motivated to regain the movement they saw in the operating room.

ADVANTAGES OF WALANT VERSUS SEDATION AND TOURNIQUET IN UCL REPAIR

- You can check the stability of the reconstructed MP joint by observing active movement during the surgery.

- You can check the stability of implants with active movement if you have inserted one.

- You can make sure that MP and interphalangeal (IP) thumb active movement is optimal after you reconstruct the adductor aponeurosis.

WHERE TO INJECT THE LOCAL ANESTHETIC FOR THUMB MP JOINT FUSION AND UCL REPAIR

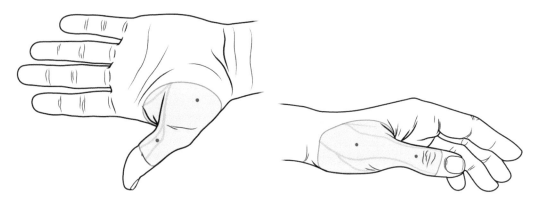

Fig. 37.1 and Fig. 37.2 Injection of the hand for thumb metacarpophalangeal (MP) joint fusion and ulnar collateral ligament (UCL) repair. *Volar injection*: Inject 12 mL of 1% lidocaine with 1:100,000 epinephrine (buffered with 10 mL lido/epi:1 mL of 8.4% sodium bicarbonate). *Dorsal injection*: Inject 12 mL of 1% lidocaine with 1:100,000 epinephrine (buffered with 10 mL lido/epi:1 mL of 8.4% sodium bicarbonate).

SPECIFICS OF MINIMALLY PAINFUL INJECTION OF LOCAL ANESTHETIC IN THESE OPERATIONS

Video 37.1 Local anesthetic injection for thumb metacarpophalangeal (MP) fusion (see surgery for this patient in Video 37.3) (Lalonde, Canada).

- ▶ Video 37.1 shows injection of local anesthetic for thumb MP fusion. (See the surgery for this patient in ▶ Video 37.3.)

- Local anesthesia injection should barely hurt at all if you follow the simple rules of Chapter 5 for hints to minimize injection pain. The patients will think you are magical.

- Inject 10 mL of the mixture under the skin on each of the volar and dorsal sides of the middle of the thumb metacarpal. Then inject 2 mL under the skin on each of the volar and dorsal sides of the middle of the thumb proximal phalanx.

- We inject the anesthetic solution a minimum of 30 minutes before surgery to allow the epinephrine to take optimal effect and provide an adequately dry working field as outlined in Chapter 4.

- We inject supine patients lying down on stretchers in a waiting area before they come into the operating room to decrease the risk of their fainting (see Chapter 6).

- In this operation, inject the first 10 mL in the most proximal part of the palmar thumb first, and then inject the next 10 mL in the most proximal part of the dorsal thumb right after that. Follow with the distal injections on the palmar and dorsal proximal phalanx, which are for the epinephrine vasoconstriction effect.

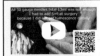

Video 37.2 Local anesthetic injection for thumb ulnar collateral ligament (UCL) repair (Lalonde, Canada).

TIPS AND TRICKS FOR PERFORMING THESE OPERATIONS WITH THE WIDE AWAKE APPROACH

- Have the patient look at the thumb to verify that he or she feels the position is good and that the thumb is straight after inserting temporary K-wires. If you or the patient does not like the position after watching the thumb move, simply remove and replace the K-wires after adjusting the fusion position.

- Have the patient move the other thumb and compare the two thumbs moving.

- Patients need to look at their thumb to get it to move, since they cannot feel the numbed thumb. Although most patients do not mind looking at the wound, you can cover the wound with a towel as they move the thumb if this seems appropriate.

- Consider performing MP fusion while standing instead of sitting so you can easily walk around the table and ensure that the fused or reconstructed thumb looks good flexing and extending from all positions.

- Close the skin with buried intradermal simple interrupted 5-0 Monocryl sutures as shown in detail for carpal tunnel closure in ▶ Video 26.9. Buried simple interrupted sutures of absorbable monofilament Monocryl mean that there are no sutures to remove.

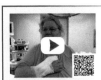

Video 37.3 Thumb metacarpophalangeal (MP) fusion of the patient in Video 37.1 (Lalonde, Canada).

Video 37.4 Thumb ulnar collateral ligament (UCL) repair surgery (Lalonde, Canada).

Video 37.5 Another thumb ulnar collateral ligament (UCL) repair without fixation of the ligament surgery. If you put both ends of the ligament inside the joint, they will heal without fixation (Lalonde, Canada).

Video 37.6 Making the diagnosis of complete ulnar collateral ligament (UCL) tear (Stener's lesion) with ultrasound and clinical examination (Lalonde, Canada).

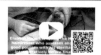

Video 37.7
Hairdresser
assesses and veri-
fies the ideal new
fusion position of
his metacarpo-
phalangeal (MP)
using his sterilized
scissors during
surgery (Hagert,
Sweden).

Video 37.8 Ulnar
collateral ligament
(UCL) repair with
internal brace.
Stability with
active movement
supports no need
for K-wire meta-
carpophalangeal
(MP) joint fixation
(Sibley, USA).

Video 37.9 Ulnar
collateral ligament
(UCL) repair with
internal brace
(Gueffier, France).

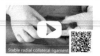

Video 37.10 Ulnar
collateral ligament
(UCL) repair with
bone anchors
(Apard, France).

Video 37.11 Radial
collateral ligament
repair (Ahmad,
Malaysia).

Video 37.12
Metacarpophalan-
geal (MP) fusion:
patient can see
interphalangeal
(IP) flexes and
extends at end of
surgery (Brutus,
Canada).

Reference

1. Takagi T, Watanabe M. Ulnar collateral ligament reconstruction of thumb metacarpophalangeal joint with adductor pollicis tendon using the wide-awake approach. J Hand Surg Am 2019;44(5):426.e1–426.e5

CHAPTER 38

TRAPEZIECTOMY WITH OR WITHOUT LIGAMENT RECONSTRUCTION FOR THUMB BASAL JOINT ARTHRITIS

Donald H. Lalonde, Julian Escobar, Xavier Gueffier, Thomas Apard, Jean Paul Brutus, Peter C. Amadio, and Geoffrey Cook

ADVANTAGES OF WALANT VERSUS SEDATION AND TOURNIQUET IN TRAPEZIECTOMY

- All of the general advantages listed in Chapter 2 apply to both the surgeon and the patient (no nausea, no tourniquet pain or let-down bleeding, decreased cost without sedation, safer surgery without sedation, etc.).[1]

- Many patients with thumb arthritis are older patients with medical comorbidities, which can be a problem when you sedate patients. It is safer for these patients to have no sedation. They just get up and go home after surgery, like when they have had a filling at the dentist.

- You can hear the thumb move through a full active range of motion after you remove the trapezium. You will sometimes hear remaining osteophytes grinding through the open wound with active movement. You can then find and remove them.

- After you remove the trapezium, you can see whether the base of the metacarpal impinges on the scaphoid when you ask the patient to move the thumb all around. If it does, you can then add a ligament reconstruction in any way that you choose—with the abductor pollicis longus (APL), flexor carpi radialis (FCR), sutures, tightrope, and so on. After the suspension or ligament repair, you can verify that the reconstruction is keeping the metacarpal away from the scaphoid when you ask the patient to move the thumb again before you close the skin.

- ▶ Video 38.1 discusses intraoperative decision-making about simple trapeziectomy versus a ligament reconstruction and tendon interposition (LRTI) based on what you see with active movement. (Also see the videos in the Tips and Tricks for Performing a Trapeziectomy with the Wide Awake Approach section of this chapter showing both impinging and nonimpinging metacarpals.)

- Movement without impingement after the trapeziectomy may help you to decide to stop there and close the skin without ligament reconstruction.

Video 38.1
Intraoperative decision-making about ligament reconstruction based on active movement (Lalonde, Canada).

- After you finish with the basal joint work, you can assess the position and active movement of the thumb metacarpophalangeal (MP) joint. If the MP joint is still hyperextending, you can surgically correct that if you choose to while the patient's hand is numbed. You can then ask the patient to move the thumb again after whichever MP joint surgery you choose. You can be sure both the basal and MP joints are actively moving well before you close the skin.

- Patients get to see that the thumb will be able to move through a full range of motion before you close the skin. They know that all can work well once they get past the postoperative discomfort and stiffness.[2,3,4,5]

WHERE TO INJECT THE LOCAL ANESTHETIC FOR A TRAPEZIECTOMY

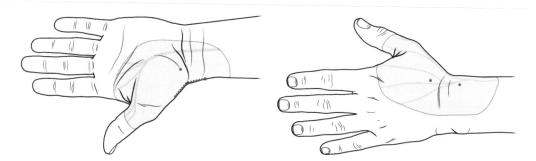

Fig. 38.1 and Fig. 38.2 Inject a mixture of 50 mL of saline solution plus 50 mL of 1% lidocaine with 1:100,000 epinephrine (buffered with 5 mL lido/epi:1 mL of 8.4% sodium bicarbonate). Injection of 50 to 70 mL usually suffices for simple trapeziectomy with or without abductor pollicis longus (APL) ligament reconstruction. Be sure to inject 10 mL under the volar forearm fascia to bathe the median nerve without eliciting paresthesias. You can start with 20 to 40 mL of local anesthetic along the volar forearm incision from proximal to distal if you are performing flexor carpi radialis (FCR) ligament reconstruction as in ▶ Fig. 38.3.

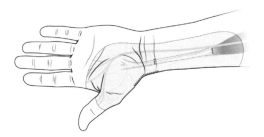

Fig. 38.3 If you are using flexor carpi radialis (FCR) for ligament reconstruction, start injections in the proximal volar forearm 2 cm above where you will be dissecting. Injecting 20 to 30 mL over the FCR tendon 30 minutes before cutting will numb this area nicely.

SPECIFICS OF MINIMALLY PAINFUL INJECTION OF LOCAL ANESTHETIC IN A TRAPEZIECTOMY

- ▶ Video 38.5 shows cannula injection of local anesthetic for a trapeziectomy with a 40-mm-long, blunt-tipped, 25-gauge cannula in a hole made with a 20-gauge needle (also see Chapter 5).

- Local anesthesia injection should barely hurt at all if you follow the simple rules of Chapter 5 for hints to minimize injection pain. The patients will think you are magical. For example, inject with a long 27-gauge needle and pinch the skin into the needle to add sensory "noise" of pressure to decrease the pain.

- Always err on the side of too much local anesthesia instead of not enough. You are aiming for patients only feeling a small sting when you insert the first local anesthesia needle. They should feel no pain for the rest of the injections or during the surgery.

- We inject the anesthetic solution a minimum of 30 minutes before surgery to allow the epinephrine to take optimal effect and provide an adequately dry working field, as outlined in Chapter 3 and Chapter 4.

- We inject supine patients lying down on stretchers in a waiting area to decrease the risk of their fainting (see ▶ Video 6.1).

- Start by injecting 10 mL of the mixture under the skin at the proximal trapeziectomy incision red dot injection point without moving the needle. Let the local anesthesia diffuse where it wants to go in a painless fashion.

- After the first 10 mL, inject another 10 mL on the dorsal side of the trapezium, staying near the metacarpal base.

- After the second 10 mL on the dorsal side, inject another 10 mL on the volar side of the trapezium, staying near the metacarpal base.

- Always alternate from dorsal to volar and back. This gives the local time to work before you reinsert the needle so it does not hurt. After the third 10 mL on the volar side, inject a fourth 10 mL slowly between the thumb and index metacarpal bases going from the dorsal articulation to the volar side where the metacarpals meet the trapezium, staying near the bone.

- Finally, distract (pull on) the thumb and inject 5 mL into the basal metacarpal trapezial joint. This last 5 mL can also be injected into the joint capsule under direct vision after the skin incision during the surgery.

- If performing an LRTI with the flexor carpi radialis, inject 20 to 40 mL of the mixture from proximal to distal so there is at least 2 cm of visible or palpable local anesthetic beyond everywhere you will dissect.

- If performing an LRTI with the abductor pollicis longus, you may need another 10 mL of the mixture over the proximal APL so there is at least 2 cm of visible or palpable local anesthetic outside of everywhere you will dissect. In ▶ Video 38.5, an APL reconstruction, no further local anesthetic was needed after the original 50 mL.

Video 38.2 Real-time 8-minute injection of a patient for trapeziectomy and abductor pollicis longus (APL) ligament reconstruction (surgery in ▶ Video 38.6) (Lalonde, Canada).

Video 38.3 How to inject local anesthesia for basal joint arthroplasty (accelerated to 1 minute) (same patient as 38.2 but on her other hand) (Lalonde, Canada).

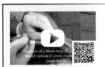

Video 38.4 Cannula injection of local anesthetic for a trapeziectomy (Lalonde, Canada).

TIPS AND TRICKS FOR PERFORMING A TRAPEZIECTOMY WITH THE WIDE AWAKE APPROACH

- Patients must look at the thumb to get it to move, because they cannot feel the numbed thumb. Although most patients don't mind looking at the wound, you can cover the wound with a towel as they move the thumb if they do mind looking at it (see ▶ Video 38.1).

- If you see the thumb metacarpal impinging on the scaphoid, you can perform a ligament reconstruction, as in the APL reconstruction in ▶ Video 38.5.

- Close the skin with buried intradermal simple interrupted 5-0 Monocryl sutures as shown in detail for carpal tunnel closure in ▶ Video 26.9. Buried simple interrupted sutures of absorbable monofilament Monocryl mean that there are no sutures to remove.

Video 38.5 Ligament reconstruction with abductor pollicis longus (APL) in the patient injected in ▶ Video 38.2 (Lalonde, Canada).

Video 38.6 Flexor carpi radialis (FCR) ligament reconstruction (Gueffier, France).

Video 38.7 Simple trapeziectomy rescue after failed fusion of trapeziometacarpal joint (Escobar, Columbia).

Video 38.8 Tendon transfer of extensor indicis (EI) to extensor pollicis longus (EPL) and trapezial implant reconstruction (Apard, France).

Video 38.9 Making sure the implant is stable in implant basal joint arthroplasty (Brutus, Canada).

Video 38.10 Intraoperative X-ray video fluoroscopy of active movement compared to 6 months postoperative video fluoroscopy of same patient where no ligament reconstruction was required (Lalonde, Canada).

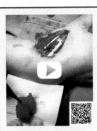

Video 38.11
Trapeziectomy
involving bony
giant cell tumor
in ASA3 patient
(Escobar,
Columbia).

Video 38.12
Severe deformity
treated by simple
trapeziectomy
(Escobar,
Columbia).

Video 38.13
Veterinary
surgeon's
impression of
surgery (entire
local injection and
surgery of her case
available at open
access reference[2])
(Lalonde, Canada).

- Many patients are interested in looking at the joint to understand the nature of their problem. You can put a mask on the patient's face and show him or her the joint move. Many patients love this. Some patients will tell others it is something they need to put on their bucket list!

References

1. Larsen LP, Hansen TB. Total trapeziometacarpal joint arthroplasty using wide awake local anaesthetic no tourniquet. J Hand Surg Eur Vol 2021;46(2):125–130
2. Farhangkhoee H, Lalonde J, Lalonde DH. Wide-awake trapeziectomy: video detailing local anesthetic injection and surgery. Hand (N Y) 2011;6(4):466–467
3. Mckee D, Lalonde D. Wide awake trapeziectomy for thumb basal joint arthritis. Plast Reconstr Surg Glob Open 2017;5(8):e1435
4. Takagi T, Weiss AC. Suture suspension arthroplasty with trapeziectomy for thumb carpometacarpal arthritis using a wide-awake approach. Tech Hand Up Extrem Surg 2020;24(2):66–70
5. Teo I, Lam W, Muthayya P, Steele K, Alexander S, Miller G. Patients' perspective of wide-awake hand surgery—100 consecutive cases. J Hand Surg Eur Vol 2013;38(9):992–999

CHAPTER 39

WRIST ARTHROSCOPY

Elisabet Hagert, Celso R. Folberg, Chris Chun-Yu Chen, and Donald H. Lalonde

ADVANTAGES OF WALANT VERSUS SEDATION AND TOURNIQUET IN WRIST ARTHROSCOPY

- All of the general advantages listed in Chapter 2 apply to both the surgeon and the patient (no nausea, no tourniquet pain or let-down bleeding, decreased cost without sedation, safer surgery without sedation, etc.).

- Watching an awake patient move the wrist during WALANT wrist arthroscopy and seeing the bones move actively provide information not available from magnetic resonance imaging (MRI) or from a sedated patient. It can be more useful as both a diagnostic and a therapeutic tool.

- Intraoperative active motion of the wrist can give you better information about the degree of ligament injury in situations such as a scapholunate or lunotriquetral injury. A cooperative, pain-free patient provides an "active" Geissler evaluation.[1]

- By performing dry or wet wrist arthroscopy using WALANT, patients can participate in the diagnosis and decision-making. This enhances their ability to take an active part in their treatment.

- You do not infuse water into the joint in dry wrist arthroscopy. This has advantages that make it valuable in diagnostic arthroscopy.[2] WALANT works well for this technique. The advantage with WALANT in dry arthroscopy is that detailed imaging of the wrist may be obtained to both diagnose and educate the patient during surgery.

WHERE TO INJECT THE LOCAL ANESTHETIC FOR WRIST ARTHROSCOPY

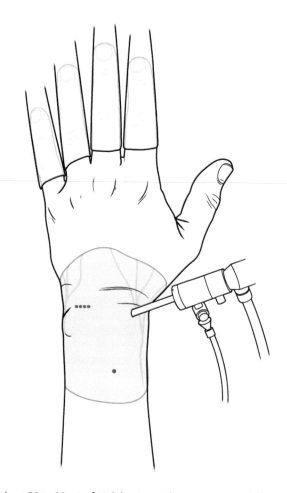

Fig. 39.1 Inject at least 20 to 30 mL of 1% lidocaine with 1:100,000 (available in North America) or 1:200,000 (available in Sweden) epinephrine (buffered with 10 mL lido/epi:1 mL of 8.4% sodium bicarbonate). Note that higher concentration of epinephrine will increase the hemostatic effect and prolong the duration of anesthesia (see Chapter 4).

SPECIFICS OF MINIMAL PAIN INJECTION OF LOCAL ANESTHETIC IN WRIST ARTHROSCOPY

- Local anesthesia injection should barely hurt at all if you follow the simple rules of Chapter 5 for hints to minimize injection pain. The patients will think you are magical.

- It is important to block the nerve branches innervating the dorsal wrist capsule so you can access the portals without pain.

- We inject patients lying down on stretchers in a waiting area before they come into the operating room to decrease the risk of their fainting (see ▸ Video 6.1).

- Slowly infiltrate at least 20 to 30 mL of buffered lidocaine with epinephrine to the dorsal aspect of the wrist to block the sensory branches of the radial, ulnar, and posterior interosseous nerves.[1] The infiltration should cover the area from the level of Lister's tubercle to the carpometacarpal joints.

- The goal of the injection is to bathe local anesthetic 2 cm beyond wherever you think you have even a small chance of dissecting in the wrist or forearm.

- To minimize the pain of injection, start with a 27-gauge needle (not a 25 gauge) in the most proximal red dot injection point.

- Ask the patient to look away. Press with a fingertip just proximal to the injection site before you put in the needle to add the sensory "noise" of pressure to decrease the pain.

- Insert the first needle perpendicularly into the subcutaneous fat. Stabilize the syringe with two hands and have your thumb ready on the plunger to avoid the pain of needle wobble until the skin needle site is numb. Inject the first visible 0.5-mL bleb and then pause. Wait 15 to 45 seconds until the patient tells you that all the needle pain is gone. Inject the rest of the first 10 mL slowly (over 2 minutes) without moving the needle.

- Reinsert the needle farther distally into skin that is within 1 cm of clearly vasoconstricted white skin that has functioning lidocaine and epinephrine so that needle reinsertion is pain-free.

- Continue injecting from proximal to distal, blowing the local anesthetic slowly ahead of the needle so that there is always at least 1 cm of visible or palpable local anesthetic ahead of the sharp needle tip the patient would feel if you advanced it into "live" nerves. "Blow slow before you go." (See Chapter 5 for further tips on how to inject local anesthetic with minimal pain.)

- Following the subcutaneous infiltration, inject at least 2 mL of lidocaine–epinephrine into the radiocarpal joint to ensure anesthesia of the volar wrist capsule should shaving manipulation of the joint proves necessary.

- A technique using portal site anesthesia alone has been described in which each portal is marked and injected with an average of 5 to 6 mL of local anesthetic.[3] Blocking the entire dorsal aspect of the wrist

Video 39.1 Portal site injection of local anesthesia for wrist arthroscopy combined with other procedures such as triangular fibrocartilage complex (TFCC) repair and distal radius fractures (Chen, Taiwan).

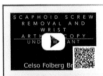

Video 39.2 Injection of local anesthesia for wrist arthroscopy and scaphoid screw removal (Folberg, Brazil).

ensures a pain-free procedure and retains the option to convert from arthroscopic to open surgery with good anesthesia and hemostasis.

- We seldom use volar wrist portals. If you plan to use these, you must infiltrate subcutaneous volar anesthetic as well.[4]

- If you are going to manipulate the palmar structures as well, you should inject an additional 10 mL under the forearm fascia between the median and ulnar nerves on the palmar side 1 cm proximal to the wrist crease.

TIPS AND TRICKS FOR PERFORMING WRIST ARTHROSCOPY WITH THE WIDE AWAKE APPROACH

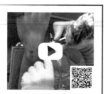

Video 39.3 Wrist arthroscopy (Hagert, Sweden).

- Patients will still have sensation in their fingers. We recommend plastic finger traps for wrist traction because the metal traps may be uncomfortable.

- Pad the upper arm to make it comfortable as well in the awake patient (▶ Video 39.1).

- Finger traction is not painful in itself; however, the patient will feel as though the fingers are cold and a little numb toward the end of the surgery. This will resolve as soon as the finger traps are removed.

- When arthroscopic shaving is done, the patient will feel the vibrations but will not feel pain. Explain this to your patient before you start shaving to reduce the patient's stress that may be caused by the sensation of vibrations.

References

1. Hagert E, Lalonde DH. Wide-awake wrist arthroscopy and open TFCC repair. J Wrist Surg 2012;1(1):55–60
2. del Piñal F. Dry arthroscopy and its applications. Hand Clin 2011;27(3):335–345
3. Ong MT, Ho PC, Wong CW, Cheng SH, Tse WL. Wrist arthroscopy under portal site local anesthesia (PSLA) without tourniquet. J Wrist Surg 2012;1(2):149–152
4. Slutsky DJ, Nagle DJ. Wrist arthroscopy: current concepts. J Hand Surg Am 2008;33(7):1228–1244

CHAPTER 40

WRIST ARTHRITIS SURGERY

Carlos Ramos de Pina and Donald H. Lalonde

ADVANTAGES OF WALANT VERSUS SEDATION AND TOURNIQUET IN WRIST ARTHRITIS SURGERY

- All of the general advantages listed in Chapter 2 apply to both the surgeon and the patient (no nausea, no tourniquet pain or let-down bleeding, decreased cost without sedation in minor procedure room, safer surgery without sedation, etc.).

- At the end of the case, patients can see the best possible range of active motion they can get after the reconstruction, so they leave the operating room with realistic expectations. They also have a visual goal of how much they might be able to move if they attend rehabilitation.

- Adjustments in the reconstruction to improve active movement of the wrist can be accomplished before the skin is closed as in the proximal row carpectomy case in ▶ Video 40.3.

WHERE TO INJECT THE LOCAL ANESTHETIC FOR WRIST ARTHRITIS SURGERY

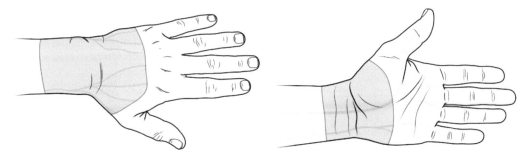

Fig. 40.1 and Fig. 40.2 Inject up to 80 to 100 mL of 0.5% lidocaine with 1:200,000 epinephrine (buffered with 5 mL of 8.4% sodium bicarbonate per 50 mL of 1% lidocaine with 1:100,000 epinephrine).

Video 40.1a
Injection of local anesthesia for wrist arthritis surgery (de Pina, Portugal).[1,2]

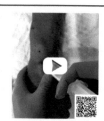

Video 40.1b
A second case injection of local anesthesia for wrist arthritis surgery narrated by the author (de Pina, Portugal).

SPECIFICS OF MINIMALLY PAINFUL INJECTION OF LOCAL ANESTHETIC FOR WRIST ARTHRITIS SURGERY

- Local anesthesia injection should barely hurt at all if you follow the simple rules of Chapter 5 for hints to minimize injection pain. The patients will think you are magical.

- Inject the anesthetic solution a minimum of 30 minutes before surgery to allow the epinephrine to take optimal effect and provide an adequately dry working field as outlined in Chapter 4. We inject patients outside the operating room before they come in.

- Always inject from proximal to distal to decrease the pain of local injection.

- Most patients will require about 80 mL to numb up the whole wrist, so you could prepare 100 mL of 0.5% lidocaine with 1:200,000 epinephrine to stay under 7 mg/kg of lidocaine with epinephrine.

- We start with 10 mL tumescent injection 7 cm proximal to radial styloid near the radial nerve, but always at least 5 mm away from it. Never elicit paresthesia which would mean possible nerve injury.

- Inject 10 mL of tumescent dorsal to Lister's tubercle and another 10 mL at the radius periosteal level ulnar to Lister's tubercle.

- Inject 5 to 10 mL dorsally above and in the capitolunate joint.

- Inject 8 to 10 mL dorsally above and in the radiocarpal joint.

- Inject 5 to 7 mL dorsally above and in midcarpal joint.

- We use 5 mL dorsally directly in contact with the capitate and triquetrum periosteum/bone.

- Using the same needle entry site as you do for the bone triquetral tumescence, inject 5 mL in the vicinity of the dorsal cutaneous branch of the ulnar nerve.

- Volar injection over the scaphoid tuberosity will be helpful in proximal row carpectomy or scaphoid reconstructions.

- If radius graft harvest is anticipated, such as in the case of partial carpal fusions, add an additional 5 to 10 mL of distal radial volar periosteal local anesthesia.

- We do not routinely have to perform median or ulnar nerve blocks with these procedures, but they may be helpful in some cases.

- We always inject all patients while they are lying down to decrease the risk of their fainting (see ▶ Video 6.1).

TIPS AND TRICKS FOR PERFORMING WRIST ARTHRITIS SURGERY WITH THE WIDE AWAKE APPROACH

- Expect some blood in the field at the beginning of the surgery; this is not bloodless tourniquet surgery. Suction may be helpful as you see in the videos.

- The patient needs to look at the hand to properly move the reconstructed wrist, since he or she cannot feel the numbed digit. Although most patients don't mind looking at the wound, you can cover the wound with a towel as the patient flexes all fingers together while looking at them. You need to take the sterile drape down so they can see their hand move.

- Close the skin with buried intradermal simple interrupted 5-0 Monocryl sutures as shown in detail for carpal tunnel closure in ▶ Video 26.9. Buried simple interrupted sutures of absorbable monofilament Monocryl mean that there are no sutures to remove.

- For longer procedures, patients may become uncomfortable lying on their back with their shoulder abducted, especially if they also have shoulder problems. Offer to the patients to lie on their side or partially on their side to give their shoulder relief. You will still see very well.

- Offer a restroom visit just before you take the patient into the operating room, so they have an empty bladder for comfort. We also do not give the patients intravenous fluid as they don't need it and it will only give them an urge to void.

- You can educate the patient about best postoperative activities during the local anesthetic injection, the surgery, and bandage application. This will serve to decrease your complication rate because your patients will understand why they should keep their hand elevated and how to take postoperative pain medications (see Chapter 8).

- These patients will be sore after surgery when the local anesthesia wears off. One of the best strategies to help postoperative pain is intraoperative education about keeping the hand elevated until all local anesthesia is worn off and until they are off all pain medications (Chapter 8). You can inject long-lasting local anesthesia such as bupivacaine or ropivacaine, but remember that there are problems with long-lasting agents (outlined in Chapter 4, Why Not Use Long-Acting Local Anesthetics Like Bupivacaine all the Time?).

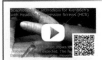

Video 40.2
Kienbock and scaphocapitate fusion (de Pina, Portugal).

Video 40.3
Proximal row carpectomy and triquetral osteochondral transfer to the capitate (de Pina, Portugal).

Video 40.4
Scaphoid excision, three corner fusion, and osteoplasty to improve active movement (de Pina, Portugal).

References

1. Ahmad AA, Yi LM, Ahmad AR. Plating of distal radius fracture using the wide-awake anesthesia technique. J Hand Surg Am 2018;43(11):1045.e1–1045.e5
2. Müller CT, Christen T, Heidekruger PI, et al. Wide-awake anesthesia no tour-niquet trapeziometacarpal joint prosthesis implantation. Plast Reconstr Surg Glob Open 2018;6(4):e1714

CHAPTER 41

FINGER FRACTURES

*Donald H. Lalonde, Lisa Flewelling, Geoffrey Cook,
Thomas Apard, Ahsan Akhtar, Chye Yew Ng,
Chris Chun-Yu Chen, Xavier Gueffier, Gökhan Tolga
Akbulut, and Amir Adham Ahmad*

ADVANTAGES OF WALANT VERSUS SEDATION AND TOURNIQUET FOR FINGER FRACTURE REDUCTION

- All of the general advantages listed in Chapter 2 apply to both the surgeon and the patient (no nausea, no tourniquet pain[1] or let-down bleeding, decreased cost without sedation in minor procedure room, safer surgery without sedation, etc.).

- One of the most important ways to decrease postoperative complications like stiffness is to educate the patient during the surgery. In WALANT patients, the education can start during the preparation of the wound before K-wire insertion.

- When you see full flexion and extension of the finger you have K-wired at surgery and see that your reduction is stable with fluoroscopy, you will feel a lot more comfortable about starting early protected movement for these fingers, just as in flexor tendon injuries.[2,3]

Video 41.1
Intraoperative patient education starts during local anesthesia injection or while prepping and draping of the patient.

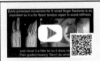

Video 41.2
Functionally stable fixation with K-wires tested with full-fist active flexion and extension at surgery permits pain-guided early protected movement at 3 to 5 days after surgery.

Video 41.3
The principles of functionally stable fixation and early protected movement of K-wired finger fractures to prevent postoperative stiffness in less than 2 minutes (Lalonde, Canada) (see Postoperative Therapy Tips after K- Wiring Finger Fractures for more details).

- You can see whether the K-wires are interrupting active finger movement by impinging on ligaments or tendons in their current location. You have the opportunity to change the K-wire location to optimize postoperative early active movement before the end of the operation.

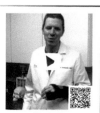

Video 41.4
Hand surgeon appreciates advantages of WALANT K-wiring of his own fractured finger in a hand surgeon's office (Domanski, USA).

- A major advantage of eliminating sedation for finger fractures is that you do not need to perform the reduction in the main operating room (see Chapter 10 and Chapter 16). If patients need internal fixation, you can perform closed reduction and K-wire insertion in minor procedure rooms in the clinic outside the main operating room Monday to Friday, 9 AM to 5 PM (see ▶ Video 41.3). You no longer need to do these at night to suit the main operating room and anesthesiologist's schedules. You are more likely to do better surgery with a clear head at 1 PM than when you are tired at 1 AM. You no longer have to admit patients to the hospital because of their medical comorbidities; these issues are only a problem when you use sedation.

Video 41.5
Augmented field sterility option for open reduction and K-wire fixation in a minor procedure room (Lalonde, Canada).

- Because you can perform these operations in minor procedure rooms outside the main operating room with either simple field sterility or augmented field sterility (see Chapter 10), your hand therapists can see how much active finger movement is possible during the surgery. You can discuss the safe early protected movement plan with therapists during and after the surgery (see Chapter 15).

- Patients have been looking at their fingers for many years. They can tell immediately if their crooked broken finger is straight after you reduced it or not.

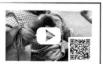

Video 41.6
Ask the patient if the K-wire reduced finger is still crooked or not. They will frequently know better than the surgeon if the finger is still crooked (final result in ▶ Video 41.TT6) (Lalonde, Canada).

WHERE TO INJECT THE LOCAL ANESTHETIC FOR FINGER FRACTURE REDUCTION

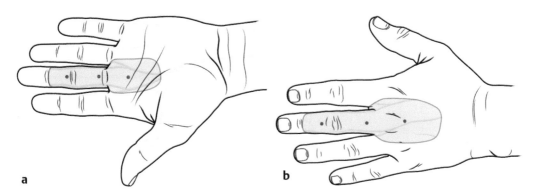

a   b

Fig. 41.1 (a) *Palmar injections*: Inject 5 to 10 mL of 1% lidocaine with 1:100,000 epinephrine (buffered with 0.5–1.0 mL of 8.4% sodium bicarbonate) in the most proximal red injection point on the palmar side. Do the most proximal dorsal injection next, and then inject 2 mL in the middle of each of the palmar proximal and middle phalanges in the subcutaneous fat. **(b)** *Dorsal injections*: Inject 4 to 5 mL of 1% lidocaine with 1:100,000 epinephrine (buffered with 0.4–0.5 mL of 8.4% sodium bicarbonate) in the proximal red injection dot on the dorsal hand. Do the two palmar injections next, and then inject 2 mL in the middle of each of the dorsal proximal and middle phalanges in the subcutaneous fat.

SPECIFICS OF MINIMALLY PAINFUL INJECTION OF LOCAL ANESTHETIC FOR FINGER FRACTURE REDUCTION

- Local anesthesia injection should barely hurt at all if you follow the simple rules of Chapter 5 for hints to minimize injection pain. The patients will think you are magical.

- Inject just under the skin. There is no need to inject into the sheath; this would only add unnecessary pain.

- Inject the anesthetic solution a minimum of 30 minutes before surgery to allow the epinephrine to take optimal effect and provide an adequately dry working field, as outlined in Chapter 4.

- Inject patients in a waiting area before they come into the procedure room to give the local anesthetic time to work (see Chapter 4 and Chapter 14).[4]

- We inject supine patients lying down on stretchers to decrease the risk of their fainting (see Chapter 6).

- If convenient, wait 15 to 30 minutes before injecting distally on the palmar side and dorsal sides so that the next two digital palmar and dorsal injections will not be painful. This waiting period can be used productively to see other patients.

- If you are only using K-wires for a percutaneous reduction and not cutting through the skin, it is still worth having epinephrine in the soft

Video 41.7
Minimal pain local anesthetic injections for proximal phalanx fractures (final result in ▶ Video 41.TT6) (Lalonde, Canada).

tissue around the bone you are K-wiring, even if that tissue is numb from proximal blocks. Epinephrine will provide less internal bleeding in the periosteal tissue, which means less callus and less scar for the patient to work through later.

TIPS AND TRICKS FOR PERFORMING FINGER FRACTURE REDUCTION WITH THE WIDE AWAKE APPROACH

- Patients need to look at their fingers or thumb to help them move the digit after you reduce the fracture, since they cannot feel the numbed digit move. Take down drapes so they can see the finger if you are asking them to move it. Although most patients do not mind looking at the wound, you can cover it with a towel as they flex and extend the tip of the finger or thumb.

- Take advantage of the fact that the patient is not sedated to give him or her clear instructions on postoperative activity. You can get better patient cooperation for postoperative hand elevation and care because the patient is able to listen and remember your advice right at the end of surgery. This can decrease your complication risk (see ▶ Video 41.8 and ▶ Video 41.9).

- See Chapter 8 for other videos on intraoperative advice for patients.

- You can test the stability of your internal fixation and the active mobility of the tendons and joints intraoperatively in complex malunion reduction cases (see ▶ Video 41.10).

- For comminuted intraarticular posterior interphalangeal (PIP) and metacarpophalangeal (MP) fractures that require distraction splinting, consider inserting K-wires for distraction splinting in the clinic. We have the therapists apply a banjo distraction splint while the patient's hand is still numb. You can then assess the joint in the splint with fluoroscopy while the patient is still numb, as in ▶ Video 41.13.

Video 41.8 Advice at the end of the surgery to decrease pain and other complications (final result in ▶ Video 41.TT6) (Lalonde, Canada).

Video 41.9 More advice at the end of the surgery to decrease pain and other complications in another patient (Lalonde, Canada).

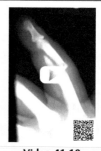

Video 41.10 A 4-week-old maluniting middle phalanx open reduction K-wire fixation (Lalonde, Canada).

Video 41.11 Posterior interphalangeal (PIP) fracture dislocation with distraction K-wires (Apard, France).

- Mallet fractures involving 50 to 60% of the joint but with congruous or parallel joint surfaces (not subluxated) can be treated with mallet splinting only.
- Not all fracture boutonnieres need surgery (see ▶ Video 41.20).

Video 41.12
Dynamic external fixation for posterior interphalangeal (PIP) fracture dislocation (Gueffier, France).

Video 41.13
Banjo splint for comminuted metacarpophalangeal (MP) and posterior interphalangeal (PIP) fractures (Lalonde, Canada).

Video 41.14
Checking active movement after plate fixation of proximal phalanx (Chen, Taiwan).

Video 41.15
Checking active movement after plate fixation of proximal phalanx (Ahmad, Malaysia).

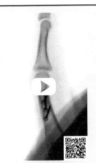

Video 41.16
Checking active movement after lag screw fixation (Ng, England).

Video 41.17 Mallet fracture dislocation reduction with K-wire (Cook, Canada).

Video 41.18 Not all mallet fracture dislocations in one-third of the joint need surgery (Lalonde, Canada).

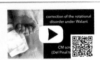

Video 41.19
Rotation osteotomy of middle phalanx: (1) insert centromedullary K-wire through both cortices, (2) insert screw into distal cortex, (3) remove screw, (4) laterodorsal approach osteotomy, and (5) replace screw (Apard, France).

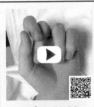

Video 41.20
Centromedullary screw after rotation osteotomy for maluniting proximal phalanx fracture (Apard, France).

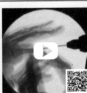

Video 41.21
Testing active movement for early protected movement after dorsal blocking K-wire for fracture dorsal dislocation of posterior interphalangeal (PIP) joint (Lalonde, Canada).

Video 41.22
Fracture boutonniere treated successfully only with a relative motion flexion splint and no surgery (Lalonde, Canada) (also see ▶ Video 54.10 for another example).

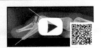

Video 41.23
Ultrasound and illustrated video of mallet fracture Ishiguro (Gueffier, France).

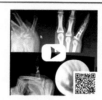

Video 41.24
Postoperative
movement
checking of
complex plates
and screws in
proximal phalanx
fracture (Tolga,
Turkey).

Video 41.25
Checking
movement after
three screws in
proximal phalanx
(Tolga, Turkey).

POSTOPERATIVE THERAPY TIPS AFTER K-WIRING FINGER FRACTURES

- Early protected movement in K-wired finger fractures is just as important as early protected movement in flexor tendon repair. We will show you how and why below.

- Education is key (see ▶ Video 41.1 and video below for how we educate patients before, during, and after surgery so they know how to behave properly after surgery to get a better result).

Video 41.TT1 Dr Lalonde starts early protected movement 4 days postoperatively in patient with K-wired proximal phalanx by explaining how this works (Lalonde, Canada).

Video 41.TT2 Dr Lalonde starts early protected movement 3 days postoperatively on a different patient with K-wired middle phalanx (Lalonde, Canada).

Video 41.TT3 Dr Lalonde starts early protected movement 4 days postoperatively for K-wiring of proximal phalanx fracture with advice on pain-guided therapy (final result in ▶ Video 41.TT6) (Lalonde, Canada).

Video 41.TT4 Patient advice 2 weeks after proximal phalanx K-wiring (Lalonde, Canada).

Video 41.TT5 How to tell if a K-wired fracture (or any finger fracture) is healed. When there is no pain on palpation of the fracture site (not pressing on the pins), the fracture is healed. When there is no pain on palpation of the fracture site, you can stop protective splinting. When there is no pain on palpation of the fracture site, you can remove the K-wires (Lalonde, Canada).

Video 41.TT6 Final resulting movement at 4 weeks after K-wire surgery and 1 week after K-wire removal (Lalonde, Canada).

Video 41.TT7 Closer look at the protective splint built for early protected movement for the same patient seen in ▶ Videos 41.1, 41.8, 41.TT3, 41.TT4, 41.TT5, 41.TT6, and 41.TT7 (Flewelling, Canada).

Video 41.TT8 We let this difficult unstable posterior interphalangeal (PIP) fracture get "sticky" for 2 weeks before starting pain-guided movement. We used a percutaneous K-wired guided bone clamp to reduce the fracture. Surgery and therapy (Lalonde, Canada).

- Education is key. See the above videos for examples of how we educate patients during and after surgery about the postoperative therapy plan to decrease stiffness and get better results.

- For the first 3 to 5 days after surgery, the K-wired hand is kept elevated and mostly immobilized. This permits time for the patient to get off all pain killers, so that he or she knows what hurts. This also lets the swelling to come down. It allows bleeding in the fracture site to stop to avoid adding more callus and scar which lead to stiffness. Totally avoiding pain killers and pain-guided movement will also prevent skin infection around K-wire sites.

- Teach your patient where their fracture site is.

- Ensure that patients understand they should not be taking pain medication.

- Teach your patient to do pain-free exercise, at least every hour. "Do little bits really often, using pain as your guide."

- Teach your patients that their daily activities should not cause pain in their fracture site.

- Educated patients feel confident they can do their exercises. They are empowered to own their therapy process.

- Learn about what activities your patients have to do during their day. This will help determine how much support they will need from their splint. The splint is mostly there to protect them during dangerous activity and while sleeping. We let them take it off to shower starting at 3 to 5 days after K-wiring.

- Knowing your patients' activity level lets you have honest discussions on when they can resume certain activities.

- At the first therapy visit, 3 to 5 days post K-wire or open reduction and internal fixation (ORIF), patients will probably find supported, isolated joint movements are easier to complete with no pain.

- Complex or multijoint movements such as interphalangeal tuck can begin as the patient's pain improves, typically at 10 to 14 days postoperatively.

- Exercises can be taught in or out of the splint.

- See Chapter 19 for more detailed similar therapy tips. The concepts of early protected movement for flexor tendon repair are like those of early protected movement for K-wired finger fractures.

References

1. Gunasagaran J, Sean ES, Shivdas S, Amir S, Ahmad TS. Perceived comfort during minor hand surgeries with wide awake local anaesthesia no tourniquet (WALANT) versus local anaesthesia (LA)/tourniquet. J Orthop Surg (Hong Kong) 2017;25(3):2309499017739499

2. Gregory S, Lalonde DH, Fung Leung LT. Minimally invasive finger fracture management: wide-awake closed reduction, K-wire fixation, and early protected movement. Hand Clin 2014;30(1):7–15

3. Jones NF, Jupiter JB, Lalonde DH. Common fractures and dislocations of the hand. Plast Reconstr Surg 2012;130(5):722e–736e

4. McKee DE, Lalonde DH, Thoma A, Glennie DL, Hayward JE. Optimal time delay between epinephrine injection and incision to minimize bleeding. Plast Reconstr Surg 2013;131(4):811–814

CHAPTER 42

METACARPAL FRACTURES

Shu Guo Xing, Susan Kean, Jin Bo Tang, Xavier Gueffier, Julian Escobar, Paul Sibley, Celso R. Folberg, Thomas Apard, Nikolas Alan Jagodzinski, Amir Adham Ahmad, and Donald H. Lalonde

ADVANTAGES OF WALANT VERSUS SEDATION AND TOURNIQUET IN REDUCTION AND INTERNAL FIXATION OF METACARPAL FRACTURES

- All of the general advantages listed in Chapter 2 apply to both the surgeon and the patient (no nausea, no tourniquet pain or let-down bleeding, decreased cost without sedation, safer surgery without sedation, etc.).

- You can see that you have solved the scissoring problem by watching your patient take the fingers through a full range of active motion before you close the skin.

- You can ask your patients if they think their scissoring is gone after you reduce the fracture. They can tell immediately if their fingers are crooked or not. They have been looking at those fingers their entire lives.

- Patients see the reduction of their bone on fluoroscopy. They watch themselves achieve a full range of flexion and extension of their fingers during the surgery. They remember this and know that this will be achievable if they stick with therapy and exercise after the surgery.

- You can educate wide awake patient during the operation to decrease the risk of postoperative complications.

- Patients can practice postoperative movement in a pain-free state during surgery.

- You can check the stability of the bone fixation with full flexion and extension during the surgery. This helps you to decide whether or not to allow early protected movement after surgery.[1]

Video 42.1 You can decrease postoperative complication rate with intraoperative education (Lalonde, Canada).

Video 42.2 You can watch the stability of the fracture on fluoroscopy with active movement to help determine suitability for early protected movement (Folberg, Brazil).

WHERE TO INJECT THE LOCAL ANESTHETIC FOR BENNETT'S FRACTURE

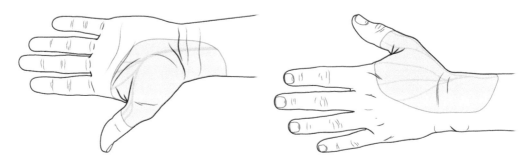

Fig. 42.1 and Fig. 42.2 Inject 40 to 60 mL of buffered 1% lidocaine with 1:100,000 epinephrine to bathe the entire radial hand at the base of the thumb and wrist joints (see ▶ Video 42.1).

WHERE TO INJECT THE LOCAL ANESTHETIC FOR REDUCTION AND INTERNAL FIXATION OF FOURTH AND FIFTH METACARPAL FRACTURES

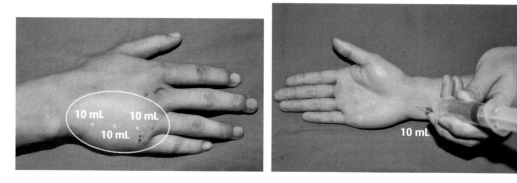

Fig. 42.3 and Fig. 42.4 Inject a total of 30 to 40 mL of 1% lidocaine with 1:100,000 epinephrine (buffered with 10 mL lido/epi:1 mL of 8.4% sodium bicarbonate). The figures showing the injection method for the fourth and fifth metacarpal fracture. On the palmar side, inject 10 mL near but not in the ulnar nerve (do NOT elicit paresthesia to avoid nerve damage) (see ▶ Video 42.2).

SPECIFICS OF MINIMALLY PAINFUL INJECTION OF LOCAL ANESTHETIC IN REDUCTION AND INTERNAL FIXATION OF METACARPAL FRACTURES

- Local anesthesia injection should barely hurt at all if you follow the simple rules of Chapter 5 for hints to minimize injection pain. The patients will think you are magical.

- For a Bennett's fracture you flood the radial side of the hand with 40 to 60 mL of buffered lidocaine with epinephrine, as shown in ▶ Video 42.2.

- Inject with a long 27-gauge needle and pinch the skin into the needle to add the sensory "noise" of pressure to decrease the pain.

- Always err on the side of too much local anesthesia instead of not enough. You are aiming for patients only feeling a small sting when you insert the first local anesthesia needle. They should feel no pain for the rest of the injections or during the surgery.

- We inject the anesthetic solution a minimum of 30 minutes before surgery to allow the epinephrine to take optimal effect and provide an adequately dry working field, as outlined in Chapter 3, Chapter 4, and Chapter 14.

- We inject supine patients lying down on stretchers in a waiting area to decrease the risk of their fainting (see Chapter 6).

- Start by injecting 10 mL of the mixture under the skin at the base of the thumb without moving the needle. Let the local anesthesia diffuse where it wants to go in a painless fashion.

- After the first 10 mL, inject another 10 mL on the dorsal side of the thumb base.

- After the second 10 mL on the dorsal side, inject another 10 mL on the volar side of the metacarpal base.

- Always alternate from dorsal to volar and back. This gives the local time to work before you reinsert the needle, so it does not hurt. After the third 10 mL on the volar side, inject a fourth 10 mL slowly between the thumb and index metacarpal bases going from the dorsal articulation to the volar side where the metacarpals meet the trapezium, staying near the bone.

- The local anesthetic for fracture dislocations of the fourth and fifth metacarpal bases is 40 mL of buffered lidocaine and epinephrine, flooding the ulnar side of the distal wrist and base of the hand, as shown in ▶ Video 42.3.

- The first dorsal 10 mL goes into the most proximal location that you will dissect. Inject the second 10 mL of local anesthetic in the center of the incision site with the needle inserted into clearly vasoconstricted white skin that has functioning lidocaine and epinephrine so that needle insertion is pain-free. You should have tumescent local anesthetic (Chapter 4) diffused at least 2 cm on either side of the incision. Inject the third 10 mL in the distal third of the incision (▶ Fig. 42.1).

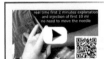

Video 42.3 How to inject minimally painful local anesthesia to K-wire a Bennett's fracture (Lalonde, Canada).

Video 42.4 How to inject local anesthesia for open reduction and plating fourth and fifth metacarpal fractures (Xing, China).

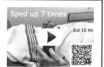

Video 42.5 How to inject local anesthesia for a fracture dislocation at the base of the fifth metacarpal (Lalonde, Canada).

Video 42.6 Local anesthetic injection for WALANT metacarpal plate removal (Lalonde, Canada).

- You can inject an additional 10 mL between the median and ulnar nerves under the forearm fascia at the volar wrist to block those nerves with tumescent local anesthetic.

- The goal of the injection is to bathe local anesthetic all around the metacarpal where dissection or internal fixation will occur, including the palmar side and between the metacarpals. You may want to add additional local anesthetic in the lateral and volar aspects of the metacarpal with a fifth 10 mL syringe.

- For plate removal, bathe the entire surgical dissection area with ample local anesthetic from proximal to distal on both sides of the surgical scar. Let the local anesthetic diffuse into the scar on its own. You should have 2 cm of local anesthetic all around the planned dissection area (see ▶ Video 42.5).

- First inject 10 mL subcutaneously proximal to the scar, then work your way around each side of the scar. Then inject distal to the scar. Inject under the scar last.

TIPS AND TRICKS FOR PERFORMING REDUCTION AND INTERNAL FIXATION OF METACARPAL FRACTURES WITH THE WIDE AWAKE APPROACH

- Ask the patients if their fingers are straight after you reduce the fracture(s). They have been looking at those fingers their whole life. They can tell you at once if their fingers are still crooked or not. They are a great judge of fracture reduction.

- After you have provisional reduction, ask the patient to make a fist and extend the fingers to test the stability of your internal fixation. You will see whether there is enough stability in the fixation to support early protected movement or whether you need to insert additional fixation.

- A dynamic compression bone clamp provides enough temporary rigid fixation in transverse metacarpal fractures so that you can test full flexion and full extension of the clamp-held reduced fractures to make sure there is no malrotation before you drill screw holes.

- After local anesthetic injection, waiting for a minimum of 30 minutes before surgery can allow the epinephrine to take optimal effect and provide an adequately dry working field. However, Drs Tang and Xing typically wait only 10 to 15 minutes to start the surgery (▶ Fig. 42.2). They have found that there is no need to wait for 20 to 30 minutes to begin surgery in these patents. During these 10 to 15 minutes, they perform preoperative preparation by cleansing the skin and draping the area.

- Close the skin with buried intradermal simple interrupted 5-0 Monocryl sutures as shown in detail for carpal tunnel closure in ▶ Video 26.9. Buried simple interrupted sutures of absorbable monofilament Monocryl mean that there are no sutures to remove.

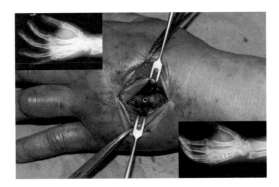

Fig. 42.5 We waited only about 10 minutes to start the surgery for this patient. By the time we got to the important part of this procedure, the bleeding was minimal. We use a hemostat on bigger vessels for a few minutes till they clot, or we simply tie them off. We no longer use cautery for most cases. The inserted pictures are preoperative and postoperative radiographs. Inserted X-ray images show the fracture before and after screw fixation.

- For articular fractures, inject 2 to 4 mL local anesthesia into the joint cavity and in the soft tissues around the joint (▶ Fig. 42.6).

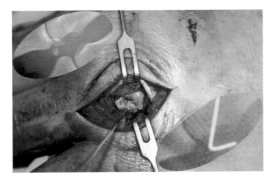

Fig. 42.6 Open reduction and internal fixation with K-wire for the third metacarpal head fracture under WALANT. Another 3 mL buffered lidocaine and epinephrine was injected into the joint. The inserted X-ray pictures are preoperative (left showing avulsion fracture) and postoperative (right showing K-wired avulsion fracture) radiographs.

Video 42.7
How to reduce a Bennett's fracture dislocation (thumb metacarpal base) so you can K-wire it without having to open it (Lalonde, Canada).

Video 42.8
Closed reduction and K-wiring of Bennett's fracture with field sterility outside the main operating room (Lalonde, Canada) (see Chapter 10 for evidence on safety of field sterility for K-wire insertion).[1,2,3,4,5]

Video 42.9
Operative reduction of fourth and fifth metacarpal fractures in the patient injected with local anesthetic seen in ▶ Video 42.2 (Xing, China).

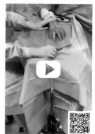

Video 42.10
Simple distraction method for transverse fractures (Gueffier, France).

Video 42.11
Testing stability of open compression screw fixation (Escobar, Columbia).

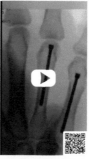

Video 42.12 Two metacarpal shaft fractures headless compression screw (Sibley, USA).

Video 42.13
Suture fixation of metacarpal fracture with testing of stability of suture (Apard, France).

Video 42.14
Check scissoring correction after dynamic compression bone clamp reduction of transverse metacarpal fracture before plating (Lalonde, Canada).[6]

Video 42.15
Plating after correction of metacarpal malunion fracture (Lalonde, Canada).

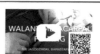

Video 42.16
Plating after correction of metacarpal malunion fracture (Jagodzinski England).

Video 42.17
Verifying no scissoring of plate metacarpal (Ahmad, Malaysia).

THERAPY TIPS FOR EARLY PROTECTED MOVEMENT AFTER K-WIRED METACARPAL FRACTURE

- Active tendon gliding exercises in isolated and composite positions are initiated approximately 4 days postsurgery.

- Active motion is performed to maintain joint mobility and tendon glide through the surgical zone.

- The patient is educated that range of motion is performed within pain-free limits.

- The exercises are demonstrated to the patient by the therapist with education on hand position, repetitions, and frequency that should be continued independently at home.

- The patient performs the exercises with the therapist and corrections are made in real time to ensure they are completed appropriately.

- The session can be videoed on the patient's cell phone for future reference if appropriate.

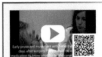

Video 42.TT1
Early protected movement after open reduction and K-wire fixation of maluniting fracture at 4 weeks post injury (includes detailed surgery) (Kean, Canada).[7]

References

1. Dua K, Blevins CJ, O'Hara NN, Abzug JM. The safety and benefits of the semi-sterile technique for closed reduction and percutaneous pinning of pediatric upper extremity fractures. Hand (N Y) 2019;14(6):808–813

2. Garon MT, Massey P, Chen A, Carroll T, Nelson BG, Hollister AM. Cost and complications of percutaneous fixation of hand fractures in a procedure room versus the operating room. Hand (N Y) 2018;13(4):428–434

3. Starker I, Eaton RG. Kirschner wire placement in the emergency room. Is there a risk? J Hand Surg [Br] 1995;20(4):535–538

4. Gillis JA, Williams JG. Cost analysis of percutaneous fixation of hand fractures in the main operating room versus the ambulatory setting. J Plast Reconstr Aesthet Surg 2017;70(8):1044–1050

5. Steve AK, Schrag CH, Kuo A, Harrop AR. Metacarpal fracture fixation in a minor surgery setting versus main operating room: a cost-minimization analysis. Plast Reconstr Surg Glob Open 2019;7(7):e2298

6. Lalonde DH. Dynamic compression bone clamp for transverse fractures. Can J Plast Surg 2000;8(2):78–80

7. Hyatt BT, Rhee PC. Wide-awake surgical management of hand sractures: technical pearls and advanced rehabilitation. Plast Reconstr Surg 2019;143(3):800–810

CHAPTER 43

WRIST FRACTURE AND LIGAMENT INJURIES

Celso R. Folberg, Xavier Gueffier, Carlos Ramos de Pina, Donald H. Lalonde, Nikolas Alan Jagodzinski, Elisabet Hagert, Thomas Apard, and Amir Adham Ahmad

ADVANTAGES OF WALANT VERSUS SEDATION AND TOURNIQUET IN WRIST FRACTURE SURGERY

- All of the general advantages listed in Chapter 2 apply to both the surgeon and the patient (no nausea, no tourniquet pain or let-down bleeding, decreased cost without sedation in minor procedure room, safer surgery without sedation, etc.).

- You can see active wrist and finger movement during the surgery both before and after fracture fixation.

- After reductions of fractures and dislocations, provisional or definite correction of malalignment of carpal bones, and final implants, you can test the full range of active motion by the unsedated patient. You can see the reconstructed bone and joint active movement anatomy. You can adjust bony (such as osteophytes) or soft tissue impairments to full range of motion.

- After reconstruction, you can see how strong your fixation is when the patient takes the hand and wrist through a full range of motion. You can decide if you need to augment or change your method of fixation.

- At the end of the case, patients can see the best possible range of active motion they can do after the reconstruction, so they leave the operating room with realistic expectations. They also have a visual goal of how much they might be able to move if they attend rehabilitation.

WHERE TO INJECT THE LOCAL ANESTHETIC

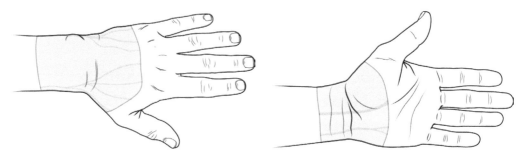

Fig. 43.1 and Fig. 43.2 For major wrist trauma, as in everywhere else, too much volume of local anesthesia is better than not enough local anesthesia. Up to 100 mL of 0.5% lidocaine with 1:200,000 epinephrine will numb the whole wrist region. Smaller areas can be tumesced so that all dissected areas are injected as shown in Videos 43.1 to 43.10.

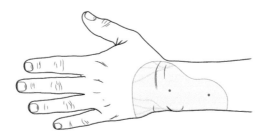

Fig. 43.3 Local injection for triangular fibrocartilage complex (TFCC) repair. Inject 40 mL of buffered 1% lidocaine with 1:100,000 epinephrine. Begin the injection 5 to 7 cm proximal to the distal radioulnar joint (DRUJ), along the ulnar border of the forearm. Slowly inject 20 mL along the ulnar border and dorsal distal ulna. Inject about 10 mL along the dorsal wrist, making sure to add 2 mL in the area of the posterior interosseous nerve (PIN) at the level of Lister's tubercle. Finally, inject the remaining 5 to 10 mL in the ulnocarpal region, with a few milliliters into the ulnocarpal joint.

 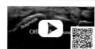 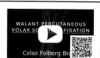

Video 43.1 Injection of local anesthesia for major wrist trauma such as perilunate dislocation (de Pina, Portugal).[1,2]

Video 43.2 Scaphoid screw local anesthesia, preoperative ultrasound, and surgery (Gueffier, France).

Video 43.3 Local anesthesia injection for volar percutaneous screw scaphoid fracture (Jagodzinski, England).

Video 43.4 Local anesthesia injection for volar percutaneous screw scaphoid fracture (Folberg, Brazil).

Video 43.5a Local injection and surgery for dorsal screw scaphoid fracture (Ahmad, Malaysia).

Video 43.5b Open dorsal screw for scaphoid fracture (Apard, France).

Video 43.6 Local anesthesia injection and dorsal percutaneous screw for scaphoid fracture (Folberg, Brazil).

SPECIFICS OF MINIMALLY PAINFUL INJECTION OF LOCAL ANESTHETIC FOR WRIST TRAUMA AND LIGAMENT SURGERY

- Local anesthesia injection should barely hurt at all if you follow the simple rules of Chapter 5 for hints to minimize injection pain. The patients will think you are magical.

- Inject the anesthetic solution a minimum of 30 minutes before surgery to allow the epinephrine to take optimal effect and provide an adequately dry working field, as outlined in Chapter 4 and Chapter 14. We inject patients outside the operating room before they come in.

- After you finish your injections the patient must be pain-free with active and passive motion of the injured area which is a good sign of adequate local anesthesia.

- Always have spare local anesthesia for possible reinforcement during the procedure, although the goal is painless surgery with no need of reinforcements.

- Volar injection over the scaphoid tuberosity will be helpful in scaphoid reconstructions.

- If radius graft harvest is anticipated, inject an additional 10 to 15 mL local anesthesia to distal radial volar periosteal.

- We do not have to perform median or ulnar nerve blocks routinely with these procedures, but they may be helpful as part of tumescent local anesthesia in some cases.

- We always inject all patients while they are lying down to decrease the risk of their fainting (see Chapter 6).

TIPS AND TRICKS FOR PERFORMING WRIST FRACTURE SURGERY WITH THE WIDE AWAKE APPROACH

- Expect some blood in the field at the beginning of the surgery; this is not bloodless tourniquet surgery. Suction may be helpful.

- The patients need to look at the hand to properly move the reconstructed wrist, since they cannot feel the hand and wrist joints. Although most patients don't mind looking at the wound, you can cover the wound with a towel as the patients flex all fingers together while looking at them. You need to take the sterile drape down so they can see their hand move.

- Close the skin with buried intradermal simple interrupted 5-0 Monocryl sutures as shown in detail for carpal tunnel closure in ▶ Video 26.9. Buried simple interrupted sutures of absorbable monofilament Monocryl mean that there are no sutures to remove.

- During longer procedures, patients may become uncomfortable lying on their back with their shoulder abducted, especially if they also have shoulder problems. Offer to the patients to lie on their side or partially on their side to give their shoulder relief. You will still see very well.

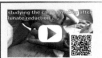

Video 43.7
Studying active movement of the carpus after reduction of the lunate in perilunate dislocation (de Pina, Portugal).

Video 43.8
Studying active movement after triangular fibrocartilage complex (TFCC) repair (Hagert, Sweden).[3]

Video 43.9
Surgery for scaphoid lunate separation (de Pina, Portugal).

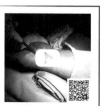

Video 43.10 Volar percutaneous screw fixation for scaphoid fracture (de Pina, Portugal).

- Offer a restroom visit just before you take the patients into the operating room so they have an empty bladder for comfort. We also do not give the patients intravenous fluid as they don't need it and it will only give them an urge to void.

- You can educate the patient about best postoperative activities during the local anesthetic injection, the surgery, and bandage application. This will serve to decrease your complication rate because your patients will understand why they should keep their hand elevated and how to take postoperative pain medications (see Chapter 8).

References

1. Ahmad AA, Yi LM, Ahmad AR. Plating of distal radius fracture using the wide-awake anesthesia technique. J Hand Surg Am 2018;43(11):1045.e1–1045.e5
2. Müller CT, Christen T, Heidekruger PI, et al. Wide-awake anesthesia no tourniquet trapeziometacarpal joint prosthesis implantation. Plast Reconstr Surg Glob Open 2018;6(4):e1714
3. Hagert E, Lalonde DH. Wide-awake wrist arthroscopy and open TFCC repair. J Wrist Surg 2012;1(1):55–60

CHAPTER 44

DISTAL RADIUS AND FOREARM FRACTURES

Amir Adham Ahmad, Paul Sibley, Kamal Rafiqi, Chris Chun-Yu Chen, Julian Escobar, Celso R. Folberg, Steven Koehler, Nikolas Alan Jagodzinski, Xavier Gueffier, Gökhan Tolga Akbulut, and Donald H. Lalonde

ADVANTAGES OF WALANT IN DISTAL RADIUS AND FOREARM FRACTURES

- All of the general advantages listed in Chapter 2 apply to both the surgeon and the patient (no nausea, no tourniquet pain or let-down bleeding, decreased cost without sedation, affordable surgery in developing nations, safer surgery without sedation, fewer complications, etc.).[1,2,3,4,5,6,7]

- After reduction and fixation of the fracture, the patient who is awake and comfortable can show you the movements of his or her wrist joint. This allows you to see it moving well and to assess the stability of the fixation in active motion.

- When you see full active motion of the wrist and observe the stability of the fixation with fluoroscopy, you will be more confident to initiate earlier active range of movement exercises for the wrist.

- It may lead to less protection after surgery based on intraoperative assessments.

- You can assess flexor pollicis longus contact with the plate in active motion.

- Skin closure is easier when you plate the radius with WALANT. Since there is minimal tissue bleeding without tourniquet let down, the tissues are less swollen.

- No sedation is safer in older patients with heart or lung comorbidities.

- Patients with distal radius fracture plated with WALANT experience less pain and stay in hospital for less time than those fixed with traditional general anesthesia. Part of the reason for this is the removal of the tourniquet and the intraoperative education about keeping the hand elevated which starts as soon as the patient sits up from the surgery.[4] This is a good thing because pain is one of the most common reasons for readmission after distal radius fracture.[8]

- In two level III evidence papers, patients with wide awake distal radius plated fracture recovered and returned to work sooner than locoregional anesthesia patients.[9,10]

- It is possible to plate both radius and ulna fractures in "both bone fractures" of the forearm in children as demonstrated by Dr Stephen Koehler from New York (see ▶ Video 9.10).

WHERE TO INJECT THE LOCAL ANESTHETIC FOR DISTAL RADIUS FRACTURES

Video 44.1
Local anesthesia injection for WALANT distal radius fracture injection (Ahmad, Malaysia).

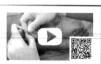

Video 44.2
Alternative method of local anesthesia injection for WALANT distal radius fracture surgery starts with a hematoma block followed by subcutaneous and other injections (Chen, Taiwan).

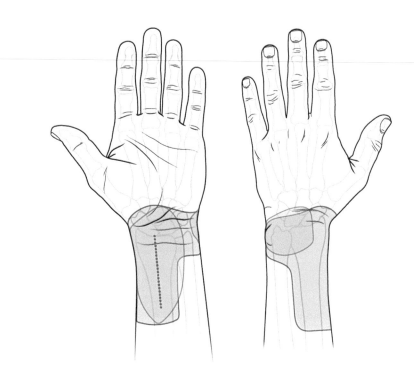

Fig. 44.1 Prepare up to 100 mL of tumescent local anesthesia with 50 mL of 1% lidocaine with 1:100,000 epinephrine added to 5 mL of 8.4% bicarbonate and 50 mL of saline. Inject 10 to 20 mL of buffered 0.5% lidocaine with 1:200,000 epinephrine subcutaneously (*blue*) along the incision site. Bathe the radius with 30 to 50 mL periosteally (*pink*) along the radial aspect of the distal radius. Inject 10 to 30 mL into the distal radioulnar joint and ulnar wrist area so the whole area of dissection or moving torn ligaments or broken bones is tumesced with visible, palpable local anesthesia.

WHERE TO INJECT THE LOCAL ANESTHETIC FOR MID FOREARM RADIUS AND ULNA FRACTURES

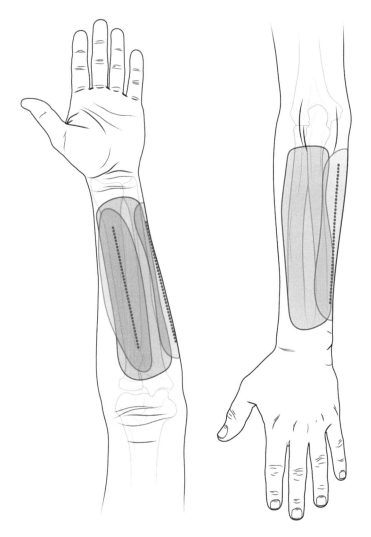

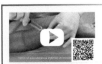

Video 44.3 Local anaesthesia injection for WALANT both mid radius and ulna bone fractures injection (Ahmad, Malaysia).

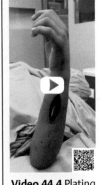

Video 44.4 Plating mid forearm radius and ulna fractures surgery (Ahmad, Malaysia).

Fig. 44.2 Prepare up to 150 mL of tumescent local anesthesia with 50 mL of 1% lidocaine with 1:100,000 epinephrine added to 5 mL of 8.4% bicarbonate and 100 mL of saline. Now inject 10 to 20 mL of the buffered 0.33% lidocaine with 1:300,000 epinephrine subcutaneously (*blue*) at each of the two incision sites. Bathe all involved areas of the radius and ulna with 30 to 50 mL each periosteally (*pink*).

- Also see ▶ Video 9.10 in Chapter 9 local anesthesia and plating both radius and ulna fractures in "both bone fractures" of the forearm in a 12-year-old by Steven Koehler, USA.

SPECIFICS OF MINIMALLY PAINFUL INJECTION OF LOCAL ANESTHETIC IN DISTAL RADIUS AND FOREARM FRACTURES

- Local anesthesia injection should barely hurt at all if you follow the simple rules of Chapter 5 for hints to minimize injection pain. The patients will think you are magical. For example, inject with a long 27-gauge needle and pinch the skin into the needle to add sensory "noise" of pressure to decrease the pain.

- Always err on the side of too much local anesthesia instead of not enough. You are aiming for patients only feeling a small sting when you insert the first local anesthesia needle. They should feel no pain for the rest of the injections or during the surgery.

- There are two types of injections for fractures. The first injection is the subcutaneous injection when you inject at the incision site. The second injection is the periosteal injection when you inject along the proximal, middle, and distal aspects of the periosteum to bathe the entire area where dissection or noxious stimuli will happen.

- To minimize the injection pain, inject with a long 27-gauge needle for the subcutaneous injection and periosteal injections.

- Pinch the skin into the needle to add sensory "noise" of pressure to decrease the pain. (See Chapter 5 for other hints on how to decrease the pain of local injection.)

- Always inject proximal to distal in both subcutaneous and periosteal injections to avoid sharp needle penetration of nonanesthetized tissue.

- For periosteal injection, start the injection at the side where the bone is easily palpable (radially for radius and ulnarly for ulna).

- Start by injecting the first 10 to 20 mL subcutaneously along the incision site (zone 1 in ▶ Fig. 44.3).

- Then proceed with the periosteal injections. You will need a needle long enough to reach across the radius. Start at the radial border 2 cm proximal to the proximal edge of the plate.

- Insert the needle perpendicularly at the radial border and go deep to the periosteum. Start by injecting 3 mL at the radial border (zone 2 in ▶ Fig. 44.3). Do not remove the needle as you need to "walk the bone" to go to the volar and dorsal aspect of the radius. Inject 5 mL volarly and 5 mL dorsally across the radius. Inject the same 3 mL at the radial border and 5 mL volarly and 5 mL dorsally at the mid dissection level (zone 3 in ▶ Fig. 44.3). Inject the same 3 mL at the radial border and 5 mL volarly and 5 mL dorsally at the distal dissection level (zone 4 in ▶ Fig. 44.3).

- The same technique is used for midshaft radius and ulna fracture fixation seen in ▶ Fig. 44.2.[5]

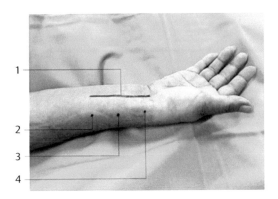

Fig. 44.3 Schematic outline of the injection technique: (1) Inject 10 to 20 mL subcutaneously along the skin incision. (2) Inject 13 to 15 mL periosteally proximal to fracture site. (3) Inject 13 to 15 mL periosteally at the fracture site. (4) Inject 13 to 15 mL at the distal radius.

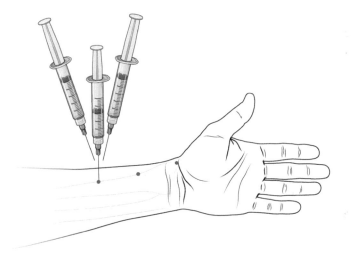

Fig. 44.4 In each of the three injection sites shown in ▶ Fig. 44.3 and ▶ Fig. 44.4, 3 mL is injected at the radial border of the radius and 5 mL each in the volar and dorsal aspects of the distal radius, staying on the bone.

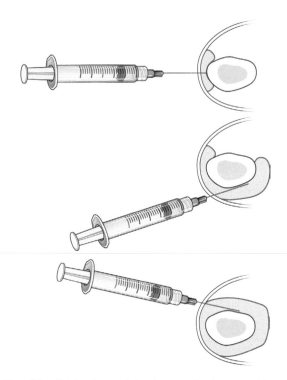

Fig. 44.5 Cross-section of the distal radius and ulna (or any other long bone) for injection at the periosteal layer. Only one skin needle entry site is required in each of the three injection sites. The skin can be pushed volarly and dorsally with the needle to keep the needle tip at the periosteal level.

- Inject 10 to 30 mL into the distal radioulnar joint and ulnar wrist area so the whole area of dissection or moving torn ligaments or broken bones is tumesced with visible, palpable local anesthesia.

- In cases with concurrent ulna styloid fracture, be sure the distal ulna is bathed with tumescent local anesthesia to avoid pain while fixing the distal radius.

- For injections to the distal radius, injury to the radial artery can be avoided by palpating the radial artery and injecting lateral to the radial artery where the radial border of the radius is easily palpable. The needle should then follow the periosteum.

- Without removing the needle, guide it toward the dorsal and volar side of the radius to ensure the local anesthesia is bathing the entire distal radius circumferentially. This is to avoid pain when manipulating the fracture at the ulnar border of the distal radius and especially during drilling the far (dorsal) cortex during fixation.

- Do not rush the injections. The whole process should take about 10 to 30 minutes. Score yourself every time you inject to try to get a hole-in-one every time. (See Chapter 5 for other hints on how to decrease the pain of local injection.)

- Inject 30 minutes before incision to allow the epinephrine to take optimal effect and provide adequately dry working field, as outlined in Chapter 4 and Chapter 14.

- Inject your patients (lying down to decrease risk of fainting) in the waiting area before going into the operating room (see ▶ Video 6.1).

TIPS AND TRICKS FOR OPERATIVE REDUCTION OF DISTAL RADIUS AND FOREARM FRACTURES WITH THE WIDE AWAKE APPROACH

- Before surgery, test the anesthetic effect by manipulating the fracture site. The pain score should be "0" during manipulation and palpation of fractures. This is a sign that the local anesthesia has taken effect and it is safe to proceed with the surgery without pain.

- Wait at least 25 to 30 minutes between injection and incision. It is more efficient to inject them on a stretcher before they come into the operating room.

- There is no need to cauterize most of the little bleeders as they will stop on their own by the time the case is done.

- Show the patients what the plate looks like before putting it in so they can see what they will have inside of them.

- Have patients see and move their wrist in all directions (flexion/extension, supination, pronation, radial/ulnar deviation, dart-throwers). Look at the bones on "cine" mode on the mini C-arm to look for fracture stability. This will be motivation if they happen to get stiff.

- Close the skin with buried intradermal simple interrupted 5-0 Monocryl sutures as shown in detail for carpal tunnel closure in ▶ Video 26.9. Buried simple interrupted sutures of absorbable monofilament Monocryl mean that there are no sutures to remove.

- You can do radius malunion cases with WALANT as is shown in the next clip by Dr Kamal Rafiqi in Morocco.[6]

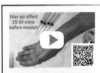

Video 44.5 Wait at least 25 to 30 minutes between injection and excision. It is best to inject patients before they come into the operating room (Sibley, USA).

Video 44.6 Radius malunion osteotomy and plating. Confirming active movement and forearm appearance at the end of the case (Rafiqi, Morocco).

Video 44.7 Check all wrist and hand movements after plating radius to assess mobility and stability with X-ray (Sibley, USA).

Video 44.8 Extensor pollicis longus (EPL) repair and distal radius fracture plating (Escobar, Columbia).

Video 44.9 Local injection and plating distal radius fracture (Rafiqi, Morocco).

Video 44.10 Ulna shaft fractures (Rafiqi, Morocco).

Video 44.11 Monteggia fracture/dislocation local anesthesia injection and end of surgery (Ahmad, Malaysia).

Video 44.12 Dorsal distal radius plating (Chen, Taiwan).

Video 44.13 Injection of local anesthesia and closed K-wiring of distal radius fracture (Folberg, Brazil).

Video 44.14
Injection of local anesthesia and minimally invasive small incision open plating of distal radius fracture (Escobar, Columbia).

Video 44.15
Injection of local anesthesia and plating of distal radius fracture (Jagodzinski, England).

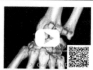

Video 44.16
Injection of local anesthesia and plating of distal radius fracture (Gueffier, France).

Video 44.17
Showing adequate local anesthesia with active and passive movement and plating of mid radius fracture (Rafiqi, Morocco).

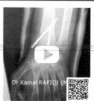

Video 44.18
Closed reduction and K-wiring of distal radius fracture (Rafiqi, Morocco).

Video 44.19
Checking stability of plate after distal radius reduction (Akbulut, Turkey).

References

1. Ahmad AA, Yi LM, Ahmad AR. Plating of distal radius fracture using the wide-awake anesthesia technique. J Hand Surg Am 2018;43(11):1045.e1–1045.e5
2. Orbach H, Rozen N, Rubin G. Open reduction and internal fixation of intra-articular distal radius fractures under wide-awake local anesthesia with no tourniquet. J Int Med Res 2018;46(10):4269–4276
3. Huang YC, Hsu CJ, Renn JH, et al. WALANT for distal radius fracture: open reduction with plating fixation via wide-awake local anesthesia with no tourniquet. J Orthop Surg Res 2018;13(1):195
4. Huang YC, Chen CY, Lin KC, Yang SW, Tarng YW, Chang WN. Comparison of wide-awake local anesthesia no tourniquet with general anesthesia with tourniquet for volar plating of distal radius fracture. Orthopedics 2019;42(1):e93–e98
5. Ahmad AA, Ikram MA. Plating of an isolated fracture of shaft of ulna under local anaesthesia and periosteal nerve block. Trauma Case Rep 2017;12:40–44
6. Rafiqi K, Kamil S, Benzmane K. Wide-awake local anesthesia for osteotomy of distal radius malunion. Hand Surg Rehabil 2020;39(4):339–340
7. Tahir M, Mehboob G, R Jamali A, Phillips AM. Use of the wide-awake local anaesthetic no tourniquet in the management of distal radius fractures. J Pak Med Assoc 2020;70(2):S42–S48
8. Sumner K, Grandizio LC, Gehrman MD, Graham J, Klena JC. Incidence and reason for readmission and unscheduled health care contact after distal radius fracture. Hand (N Y) 2020;15(2):243–251
9. Dukan R, Krief E, Nizard R. Distal radius fracture volar locking plate osteosynthesis using wide-awake local anaesthesia. J Hand Surg Eur Vol 2020;45(8):857–863
10. Tahir M, Chaudhry EA, Zaffar Z, et al. Fixation of distal radius fractures using wide-awake local anaesthesia with no tourniquet (WALANT) technique: a randomized control trial of a cost-effective and resource-friendly procedure. Bone Joint Res 2020;9(7):429–439

CHAPTER 45

SURGERY AROUND THE ELBOW

*Amir Adham Ahmad, Celso R. Folberg, Kamal Rafiqi,
and Donald H. Lalonde*

ADVANTAGES OF WALANT VERSUS SEDATION AND TOURNIQUET IN ELBOW FRACTURES

- All of the general advantages listed in Chapter 2 apply to both the surgeon and the patient (no nausea, no tourniquet pain or let-down bleeding, decreased cost without sedation in minor procedure room, safer surgery without sedation, etc.).

- After reduction and fixation of the fracture, the patient who is awake and comfortable would be able to demonstrate the movements of the elbow joint. This allows you to assess the stability of the fixation in active motion.

- When you see full active motion of the elbow and observe the stability of the fixation with fluoroscopy, you will be more confident to initiate early active range of movement exercises for the elbow.

- It may lead to less protection after surgery based on intraoperative assessments.

- You can take the advantage of the patient being awake to educate him or her during the surgery on how to move the elbow so it will not get stiff after the surgery. You should also teach the patient how to use the upper limb to protect the fracture from coming apart after the surgery.

- You will be able to assess the posterior interosseous nerve with active finger extension during surgery after plating of the radial neck/head.

- No sedation is safer in older patients with heart or lung comorbidities.

WHERE TO INJECT THE LOCAL ANESTHETIC FOR TENSION BAND WIRE/PLATING OF OLECRANON

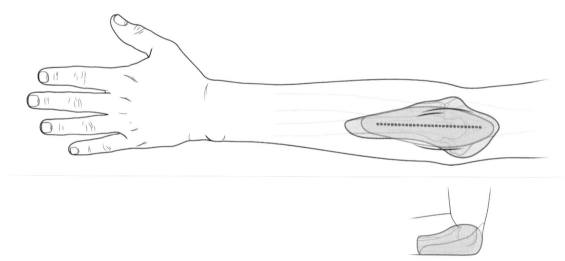

Fig. 45.1 Prepare up to 100 mL of tumescent local anesthesia with 50 mL of 1% lidocaine with 1:100,000 epinephrine added to 5 mL of 8.4% bicarbonate and 50 mL of saline. Inject 10 to 20 mL of this 0.5% lidocaine with 1:200,000 epinephrine solution subcutaneously (*blue*) along the incision site using a long 27-gauge needle. In the areas proximal and distal to the tension band wire/plate dissection as well as at the fracture site, inject an additional total of 40 to 45 mL of the same solution at periosteal level (*pink*) on the posterior, radial, and ulnar borders of the bone. *Red dotted line* is possible incision.

WHERE TO INJECT THE LOCAL ANESTHETIC FOR PLATING RADIAL NECK/HEAD FRACTURES

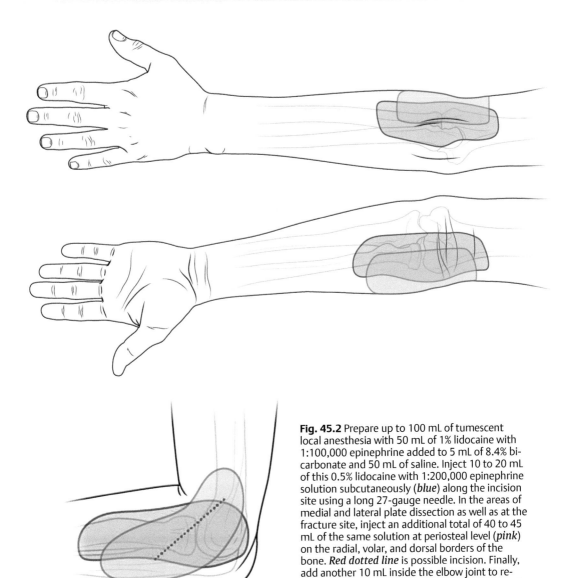

Fig. 45.2 Prepare up to 100 mL of tumescent local anesthesia with 50 mL of 1% lidocaine with 1:100,000 epinephrine added to 5 mL of 8.4% bicarbonate and 50 mL of saline. Inject 10 to 20 mL of this 0.5% lidocaine with 1:200,000 epinephrine solution subcutaneously (*blue*) along the incision site using a long 27-gauge needle. In the areas of medial and lateral plate dissection as well as at the fracture site, inject an additional total of 40 to 45 mL of the same solution at periosteal level (*pink*) on the radial, volar, and dorsal borders of the bone. *Red dotted line* is possible incision. Finally, add another 10 mL inside the elbow joint to reduce the pain while manipulating the radial head.

SPECIFICS OF MINIMALLY PAINFUL INJECTION OF LOCAL ANESTHETIC IN ELBOW SURGERY

- Local anesthesia injection should barely hurt at all if you follow the simple rules of Chapter 5 for hints to minimize injection pain. The patients will think you are magical. For example, inject with a long 27-gauge needle and pinch the skin into the needle to add sensory "noise" of pressure to decrease the pain.

- Always err on the side of too much local anesthesia instead of not enough. You are aiming for patients only feeling a small sting when you insert the first local anesthesia needle. They should feel no pain for the rest of the injections or during the surgery.

- There are two types of injections for fractures. The first injection is the subcutaneous injection where you inject at the incision site. The second injection is the periosteal injection to bathe the entire area of bone or joint where dissection or noxious stimuli will happen.

- Start by injecting the first 10 to 20 mL subcutaneously along the incision site.

- Follow subcutaneous injections with periosteal injection. The goal is to flood the periosteum circumferentially from 2 cm medial to 2 cm lateral to the area of plate fixation.

- Always inject proximal to distal in both subcutaneous and periosteal injections to avoid sharp needle penetration of nonanesthetized tissue.

- For periosteal injections, start the injection at the most proximal aspect of the subcutaneous injection (tip of olecranon for olecranon fracture and lateral epicondyle for radial neck/head fracture).

- Start by injecting at the tip of the olecranon. Do not remove the needle as you need to "walk the bone" to go to the radial and ulnar aspects of the olecranon. Do this at three or four intervals along the olecranon and proximal ulna.

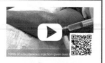

Video 45.1
Local anesthesia injection for WALANT olecranon fracture (Ahmad, Malaysia).[1]

Video 45.2
Local anesthesia injection and cancellous screw for WALANT olecranon fracture (Folberg, Brazil).

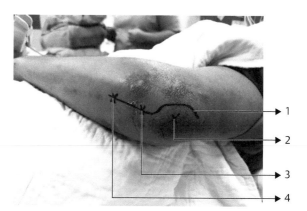

Fig, 45.3 Schematic outline of the injection technique: (1) Inject 10 to 20 mL subcutaneously along the dotted skin incision. (2) Inject 13 to 15 mL periosteally proximal to the fracture site. (3) Inject 13 to 15 mL periosteally at the fracture site. (4) Inject 13 to 15 mL distal to the fracture site.

- Start by injecting at the lateral epicondyle. Do not remove the needle as you need to "walk the bone" to go to the volar and dorsal aspects of the lateral epicondyle. Do this at three or four intervals along the radial neck/head and proximal radius.

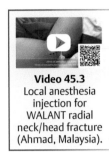

Video 45.3
Local anesthesia injection for WALANT radial neck/head fracture (Ahmad, Malaysia).

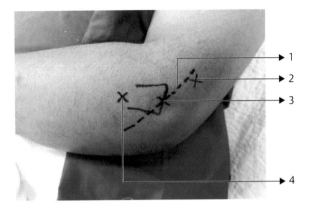

Fig. 45.4 Schematic outline of the injection technique: (1) Inject 10 to 20 mL subcutaneously along the dotted skin incision. (2) Inject 13 to 15 mL periosteally proximal to the fracture site. (3) Inject 13 to 15 mL periosteally at the fracture site. (4) Inject 13 to 15 mL distal to the fracture site.

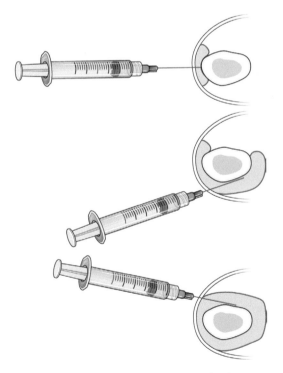

Fig. 45.5 The concept of "walking the bone" with the needle to bathe the entire involved periosteum is demonstrated.

- Do not rush the injections. The whole process should take about 10 to 30 minutes. Score yourself every time you inject to try to get a hole-in-one every time. (See Chapter 5 for other hints on how to decrease the pain of local anesthesia injection.)

- Inject 30 minutes before incision to allow the epinephrine to take optimal effect and provide adequately dry working field, as outlined in Chapter 4 and Chapter 14.

- Inject your patients (lying down to decrease risk of fainting) in the waiting area before going into the operating room (see Chapter 6).

TIPS AND TRICKS FOR OPERATIVE REDUCTION OF ELBOW FRACTURES WITH THE WIDE AWAKE APPROACH

Video 45.4 Check elbow movements after plating of olecranon to assess mobility and stability with X-ray (Ahmad, Malaysia).

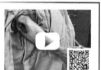

Video 45.5 Check elbow movements after tension band wiring of olecranon to assess mobility and stability with X-ray (Ahmad, Malaysia).

- Wait at least 25 to 30 minutes between injection and incision. It is more efficient to inject them on a stretcher before they come into the operating room.

- Before surgery, test the anesthetic effect by manipulating the fracture site. The pain score should be "0" during manipulation. This is a sign that the local anesthesia has taken effect and it is safe to proceed with the surgery without pain.

- As the ulnar nerve lie close to the medial side of the olecranon, extra care must be given when injecting around it. The needle should be constantly on the ulna bone before injecting the local anesthesia. This will ensure that the local anesthesia will be given periosteally. However, the diffusion of tumescent local anesthesia may cause an ulnar nerve block.

- Be careful not to inject into or injure the median, ulnar, and posterior interosseus nerves or large blood vessels near them.

- After the reconstruction, take down the drape and have patients see and move their elbow in all directions (flexion/extension, supination, pronation). Look at the bones on "cine" mode on the mini C-arm to look for fracture and fixation stability. This will be motivation if the patients happen to get stiff.

- Close the skin with buried intradermal simple interrupted 5-0 Monocryl sutures as shown in detail for carpal tunnel closure in ▶ Video 26.9. Buried simple interrupted sutures of absorbable monofilament Monocryl mean that there are no sutures to remove.

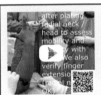

Video 45.6 Check elbow supination and pronation after plating of radial neck/head to assess mobility and stability with X-ray. We also verify finger extension to see there is no injury to the posterior interosseous nerve (Ahmad, Malaysia).

Video 45.7 Verifying movement in olecranon fracture (Rafiqi, Morocco).

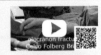

Video 45.8 Verifying movement in olecranon fracture after cannulated screw (Folberg, Brazil).

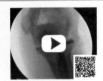

Video 45.9 Pronation and supination movement of screw in radial head fracture (Folberg, Brazil).

Reference

1. Ahmad AA, Sabari SS, Ruslan SR, Abdullah S, Ahmad AR. Wide-awake anesthesia for olecranon fracture fixation. [published online ahead of print, 2019 Jul 9] Hand (N Y) 2019;1558944719861706. doi: 10.1177/1558944719861706

CHAPTER 46

CLAVICLE AND ACROMION FRACTURES

Amir Adham Ahmad, Chris Chu-Yun Chen,
and Donald H. Lalonde

ADVANTAGES OF WALANT VERSUS SEDATION AND TOURNIQUET IN CLAVICLE FRACTURES[1]

- All of the general advantages listed in Chapter 2 apply to both the surgeon and the patient (no nausea, no tourniquet pain or let-down bleeding, decreased cost without sedation in minor procedure room, safer surgery without sedation, etc.).

- After reduction and fixation of the fracture, the patient who is awake and comfortable would be able to demonstrate the movements of the shoulder joint. This allows you to assess the stability of the fixation in active motion.

- When you see full active motion of the shoulder and observe the stability of the fixation with fluoroscopy, you will be more confident to initiate early active range of movement exercises for the shoulder.

- You can take advantage of the patient being awake to educate him or her during the surgery on how to move the shoulder so that it will not get stiff after the surgery. You should also teach the patient how to use the arm to protect the fracture from coming apart after the surgery.

WHERE TO INJECT THE LOCAL ANESTHETIC FOR PLATING CLAVICLE FRACTURES

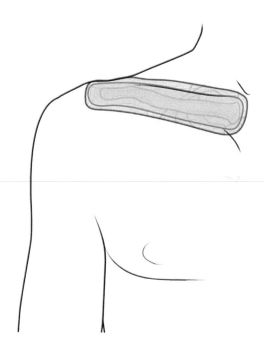

Fig. 46.1 Prepare up to 100 mL of tumescent local anesthesia with 50 mL of 1% lidocaine with 1:100,000 epinephrine added to 5 mL of 8.4% bicarbonate and 50 mL of saline. Inject 10 to 20 mL of this 0.5% lidocaine with 1:200,000 epinephrine solution subcutaneously (blue is sub-Q) along the incision site using a long 27-gauge needle. In the areas of medial and lateral plate dissection as well as at the fracture site, inject an additional total of 40 to 45 mL of the same solution at periosteal level (pink is periosteal) on the superior, anterior, and posterior borders of the bone. WARNING: Do not inject local anesthesia under (inferior to) the clavicle until you see that area with direct vision during the surgery. Large vessels directly beneath the inferior border could be a vehicle for large intravenous boluses of local anesthesia which could be toxic, especially with bupivacaine (see Chapter 4 about the dangers of bupivacaine).

SPECIFICS OF MINIMALLY PAINFUL INJECTION OF LOCAL ANESTHETIC IN CLAVICLE FRACTURES

Video 46.1
Local anesthesia injection for WALANT clavicle fracture plating (Ahmad, Malaysia).

- WARNING: We only use lidocaine and not bupivacaine in our tumescent solutions (see Chapter 4). Bupivacaine can be lethal in intravenous bolus doses. Lidocaine is much safer. Large vessels under the clavicle could be a vehicle for toxic doses of local anesthesia. Do not inject local anesthesia under (inferior to) the clavicle until you see that area with direct vision.

- Always err on the side of too much local anesthesia instead of not enough. You are aiming for patients only feeling a small sting when the first local anesthesia needle is inserted. They should feel no pain for the rest of the injections or during the surgery.

- There are two types of injections for fractures. The first injection is the subcutaneous injection when you inject at the incision site. The second injection is the periosteal injection when you inject along the superior, anterior, and posterior aspects of the clavicle to bathe the entire area where dissection or noxious stimuli will happen.

- To minimize the injection pain, inject with a long 27-gauge needle for the subcutaneous and periosteal injections.

- Pinch the skin into the needle to add sensory "noise" of pressure to decrease the pain. See Chapter 5 for other hints on how to decrease the pain of local injection.

- Start by injecting the first 10 to 20 mL subcutaneously along the incision site.

- Follow subcutaneous injections with periosteal injection. The goal is to flood the periosteum circumferentially from 2 cm medial to 2 cm lateral to the area of plate fixation.

- The periosteal injections can start from medially and end laterally.

- Start by injecting at superior clavicle as in ▶ Video 46.1. Do not remove the needle as you need to "walk the bone" to go to the anterior and posterior aspects of the clavicle. Stay on the bone to avoid large vessel penetration. Do this at three or four intervals along the clavicle. Wait until you see the inferior clavicle during the surgery to inject the inferior surface.

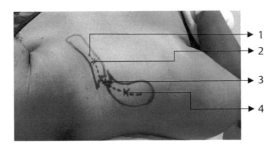

Fig. 46.2 Schematic outline of the injection technique. (1) Inject 10 to 20 mL subcutaneously along the dotted skin incision. (2) Inject 13 to 15 mL periosteally medial to the fracture site. (3) Inject 13 to 15 mL periosteally at the fracture site. (4) Inject 13 to 15 mL lateral to the fracture site.

- Do not rush the injections. The whole process should take about 10 to 30 minutes. Score yourself every time you inject to try to get a hole-in-one every time. (See Chapter 5 for other hints on how to decrease the pain of local anesthesia injection.)

- Inject 30 minutes before incision to allow the epinephrine to take optimal effect and provide adequately dry working field, as outlined in Chapter 4 and Chapter 14.

- Inject your patients (lying down to decrease risk of fainting) in the waiting area before going into the operating room (see ▶ Video 6.1).

TIPS AND TRICKS FOR OPERATIVE REDUCTION OF CLAVICLE FRACTURES WITH THE WIDE AWAKE APPROACH

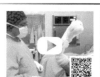

Video 46.2
WALANT clavicle fracture plating surgery (Chen, Taiwan).

- Wait at least 25 to 30 minutes between injection and incision. It is more efficient to inject the patients on a stretcher before they come into the operating room.

- Before surgery, test the anesthetic effect by manipulating the fracture site. The pain score should be "0" during manipulation. This is a sign that the local anesthesia has taken effect and it is safe to proceed with the surgery without pain.

- After your skin incisions and clear visualization of the bone and fracture, you can finish injecting the inferior surface of the clavicle under direct vision with an additional 10 to 15 mL with care to avoid intravascular bolus injection.

- Aching of the neck and shoulder girdle is commonly encountered during the procedure. If the patient complains of aching, temporarily stop the surgery to allow the patient to stretch out his or her neck and shoulder.

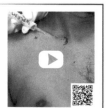

Video 46.3
WALANT clavicle local anesthesia and end of surgery (Ahmad, Malaysia).

- Careful administration of local anesthesia requires a keen familiarity of the anatomical structures surrounding the clavicle. This precaution is necessary in order to minimize the risk of injury to the lung apex lying deep to the clavicle as well as divisions of the trunks of brachial plexus and subclavian vessels passing behind the medial two-thirds of the clavicle.

- Close the skin with buried intradermal simple interrupted 5-0 Monocryl sutures as shown in detail for carpal tunnel closure in ▶ Video 26.9. Buried simple interrupted sutures of absorbable monofilament Monocryl mean that there are no sutures to remove.

LOCAL ANESTHESIA AND SURGERY FOR ACROMION FRACTURE

Video 46.4
WALANT acromion fracture local anesthesia and surgery (Ahmad, Malaysia).

Reference

1. Ahmad AA, Ubaidah Mustapa Kamal MA, Ruslan SR, Abdullah S, Ahmad AR. Plating of clavicle fracture using the wide-awake technique. J Shoulder Elbow Surg 2020;29(11):2319–2325

CHAPTER 47

FINGER AND RAY AMPUTATION

Donald H. Lalonde and Egemen Ayhan

ADVANTAGES OF WALANT VERSUS SEDATION AND TOURNIQUET FOR FINGER AND RAY AMPUTATION

- Losing a finger is a major event in a patient's life. You get a precious 1-hour opportunity during the surgery to educate the patient on what to expect for recovery and future hand function. This can go a long way toward helping the patient to adapt to the physical changes in the hand.

- All of the general advantages listed in Chapter 2 apply to both the surgeon and the patient (no nausea, no tourniquet pain or let-down bleeding, decreased cost without sedation in minor procedure room, safer surgery without sedation, etc.).

- The patient gets to see what you remove. For example, when you open a destroyed finger after removing it, you can offer to show the damaged parts to the patient. If he or she wants to see it, we have found that the individual may better understand and accept why an attempt to salvage the finger was never going to work. This can help in the "grieving" process for the amputated part.

- Patients get to see that all of the remaining parts of their hand have a full range of active movement after the amputation, at the end of the operation. After patients recover from the pain and stiffness of surgery, they realize that with therapy they can regain full movement in the remaining fingers.

- There is no higher revision rate of digit amputation in the emergency room than in the main operating room, but the cost is much less.[1]

WHERE TO INJECT THE LOCAL ANESTHETIC FOR FINGER AMPUTATION

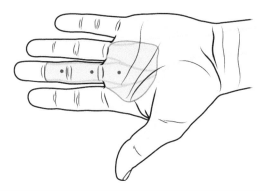

Fig. 47.1 *Palmar injections*: Inject 10 mL of 1% lidocaine with 1:100,000 epinephrine (buffered with 1 mL of 8.4% sodium bicarbonate) in the most proximal palmar red injection point. Perform the most proximal dorsal injection next, and then inject 2 mL in the middle of each of the palmar proximal and middle phalanges in the subcutaneous fat. Performing the proximal dorsal injection before the two distal palmar injections decreases distal palmar injection pain by giving time for the proximal nerve block to work.

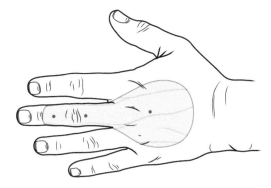

Fig. 47.2 *Dorsal injections*: Inject 4 mL of 1% lidocaine with 1:100,000 epinephrine (buffered with 0.4 mL of 8.4% sodium bicarbonate) in the proximal red injection dot on the dorsal hand. Do the two palmar injections next, and then inject 2 mL in the middle of the dorsal proximal and middle phalanges in the subcutaneous fat.

SPECIFICS OF MINIMALLY PAINFUL INJECTION OF LOCAL ANESTHETIC FOR FINGER AMPUTATION

Video 47.1
Local anesthetic injection for proximal phalanx finger amputation (Lalonde, Canada).

- Inject just under the skin. Sheath injections add unnecessary pain. The local anesthetic will diffuse into the sheath.

- Local anesthesia injection should barely hurt at all if you follow the simple rules of Chapter 5 for hints to minimize injection pain. The patients will think you are magical.

- We always inject all patients while they are lying down to decrease the risk of their fainting (▶ Video 6.1).

- To minimize the pain of injection, inject with a fine 27- or 30-gauge needle (not a 25 gauge) into the most proximal injection point (red dot).

- The distal injections are for the epinephrine vasoconstriction effect; the skin is already numb from the proximal nerve blocks.

- There is no need to inject the palm if the finger amputation is at a more distal level than the proximal phalanx, as shown in ▶ Video 47.2 of a finger amputation at the distal interphalangeal (DIP) joint.

- ▶ Video 47.2 shows a SIMPLE (single subcutaneous injection in the midline proximal phalanx with lidocaine and epinephrine) block for a distal phalanx squamous cell cancer amputation of the distal phalanx of the long finger (see Chapter 1 and Chapter 5 for details of the SIMPLE block).

Video 47.2
SIMPLE (single subcutaneous injection in the midline proximal phalanx with lidocaine and epinephrine) block for distal phalanx squamous cell cancer amputation (Lalonde, Canada).

WHERE TO INJECT THE LOCAL ANESTHETIC FOR RAY AMPUTATION

MINIMALLY PAINFUL INJECTION OF LOCAL ANESTHETIC FOR RAY AMPUTATION

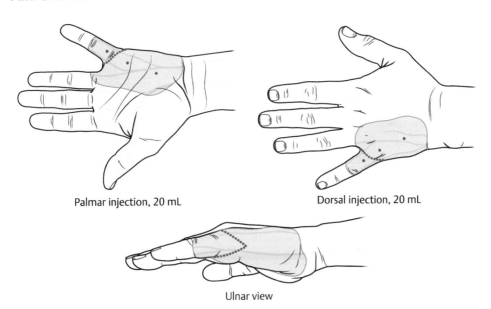

Palmar injection, 20 mL

Dorsal injection, 20 mL

Ulnar view

Fig. 47.3 For ray amputation, inject 20 mL of 1% lidocaine with 1:100,000 epinephrine (buffered with 10 mL lido/epi:1 mL of 8.4% sodium bicarbonate) on each of the palmar and dorsal sides of the ray to be amputated, for a total of 40 mL.

SPECIFICS OF MINIMALLY PAINFUL INJECTION OF LOCAL ANESTHETIC FOR RAY AMPUTATION

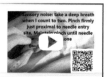

Video 47.3
Minimal pain
injection for
ray amputation
(Lalonde, Canada).

- Inject 10 mL in the most proximal palmar red dot injection point in the subcutaneous fat and under the superficial palmar fascia without moving the needle. Then inject 10 mL in the most proximal red dorsal dot of in the subcutaneous fat over the dorsal proximal hand without moving the needle. This gives time for the distal injection points to get numb before you inject them.

- If it is convenient, wait 15 to 30 minutes for the distal palmar and dorsal hand to get numb so the patient does not feel the distal injections.

- Then inject 8 mL each in the palmar and dorsal central red dot injection points at the head of the metacarpal level in the subcutaneous fat between the digital nerves without moving the needle.

- Finally, inject 2 mL in the palmar and dorsal distal red dot injection points in the subcutaneous fat of the proximal phalanx.

- To decrease the pain of injections, use the other tips discussed in Chapter 5.

TIPS AND TRICKS FOR PERFORMING FINGER AND RAY AMPUTATION WITH THE WIDE AWAKE APPROACH

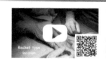

Video 47.4 Ray
amputation
surgery (Ayhan,
Turkey).

- Wait for 30 minutes after the last injection for the epinephrine to reach maximal vasoconstrictive effect, and then operate. Part of these 30 minutes can be spent bringing the patient into the operating room, prepping, draping, patient education, or other tasks.

- Warn the patient that he or she will hear sounds of bone and joint manipulation but will not feel pain. The patient may choose to listen to music on earphones.

- Get the patient to observe his or her hand going through a full range of active movement after you have cleansed the hand at the end of the operation. The patient will know that he or she can regain full movement again after the pain and stiffness of healing subside.

- Use the opportunity to educate the patient on postoperative care of the operated hand (see Chapter 8).

- Use the intraoperative opportunity while closing the skin to educate the patient on what to expect for recovery and future hand function. For example, you can discuss time out of work, phantom limb pain, etc. This can go a long way toward helping the patient adapt to his or her new hand.

- Dr Lalonde most often prefers secondary healing at all levels of finger amputation if there are enough skin and fat that will cover the bone with secondary healing. In mid middle phalanx amputations, for example, this preserves superficialis finger function which is better than shortening the bone to the posterior interphalangeal (PIP) joint to get "faster healing."[2]

References

1. Gil JA, Goodman AD, Harris AP, Li NY, Weiss AC. Cost-effectiveness of initial revision digit amputation performed in the emergency department versus the operating room. Hand (N Y) 2020;15(2):208–214
2. Krauss EM, Lalonde DH. Secondary healing of fingertip amputations: a review. Hand (N Y) 2014;9(3):282–288

CHAPTER 48

REPLANTATION

*Gökhan Tolga Akbulut, Jason Wong, Xiao Fang Shen,
Chung-Chen Hsu, and Donald H. Lalonde*

ADVANTAGES OF WALANT VERSUS SEDATION AND FOR REPLANTATION

- All of the general advantages listed in Chapter 2 apply to both the surgeon and the patient (no nausea, no tourniquet pain or let-down bleeding, decreased cost without sedation in minor procedure room, safer surgery without sedation, etc.).

- Replanting a finger is a major event in a patient's life. You get a precious uninterrupted time during the surgery to educate the patient on how to manage recovery and what to expect with future hand function. This can go a long way toward helping the patient to adapt to the replanted part with new hand function issues.

- The patient gets to see how difficult a replantation can be. This can help in the "grieving" process if the replantation is unsuccessful.

- Much less cost[1] and risk than a long general anesthetic case.

- It can be easier to find the proximal ends of the arteries without a tourniquet.

- Replanting digits quickly under WALANT demystifies the procedure and allows you to have a frank discussion with the patient at the time about letting it go if it does not appear to be salvageable.

- The patients do not have to fast, there are no side effects from general anesthesia, no invasive monitoring, they get to know their surgeon and appreciate the effort, and they recover much quicker.

WHERE TO INJECT THE LOCAL ANESTHETIC FOR FINGER REPLANTATION

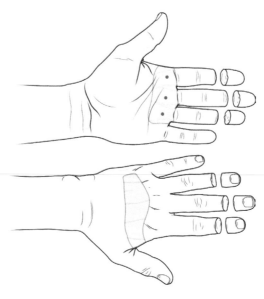

Fig. 48.1 and Fig. 48.2 Injection of local anesthesia in the palm of the hand for replantations outside of the zone of effect of the epinephrine.

SPECIFICS OF MINIMALLY PAINFUL INJECTION OF LOCAL ANESTHETIC FOR FINGER REPLANTATION

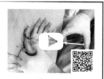

Video 48.1
Injection of
local anesthesia
for thumb
revascularization
(Akbulut, Turkey).

- Dr Gökhan Tolga Akbulut injects epinephrine 1:100,000 with lidocaine 2% and bicarbonate 1:10 where he performs the anastomosis. In this case he injected 1 mL proximal to the wound and 1 mL distal to the wound as shown in ▶ Video 48.1. He also injected 1 mL on the dorsum of the thumb, which is not shown in this video.

- Inject just under the skin. Flexor sheath injections add unnecessary pain and will send the epinephrine up into the finger.

- Local anesthesia injection should barely hurt at all if you follow the simple rules of Chapter 5 for hints to minimize injection pain. The patients will think you are magical.

- See ▶ Video 41.7 (injection for phalanx fracture) for how to inject 10 mL in the palm at the base of the finger and 6 to 7 mL on the dorsum of the hand at the base of the finger to get distal numbness to K-wire a finger. The local anesthesia injection for amputation is the same except that there is no need to inject either the volar or dorsal proximal phalanx when you are performing replantation. Palm and hand dorsum injections suffice. Finger epinephrine may interfere with arterial inflow and is not required. You can reverse the epinephrine vasoconstriction with phentolamine if this is a problem (Chapter 3). The epinephrine injected in the palm will not cause vasoconstriction in the finger if you do not inject in the flexor sheath. However, the lidocaine will provide distal sympathectomy which will make the finger hyperemic. This can be helpful in replantation.

TIPS AND TRICKS FOR PERFORMING FINGER REPLANTATION WITH THE WIDE AWAKE APPROACH

- Let the patient go to the toilet just before you begin. You may have to interrupt the surgery and wrap the hand in a sterile towel for another bathroom break. To help avoid these issues, do not run a high-volume intravenous infusion.

- Patients tend to get restless in procedures lasting over 3 hours. Consider splitting the operation up into two parts: Part one: debride, fix the fracture, repair the tendons, and harvest vein grafts if necessary. Wrap the hand up and allow the patient to go and have a bathroom break. Part two: redrape the patient, repair or graft the artery, repair the digital nerves, and repair the dorsal veins. Allow the patient to shift and change positions as you take a little break as well.

- If there is a question about inflow, injecting verapamil or phentolamine to the digits as discussed in Chapter 3 may help with the vasospasm and you may see reperfusion restored more quickly.

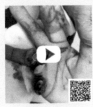
Video 48.2 Revascularization and replantation of two fingers (Akbulut, Turkey).

Video 48.3 Replantation of three fingers (Shen, China).

Video 48.4 Revascularization and cross-finger flap after ring avulsion injury (Wong, England).

Video 48.5 Revascularization with wrist vein grafts (Hsu, Taiwan).

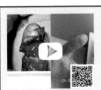
Video 48.6 Various revascularization and replantation examples (Akbulut, Turkey).

Video 48.7 Vascularization with vein graft (Wong, England).

Video 48.8 When replantation fails, WALANT is helpful in adult pollicization of the index (Lalonde, Canada).

Reference

1. Gil JA, Goodman AD, Harris AP, Li NY, Weiss AC. Cost-effectiveness of initial revision digit amputation performed in the emergency department versus the operating room. Hand (N Y) 2020;15(2):208–214

CHAPTER 49

WHAT YOU NEED TO KNOW ABOUT THE BASICS OF USING ULTRASOUND FOR WALANT HAND SURGERY

Brian Jurbala

INTRODUCTION TO ULTRASOUND

- Office-based high resolution musculoskeletal ultrasound (HRMSKUS) has gained significant popularity over the past decade for diagnosis, guiding injections, and doing procedures.

- Popularity of ultrasound has mainly been because of its low cost, portability, and its unprecedented ability to image deeply and clearly into the body.

- Ultrasound allows the operator to clearly and specifically identify underlying submillimeter soft tissue structures in real time with axial resolutions often exceeding 150 μm.

- What I have also discovered in learning about and applying this technology, in my office based upper extremity practice over the years, is that HRMSKUS has a greater field of vision than any other imaging modality (including endoscopy).

- Ultrasound allows the trained and experienced operator to easily and clearly see all structures, in all layers, from the skin to the bones and the relationships of those structures to one another, and to your surgical instruments.

- Ultrasound is very useful both in diagnosing and guiding minimally invasive surgery with WALANT.

- Procedures need less but more precisely delivered local anesthetic, through smaller, less invasive incisions with less tissue dissection. This means less postoperative pain and scarring with a faster, less complicated recovery.

- Unlike endoscopy, HRMSKUS does not require expensive and bulky video equipment. There is no need for it to be sterilized in an autoclave prior to each case. It is portable in the clinic for diagnostic purposes and for ultrasound-guided injections. It generates value when it is not in use during surgery. This means that HRMSKUS is more useful and economical to purchase and maintain in the clinic for minimally invasive WALANT surgery as compared to an endoscopy setup.

SECTION 1: RELEVANT BASICS OF HIGH-RESOLUTION ULTRASOUND

BASIC SCIENCE OF ULTRASOUND YOU SHOULD KNOW

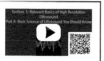

Video 49.1
Ultrasound basic science you should know.

- Ultrasound is defined as all sound frequencies above human hearing range (20 to 20 kHz). Diagnostic medical ultrasound falls in the 2.5 to 40 MHz range.

- An ultrasound unit creates a picture on a screen through a sending–receiving unit, i.e., an **ultrasound transducer** (or probe) converts an electrical signal to a pressure wave (or sound) via a **piezoelectric crystal** linear array on the surface of the probe. This pressure wave is then propagated through tissue. Some of the pressure wave is reflected (echo), some absorbed, and some scattered.

- The returning echoes are gathered by the transducer (or probe) (sending–receiving unit) and converted back to an electrical signal which then is converted to a two-dimensional picture on the screen.

- There are several modes of ultrasound but the one that we use primarily for musculoskeletal ultrasound is **B-mode** or **brightness mode ultrasound** and it recreates a two-dimensional grayscale image (**grayscale = 256 shades of gray**) of the electrical data which closely (but not exactly) represents underlying anatomy on the screen.

- Because it is a waveform, when the ultrasound beam interacts with tissue, it **obeys the laws of reflection and refraction**.

ULTRASOUND NOMENCLATURE YOU SHOULD KNOW

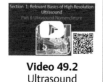

Video 49.2
Ultrasound language you should know.

- Like with any discipline, there is a specific language to describe the ultrasound image. These terms are:
    - Echogenic.
    - Anechoic.
    - Hyperechoic.
    - Hypoechoic.
    - Isoechoic.

COMMON ULTRASOUND ARTIFACTS YOU SHOULD KNOW ABOUT

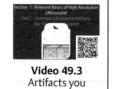

Video 49.3
Artifacts you should know.

- Because of the way ultrasound behaves as a wave and interacts with the underlying tissue it can create artifacts or image distortions. There are many of these artifacts and the most common of these artifacts that you should be familiar with are:
    - Anisotropy.
    - Signal drop off.
    - Edge artifact.
    - Ring down.
    - Posterior acoustic shadowing.
    - Posterior acoustic enhancement.
    - Reverberation.

ULTRASOUND TISSUE APPEARANCES YOU SHOULD KNOW ABOUT

- Tissue appearances differ by echogenicity (intensity of greyscale reflection) and echotexture (textured appearance of the tissue on ultrasound).

- Most tissues have unique "echogenic signatures" or appearances and the basic ones you should know for musculoskeletal ultrasound are that of tendon, bone, muscle, nerve, fat, blood, fluid, and cartilage.

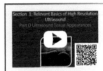

Video 49.4
Ultrasound tissue appearances.

PROBE HANDLING SKILLS AND MANEUVERS YOU SHOULD KNOW ABOUT

- Probe handling skills are supremely important and are the most important skills for you to learn to get good at ultrasound.

- Like any other skill you need to practice them outside of the "game time" situation.

- We will go over the basics here but there are things you have to do to learn and get good at:

  - Hold the probe like a pencil.
  - Rest your wrist or finger.
  - Maintain skin probe contact.
  - Use sufficient gel.
  - Always know your probe-screen orientation.
  - Always know where you are on the court.
  - Always be moving.
- The maneuvers to know:

  - Fishtail.
  - Heel toe.
  - Tilt.
  - Slide/Translate medial/Lateral.
  - Slide/Translate distal to proximal.

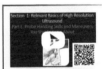

Video 49.5 Probe handling skills.

KNOBOLOGY: THE KNOBS AND BUTTONS YOU SHOULD KNOW ABOUT

- Factory Presets, Musculoskeletal Body Area Presets, Custom User Presets.

- AutoGain (Easy Button) = AutoOptimize, AutoTuning, Tissue Equalization.

- Suggested seven knobs and adjustments with recommended order.

Video 49.6
Knobology.

IMAGE ACQUISITION AND STORAGE YOU SHOULD KNOW ABOUT

- Freeze/Save, Cine or Clip, 10-second Look Back, Measure Menus

Video 49.7 Image acquisition and storage.

Video 49.8
Hardware choices and room setup.

MACHINE SELECTION DETAILS, SCANNING ACCESSORIES, AND MINOR INJECTION ROOM SETUP YOU SHOULD KNOW ABOUT

- This technology, much like computers, changes fast so you must get upgraded every 3 to 5 years to have the latest tools. Handhelds unfortunately do not meet the standard of image quality or have the variety of features useful for ultrasound-guided procedures. Stick to tablet-sized units of 16 MHz or greater or larger units.

SECTION 2: ULTRASOUND-GUIDED INJECTION OF LOCAL ANESTHETIC

Video 49.9
Ultrasound-guided local anesthetic injection.

Advantages: Less local anesthetic can be used, anesthetic can be more precisely placed, and selective nerve blocks can be performed.

Tips and tricks: Make sure you find your target first. Note the depth and slide the probe so the end nearest the planned needle path is right on the edge of target. Measure the depth and then plan an entry 2 to 2.5 times the depth back from probe. This will allow you to keep the needle 20 to 30 degrees to the probe face so that it is visible.

SECTION 3: GENERAL CONSIDERATIONS WHEN USING ULTRASOUND FOR PROCEDURE GUIDANCE IN OFFICE-BASED SURGERY

Video 49.10
General considerations for ultrasound-guided surgery and office surgery.

Advantages: Better field of vision, less dissection needed, can see anatomy preoperatively with ultrasound and make adjustments to approach accordingly, make smaller incisions in most cases to avoid complications, other pathology can be seen and addressed, and this is much more convenient for patients and surgeons.

Tips and tricks: Always do a diagnostic scan before your injection; mark your skin surface landmarks to facilitate your visualization and recognition of underlying structures, especially when you first get started; and use a needle as a preliminary guide to plan and test your incision pathways to make sure your alignment is correct.

Video 49.11
More thoughts on ultrasound by Dr Jurbala.

Room setup details: We use a minor procedure room with comforts for the patients like a big fluffy recliner, a nice music system, and a TV where they can either watch the ultrasound portion of the procedure or Netflix if they wish. We recommend (especially at first) having all the supplies necessary to complete the case in an open surgery manner if you need to convert.

CHAPTER 50

ULTRASOUND-ASSISTED UPPER EXTREMITY PROCEDURES

Brian Jurbala and Donald H. Lalonde

INTRODUCTION TO ULTRASOUND-ASSISTED PROCEDURES

- We are in a new world order. Simple hand surgeries are among the most common ailments we can more easily treat with ultrasound-guided surgery than open surgery.

- Ultrasound-guided surgery provides simpler, effective, more affordable, and more patient-friendly procedures than open surgery.

- Ultrasound-guided surgery can be performed easily in the hand surgeon's office or hospital procedure room outside of the expensive main operating room environment.

- Ultrasound-guided surgery permits patients to get back to work in days instead of weeks after open surgery.

- Ultrasound-guided surgery is easy to learn and readily available to all hand surgeons.

ULTRASOUND-ASSISTED TRIGGER FINGER RELEASE

ADVANTAGES

- This can be done easily in the clinic or office with WALANT, and therefore all of the other advantages of WALANT listed in Chapter 2 are maintained.

- It can all be done through a very extensile but tiny 3-mm skin incision.

- There are no stitches necessary for these procedures, even with the extended incisions. We use buried absorbable Monocryl suture along with benzoin and 0.25-inch skin tape to close the incision.

Video 50.1
Ultrasound-assisted trigger finger release, part 1.

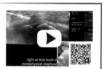

Video 50.2
Ultrasound-
assisted trigger
finger release,
part 2.

- After our first several hundred cases we switched to a phone or tele-heath follow-up only, unless there was a flexor digitorum superficialis (FDS) slip excision, patient concern, or suspected complication.

- Less than 5% of over 2,000 patients have required postoperative hand therapy.

- Multiple procedures and bilateral surgery are not a problem because of the low morbidity of this minimally invasive approach.

- Good results: The first author's series to date of over 2,000 cases show no reported infections or neurovascular complications. The only known patients in the series to underwent revision for an FDS ulnar slip excision was due to recurrent triggering at the A-2 pulley either on the table or later in postoperative period.

TIPS AND TRICKS

- Always try to insert tip of instrument at 20 degrees or less angle to the palm.

- For the middle and ring fingers, it is sometimes useful to swing the finger medially or laterally when inserting the guide tip so you can drop your hand and aim uphill. Because of the metacarpophalangeal (MP) joint, the tendon sheath is actually uphill. When entering retrograde, the trajectory is uphill.

- Use an ergonomically easy and more precise distal-to-proximal technique that ensures complete release of the A-1 pulley, preserves the A-2 pulley, and allows for simple release of the A-0 pulley (or thickened flexor retinaculum) in cases where thickening or constriction of this structure creates a loss of flexion, crepitus, or triggering more proximally after A-1 pulley release.

- Up to 25% of the proximal A-2 pulley can be released through the 3-mm incision without extending it if there is any residual triggering at the A-2, or A3 pulleys, or at the posterior interphalangeal (PIP) joint after the A-1 pulley release.

- In cases where there is still residual triggering after proximal A-2 pulley release, or if there is a flexion contracture of greater than 10 degrees, an ulnar FDS slip excision can be performed by extending the incision a few millimeters proximally and performing a second chevron incision distally at the ulnar PIP joint to isolate the ulnar slip.

- See ▶ Video 50.1 and ▶ Video 50.2 for a better understanding of the above as well as many other tips and tricks.

POSTOPERATIVE CARE

- These patients get over-the-counter pain medications without narcotic.

- Patients are instructed to keep the hand elevated for 24 hours and perform light flexion and extension of the finger/hand five times every 30 minutes.

- They are allowed to return to light activity the next day and full activity after 48 hours.

- They may remove postoperative Band-Aid at 48 hours and get incision wet in the shower or rinse hand under faucet.

- No soaking or getting hand sweaty in a glove for at least 2 weeks is recommended.

- Patients with flexion contractures that are released are given additional exercises directed at stretching the PIP and promoting full active flexion. These patients take longer to obtain full range of motion.

ULTRASOUND-ASSISTED TRIGGER THUMB RELEASE

ADVANTAGES

- This can be done easily in the clinic or office with WALANT, and therefore all of the advantages of WALANT listed in Chapter 2 and above for ultrasound-assisted trigger finger are maintained.

- The radial digital nerve can be visualized and mapped with ultrasound before the surgery.

Video 50.3
Ultrasound-assisted trigger thumb release.

- The intrasheath, ultrasound-guided technique, and safety bumpers on the knife all allow the nerve to be totally and completely avoided while completely and safely releasing the A-1 pulley with a single pass of the knife.

- Good results: The first author has performed over 300 cases of trigger thumb without neurovascular complications, revision, or reoccurrence.

Diagnostic imaging protocol: We recommend every thumb should undergo a complete diagnostic ultrasound scan as per the protocol defined in ▶ Video 50.3. This verifies the thickening of the A-1 pulley, maps the crossover of the radial digital nerve, and the location of the hook of the hamate which serves the landmark stay along the tendon sheath in the safest trajectory for the retrograde intrasheath passage of the tendon sheath knife.

Key skin surface landmarks: The proximal-proximal thumb MP flexion crease (PPTFC), the proximal-distal thumb MP crease (PDTFC), the line dividing the center axis of the thumb palmary, and a line drawn from the midline of the PPTFC. The hook of the hamate (which can also be found and marked sonographically) which serves as the tendon sheath and knife trajectory.

Key sonographic landmarks: The radial digital nerve as it crosses over the tendon sheath 1 to 2 cm proximal to the proximal-proximal thumb MP flexion crease, and the hook of the hamate.

Instrumentation: The same push knife device as described above for trigger finger.

Surgical technique: The 3-mm incision is distal to proximal and is made just distal to distal proximal thumb MP crease and just 1 to 2 mm radial to the midline of the thumb.

TIPS AND TRICKS

- You must insert the tip of the device under the distal A-1 pulley and quickly drop your hand to aim toward the hook of the hamate and up-hill. This requires you to position the instrument at a 20-degree angle to the midline of the thumb.

- Gently twist and push the tip as it finds its way between the tight flexor pollicis longus (FPL) and overlying A-1 pulley. In most cases this is a very tight space with less room than in fingers because the tendon is not split like the FDS in the finger.

- Once the guide tip is in the sheath, verify it with ultrasound and reposition as necessary.

- Once you are happy with the position, rotate the knife 180 degrees and slide forward a few millimeters in order to clear the dorsal ball tip under the skin. Make sure you maintain the alignment of 20 degrees and that your knife trajectory is toward the hook of the hamate and then gently twist and advance the knife until loss of resistance is felt. This will be approximately 1 to 2 cm proximal to the most proximal metacarpophalangeal flexion crease.

- See ▶ Video 50.3 for a better understanding of the above and many other tips and tricks.

ULTRASOUND-ASSISTED CARPAL TUNNEL RELEASE

ADVANTAGES

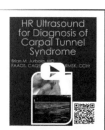

Video 50.4
Ultrasound diagnosis of carpal tunnel syndrome.

- This can be done easily in the clinic or office with WALANT, and therefore all of the advantages of WALANT listed in Chapter 2 are maintained.

- A preliminary diagnostic ultrasound examination can confirm the diagnosis promptly, painlessly, and cost effectively for the patient while allowing the surgeon to see any secondary pathology that may need to be addressed or avoided at surgery.

- This mini-open procedure reduces the usual mini-open incision from 2 cm to about 7 to 8 mm.

- Rather than using a blind technique you are able to safely position the guide proximally with ultrasound before you release the ligament.

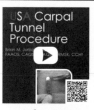

Video 50.5
Ultrasound-assisted carpal tunnel release.

- The instrumentation and guide are one-third the diameter of the typical endoscopic carpal tunnel instrumentation, eliminating the need for dilatation. This permits less crowding of the nerve by the guide which means a lower risk for a neuropraxia or damage to the nerve as compared to endoscopic surgery.

- Good results: The first author's clinical outcomes have excellent pain and early DASH scores compared to national averages and are available in real time at: **www.CarpalTunnelExpert.com/outcomes**

  Diagnostic Imaging Protocol: This protocol is designed to confirm the diagnosis, and identify secondary causes and anomalies and variations in anatomy. It employs a sector approach to scanning the entire carpal tunnel and adjacent structures. It identifies the configuration of the median nerve and its cross-sectional area (CSA) at proximal wrist crease, or at the inlet of the computed tomography (CT). It also identifies the median nerve motor branch and the dimensions of the ulnar safe zone (▸ Video 50.4).

Skin surface landmarks: The salient landmarks are Kaplan's cardinal where it intersects radial boarder of fourth ray.

Sonographic landmarks: The scaphoid tubercle and pisiform, the interval between the ulnar artery and median nerve proximally, hook of the hamate, ulnar artery and its position relative to the hook of the hamate, and the median nerve motor branch.

Instrumentation: The nondisposable instrumentation set which comes in an autoclavable cassette contains a sonographically visible guide for the proximal release, a Ragnell retractor, a modified Heiss retractor, and a pair of pickups and a scalpel handle. There is a single-use disposable tunnel tome knife that comes packaged separately.

Surgical technique: After blocking, surgical field/pathway and median nerve skin landmarks are drawn. A 5- to 7-mm incision is made using ultrasound guidance and a number 15 blade just ulnar to the median nerve halfway between the proximal wrist crease and Kaplan's cardinal line (▸ Video 50.5). Through the skin incision and under ultrasound guidance, use the knife to make a ligamentotomy about 5 mm proximal to the skin incision by gently pushing but not slicing with a slight tilt of the knife handle ulnarly to account for the curve in the transverse carpal ligament (TCL). When you feel (and see under ultrasound) the knife "pop" through the ligament, you then insert the guide in the following fashion. Guide the tip under distal exposed lip of TCL and immediately lower your hand and aim the guide toward the index finger and then push in the guide under direct ultrasound vision.

TIPS AND TRICKS

- The most common pitfall is making incision too distal. The TCL has a hump distally. If you make a ligamentotomy distal to the hump, you will not be able to place the guide in such a way that it hugs the undersurface of the TCL and squeezes out the median nerve and protects it. Therefore, pay attention to this in training.

- You need to pass the disposable knife twice to get the whole palmar proximal portion of the TCL.

- Pass the knife at least 2 cm proximal to the wrist crease.

- The distal part of the TCL is released under direct vision in order to ensure a complete safe release.

RETURN TO ACTIVITY/REHABILITATION

- Postoperative patients are instructed to keep the hand elevated for 24 to 48 hours when not in use and perform light flexion and extension of the finger/hand five times every 30 minutes.

- They are allowed to return to light activity the next day and full activity after 48 hours.

- They may remove postoperative Band-Aid at 48 hours and get incision wet in the shower or rinse hand under faucet.

- They are forbidden to lift greater than 15 pounds for 1 week; then they can gradually return to full unrestricted activity by 2 weeks postoperatively.

- They are informed that tenderness can last for 2 to 10 weeks, but after 2 weeks, they cannot damage anything and can push themselves as tolerated.

- No soaking or getting hand sweaty in a glove for at least 2 weeks is recommended.

ULTRASOUND-ASSISTED CUBITAL TUNNEL RELEASE

ADVANTAGES

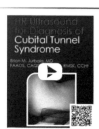

Video 50.6
Ultrasound
diagnosis of cubital
tunnel syndrome.

- This can be done easily in the clinic or office with WALANT, and therefore all of the other advantages of WALANT listed in Chapter 2 are maintained.

- Much less tissue dissection and morbidity to permit earlier range of motion and return to activity. At 24 to 48 hours after surgery, most patients can return to light work restricted to 15 pounds for the first week. They are allowed to return to full activity in the second week.

- This mini-open procedure reduces the usual long incision to about 7 to 8 mm safely.

- Ensures a complete release proximally and distally.

- Most patients return to light work in 24 to 48 hours.

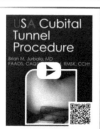

Video 50.7
Ultrasound-
assisted surgery
for cubital tunnel
release.

- This minimal morbidity approach can be combined with other procedures such as carpal tunnel release, trigger finger, etc. Bilateral release is also facilitated by the minimal morbidity.

- Ultrasound visualization helps to avoid damage to the medial antebrachial cutaneous nerve of the forearm and the motor branch of the median nerve.

Diagnostic imaging protocol: Ultrasound protocol involves short and long axis scanning from the level of the junction of the middle and distal one-third of the upper arm through the cubital tunnel and into the proximal one-third of the forearm as the ulnar nerve dives between the two heads of the flexor carpi ulnaris (FCU). The absolute value at point of maximal swelling is 8.95 mm^2 swelling ratio[1] (▶ Video 5.6).

Skin surface landmarks: The medial epicondyle, the olecranon, the humeral and ulnar attachments of the FCU, and the intervening raphe.

Sonographic landmarks: Medial epicondyle, olecranon, Osborne's fascia, medial head of triceps, humeral and ulnar head of FCU, posterior fascia of FCU, and intramuscular septum.

Instrumentation: We use the tunnel tome disposable knife with the tunnel tome instrumentation.

TIPS AND TRICKS

- Always use a needle to locate incision starting point. Release proximal first. Use ultrasound in short axis to follow tip of the guide and keep above nerve but in the external nerve sheath all the way to about 3 mm above the medial epicondyle. You may need to straighten elbow to make "turn" around the medial epicondyle.

- See ▶ Video 50.7 for surgical technique and many more tips and tricks.

  Return to activity/Rehabilitation: Ice and compression with light compression wrap for 24 hours, then return to full light activity. No lifting greater than 15 pounds for 1 week.

ULTRASOUND-ASSISTED DE QUERVAIN'S RELEASE

ADVANTAGES

- This can be done easily in the clinic or office with WALANT, and therefore all of the other advantages of WALANT listed in Chapter 2 are maintained.

Video 50.8
Ultrasound-assisted diagnosis and surgery for De Quervain's tenosynovitis.

- The limited 3-mm incision and minimal tissue dissection decreases the risk of injuring small terminal nerve branches of the superficial radial nerve or the lateral antebrachial cutaneous nerve of the forearm.

- No need to splint after surgery.

- Decreases the need for postoperative hand therapy.

- Most patient return to light activity in 24 hours.

  Diagnostic imaging protocol: Scan from junction of distal one-third and middle one-third of forearm radially to thumb MP joint. Look at the De Quervain's canal as well as the scaphoid, scaphotrapiezial joint, and thumb carpometacarpal (CMC) joints for degenerative disease, occult cysts, or other pathology to rule out other causes of pain. Also scan palmarly over radial artery to make sure there are no occult ganglions around the radial artery that could be mimicking symptoms.

  Skin landmarks: Palpate the radial styloid with your index finger, then drop into the anatomic snuff just distal and dorsal to the styloid and pinch between index and thumb the tendons of the palmar border of the first dorsal compartment tendons; the extensor pollicis brevis (EPB) dorsally and the abductor pollicis longus (APL) palmarly.

  Sonographic landmarks: The main landmarks will be the radial styloid in the long axis view (LAX) view and the tendon sheath will extend 3 to 5 mm distal to the styloid especially in the case of a dual compartment. This can create a wrenching effect on the tendons pushing them down as they drop off the styloid. The radial artery passes under the tendons halfway between the styloid and the CMC joint.

Instrumentation: We use the same version of the disposable safety knife described in the trigger finger and trigger thumb section to safely and completely effect the release.

Surgical technique: Inject starting 1.5 cm distal to the styloid right over first dorsal compartment at the level of radial artery cross under. Then inject above the compartment to 2 cm proximal. Then inject into the compartment inserting needle 1 to 2 cm proximal to styloid into compartment where in the case of dual compartment they become one. Only inject 0.5 to 1 cc of local anesthetic into compartment because more will be painful as the compartment distends with increased intracompartmental pressure. Make longitudinal 3-mm incision 1.5 cm distal to styloid and enter the desired compartment with a flat scissor tip, verify under ultrasound then exchange for tip of trigger tome micro knife and verify tip placement under ultrasound. Release compartment by gently turning knife clockwise and counterclockwise while advancing in line with tendons 1. 5 to 2 cm in retrograde fashion until loss of resistance.

TIPS AND TRICKS

- If there are two compartments, always first release the smaller, more distal, and more dorsal EPB compartment. Then you can go ahead and release the larger or more proximal and palmar APL compartment.

- The knife cannot cut the nerve easily, but you have to enter the compartments distally where the nerve branches are running laterally to De Quervain's canal. The nerves are relatively superficial. If you use an approach from proximal to distal rather than the described approach you will likely have a higher chance of transecting the dorsal branch of the superficial radial nerve where it crosses just proximal to the compartment.

Return to activity/rehabilitation: Most patients return to light activity in 24 hours, full unrestricted activity with a 15-pound restriction in 48 hours, and full activity in 7 days with no weight restrictions. The average return to work is 3 to 7 days in over 200 cases.

ULTRASOUND-ASSISTED LACERTUS RELEASE OF MEDIAN NERVE COMPRESSION AT THE ELBOW

ADVANTAGES

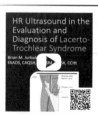

Video 50.9
Ultrasound-assisted diagnosis of lacertus syndrome.

- This can be done easily in the clinic or office with WALANT, and therefore all of the other advantages of WALANT listed in Chapter 2 are maintained.

- Reduces incision size.

- Ultrasound allows you to see the sites of compression readily before the surgery.

- Ultrasound lets you evaluate the completeness of release more extensively than when you are looking through a small surgical wound.

- Requires less dissection than open and endoscopic procedures.

    Diagnostic imaging protocol: Short and long axis views from 3 to 4 cm above humeral metaphysis distally to past the bicipital tuberosity. Verify area of pain/reproduction of symptoms with sonopalpation, absolute diameter at site of maximal swelling just proximal to lacertus which should be less than 10 mm,[2] and look for qualitative signs of nerve compression.

    Skin landmarks: Medial epicondyle, lateral border of biceps tendon and its expansion over media flexor pronator mass, medial border of biceps, and "Boomerang" extension of lacertus fascia as it swings medially and proximally to insert on medial epicondyle.

    Sonographic landmarks (short axis view [SAX] view): (at peak of humeral trochlea) Lateral to medial biceps tendon, brachial artery, median nerve, and trochlear peak with overlying brachioradialis muscle. Upper boundary of lacertus tunnel in SAX view is lacertus fascia and bottom boundary is brachioradialis muscle and humeral trochlea.

    Instrumentation: Tunnel tome nondisposable instrumentation (ultrasound-assisted carpal tunnel procedure above) and trigger tome disposable safety knife.

    Surgical technique: It is easier to go from distal to proximal on the first pass. Bluntly dissect with long Littler scissors to enter outer sheath of nerve below overlying muscle fascia and verify under ultrasound in two planes. Exchange scissors for guide and then position the guide under lacertus fascia along nerve to a level 1 cm proximal to medial epicondyle. Release with disposable tunnel tome knife.

Video 50.10
Ultrasound-assisted surgical median nerve decompression in lacertus syndrome.

TIPS AND TRICKS

Return to activity/rehabilitation: Immediate return to activity, no need for formal physiotherapy in most cases.

ULTRASOUND-ASSISTED TENNIS ELBOW RELEASE

ADVANTAGES

- Single puncture incision
- No physiotherapy
- Immediate pain relief
- Return to light activity immediately, and return to normal activity in 24 to 48 hours. Limit lifting of weight to 15 pounds for 1 week and gradually return to full racquet sports by 2 weeks.

    Diagnostic imaging protocol: LAX and SAX views over lateral epicondyle to verify diagnosis plus fine flow Doppler to document angiofibroblastic dysplasia (if any).

    Skin landmarks: Lateral epicondyle, superior border of extensor carpi radialis brevis (ECRB), inferior border of extensor carpi ulnaris (ECU), anconeus, and radial head.

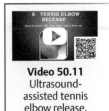

Video 50.11
Ultrasound-assisted tennis elbow release.

Sonographic landmarks: SAX or transverse view 3 to 4 cm distal to lateral epicondyle of the musculotendinous junction of the ECU, extensor digitorum communis (EDC)/ECRB (together), and extensor carpis radialis longus (ECRL) muscles.

Instrumentation: Disposable trigger tome safety knife.

Surgical technique: Locate incision site over anconeus about 0.5 cm lateral to the border of the ECU and 3 to 4 cm distal to lateral epicondyle by using a needle to locate trajectory under superficial ECU fascia. Make stab incision and use flat iris scissors to sound out entry in lateral ECU under ultrasound guidance. Then advance tips under superficial fascia and across septum under superficial fascia of EDC. Exchange scissors for trigger tome knife and release superficial fascia from lateral ECU to medial ECRB at junction with ECRL.

TIPS AND TRICKS

- Always pronate forearm to rotate posterior interosseous nerve medially.
- Always flex wrist to put tension on the superficial fascia before passing knife.
- Use "Single Pass of the Knife" through superficial fascia at the musculotendinous junction to reduce the risk of too much muscle release.
- Use scissors to sound out entry site under radial ECU and puncture through septum between ECU and EDC.
- Be careful not to go under the deep fascia because only superficial fascia needs to be released and in order to avoid underlying supinator and remote potential for injury to posterior interosseous nerve (PIN) (which is medial to, and is not in, the field).
- Verify release with tip of knife in LAX ultrasound view.

Return to activity/rehabilitation: No formal rehabilitation. Return to activity light immediately and normal in 24 to 48 hours. Limit lifting to 15 pounds for 1 week; then return to full activity, as tolerated, including sports.

References

1. Rayegani SM, Raeissadat SA, Kargozar E, Rahimi-Dehgolan S, Loni E. Diagnostic value of ultrasonography versus electrodiagnosis in ulnar neuropathy. Med Devices (Auckl) 2019;12:81–88
2. Cartwright MS, Shin HW, Passmore LV, Walker FO. Ultrasonographic reference values for assessing the normal median nerve in adults. J Neuroimaging 2009;19(1):47–51

Section IV

WALANT Lower Extremity Surgery

CHAPTER 51

PATELLA FRACTURES

Amir Adham Ahmad and Donald H. Lalonde

ADVANTAGES OF WALANT VERSUS SEDATION AND TOURNIQUET IN PATELLA FRACTURES

- All of the general advantages listed in Chapter 2 apply to both the surgeon and the patient (no nausea, no tourniquet pain or let-down bleeding, decreased cost without sedation in minor procedure room, safer surgery without sedation, etc.).

- After reduction and fixation of the fracture, the patient who is awake and comfortable can move his or her knee joint on the operating table before you close the skin. This allows you to assess the stability of the fixation in active motion.

- When you see full active motion of the knee and observe the stability of the fixation with fluoroscopy, you will be more confident to initiate early active range of movement exercises.

- Intraoperative assessment of movement and stability after fracture reduction may lead to more or less protection after surgery depending on what you see.

- You can take advantage of the patient being awake to educate him or her during the surgery on how to move the knee so it will not get stiff after the surgery. You should also teach the patient how to use the lower limb to protect the fracture from coming apart after the surgery.

- No sedation is safer in older patients with heart or lung comorbidities.

WHERE TO INJECT THE LOCAL ANESTHETIC FOR TENSION BAND WIRE OF PATELLA

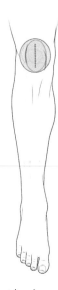

Fig. 51.1 Prepare up to 100 mL of tumescent local anesthesia with 50 mL of 1% lidocaine with 1:100,000 epinephrine added to 5 mL of 8.4% bicarbonate and 50 mL of saline. Inject 10 to 20 mL of this 0.5% lidocaine with 1:200,000 epinephrine solution subcutaneously (*blue*) along the incision site using a long 27-gauge needle. Inject an additional 40 to 45 mL of the same solution at the periosteal level covering the superior, middle, and inferior pole of the patella. *Red dotted line* is the possible incision.

SPECIFICS OF MINIMALLY PAINFUL INJECTION OF LOCAL ANESTHETIC IN PATELLA FRACTURES

- Local anesthesia injection should barely hurt at all if you follow the simple rules of Chapter 5 for hints to minimize injection pain. The patients will think you are magical. For example, inject with a long 27-gauge needle and pinch the skin into the needle to add sensory "noise" of pressure to decrease the pain.

- Always err on the side of too much local anesthesia instead of not enough. You are aiming for patients only feeling a small sting when you insert the first local anesthesia needle. They should feel no pain for the rest of the injections or during the surgery.

- There are two types of injections for fractures. The first injection is the subcutaneous injection where you inject at the incision site. The second injection is the periosteal injection to bathe the entire area of bone or joint where dissection or noxious stimuli will happen.

- Start by injecting the first 10 to 20 mL subcutaneously along the incision site.

- Follow subcutaneous injections with periosteal injection. The goal is to flood the periosteum circumferentially around the patella.

- Always inject proximal to distal in both subcutaneous and periosteal injections to avoid sharp needle penetration of nonanesthetized tissue.

- For periosteal injections, start the injection at the most proximal aspect of the subcutaneous injection (superior pole of the patella).

- Start by injecting at the superior pole of the patella. Do not remove the needle as you need to "walk the bone" to go to the medial and lateral aspects of the patella. Do this at three or four intervals along the middle and inferior pole of the patella.

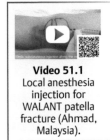

Video 51.1
Local anesthesia injection for WALANT patella fracture (Ahmad, Malaysia).

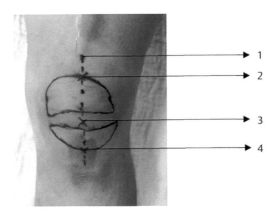

Fig. 51.2 Schematic outline of the injection technique: (1) Inject 10 to 20 mL subcutaneously along the dotted skin incision. (2) Inject 13 to 15 mL periosteally superior to the patella. (3) Inject 13 to 15 mL periosteally at the fracture site. (4) Inject 13 to 15 mL periosteally at the inferior pole of the patella.

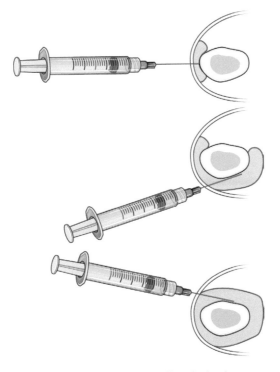

Fig. 51.3 The concept of "walking the bone" with the needle to bathe the entire involved periosteum.

- The posterior patellar surface will be numbed by the large volume of tumescent local anesthesia all around it and through the fracture site.

- Do not rush the injections. The whole process should take about 10 to 30 minutes. Score yourself every time you inject to try to get a hole-in-one every time. (See Chapter 5 for other hints on how to decrease the pain of local anesthesia injection.)

- Inject 30 minutes before incision to allow the epinephrine to take optimal effect and provide adequately dry working field, as outlined in Chapter 4 and Chapter 14.

- Inject your patients (lying down to decrease risk of fainting) in the waiting area before going into the operating room (see Chapter 2).

TIPS AND TRICKS FOR OPERATIVE REDUCTION OF PATELLA FRACTURES WITH THE WIDE AWAKE APPROACH

- Wait at least 25 to 30 minutes between injection and incision. It is more efficient to inject them on a stretcher before they come into the operating room, and it gives the epinephrine time to produce vasoconstriction.

- Before surgery, test the anesthetic effect by manipulating the fracture site. The pain score should be "0" during manipulation. This is a sign that the local anesthesia has taken effect and it is safe to proceed with the surgery without pain.

- After the reconstruction, take down the drape and have patients see and move their knee in all directions (especially in extension). This memory will be motivating if the patients happen to get stiff after surgery.

- Close the skin with buried intradermal simple interrupted 4-0 Monocryl sutures as shown in detail for carpal tunnel closure in ▶ Video 26.9. Buried simple interrupted sutures of absorbable monofilament Monocryl mean that there are no sutures to remove.

Video 51.2 Injection of local anesthesia in a second patient and checking band wire stability of the patella with active movement (Ahmad, Malaysia).

CHAPTER 52

TIBIA AND FIBULA FRACTURES

*Amir Adham Ahmad, Kamal Rafiqi,
and Donald H. Lalonde*

ADVANTAGES OF WALANT VERSUS SEDATION AND TOURNIQUET IN TIBIA AND FIBULA FRACTURES

- All of the general advantages listed in Chapter 2 apply to both the surgeon and the patient (no nausea, no tourniquet pain or let-down bleeding, decreased cost without sedation in minor procedure room, safer surgery without sedation, etc.).

- After reduction and fixation of the fracture, the patient who is awake and comfortable would be able to demonstrate the movements of the affected limb. This allows you to assess the stability of the fixation in active motion.

- When you see full active motion of the limb and observe the stability of the fixation with fluoroscopy, you will be more confident to initiate early active range of movement exercises for the foot and ankle.

- It may lead to less protection after surgery based on intraoperative assessments.

- You can take advantage of the patient being awake to educate him or her during the surgery on how to move the limb so it will not get stiff after the surgery. You should also teach the patient how to use the lower limb to protect the fracture from coming apart after the surgery.

- No sedation is safer in older patients with heart or lung comorbidities.

WHERE TO INJECT THE LOCAL ANESTHETIC FOR PLATING OF TIBIA IN MIDSHAFT TIBIA AND FIBULA FRACTURE

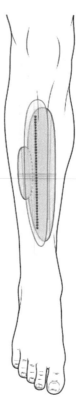

Fig. 52.1 Prepare up to 100 mL of tumescent local anesthesia with 50 mL of 1% lidocaine with 1:100,000 epinephrine added to 5 mL of 8.4% bicarbonate and 50 mL of saline. Inject 10 to 20 mL of this 0.5% lidocaine with 1:200,000 epinephrine solution subcutaneously (*blue*) along the incision site using a long 27-gauge needle. Inject an additional 40 to 45 mL of the same solution at the periosteal covering the proximal, middle, and distal aspects of the tibial fracture site. Inject an additional 10 to 20 mL at the fracture site over the fibula. *Red dotted line* is the possible incision. *Pink* is periosteal; blue is subcutaneous. Some patients with large or long legs may need 100 to 150 mL of tumescent local anesthesia. If that is the case, add 100 mL of saline to the 50 mL of 1% lidocaine with 1:100,000 epinephrine and 5 mL of 8.4% bicarbonate to make 150 mL of 0.3% lidocaine with 1:300,000 epinephrine.

SPECIFICS OF MINIMALLY PAINFUL INJECTION OF LOCAL ANESTHETIC IN TIBIA AND FIBULA FRACTURES

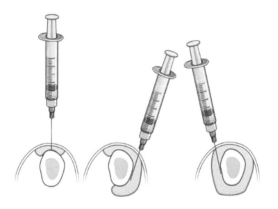

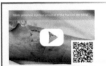

Video 52.1
Local anesthesia injection for WALANT tibia and fibula fracture (Ahmad, Malaysia).

Fig. 52.2 Cross-section of the midshaft tibia (or any other long bone) for injection at the periosteal layer. Only one skin needle entry site is required in each of the three injection sites. The skin can be pushed to one side or the other with the needle to keep the needle tip at the periosteal level.

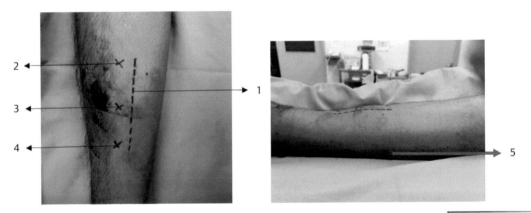

Fig. 52.3 and Fig 52.4 Schematic outline of the injection technique: (1) Inject 10 to 20 mL subcutaneously along the dotted skin incision. (2) Inject 13 to 15 mL periosteally proximal to the tibial fracture site. (3) Inject 13 to 15 mL periosteally at the fracture site. (4) Inject 13 to 15 mL periosteally distal to the tibial fracture site. (5) Inject 10 to 20 mL periosteally at the fracture site over the fibula.

Video 52.2 Test readiness of anesthesia with zero pain on manipulating the fracture site after the injection (Ahmad, Malaysia).

- Local anesthesia injection should barely hurt at all if you follow the simple rules of Chapter 5 for hints to minimize injection pain. The patients will think you are magical. For example, inject with a long 27-gauge needle and pinch the skin into the needle to add sensory "noise" of pressure to decrease the pain.

- Always err on the side of too much local anesthesia instead of not enough. You are aiming for patients only feeling a small sting when the first local anesthesia needle is inserted. They should feel no pain for the rest of the injections or during the surgery.

- There are two types of injections for fractures. The first injection is the subcutaneous injection where you inject at the incision site. The second injection is the periosteal injection to bathe the entire area of bone or joint where dissection or noxious stimuli will happen.

- Start by injecting the first 10 to 20 mL subcutaneously along the incision site.

- Follow subcutaneous injections with periosteal injection.

- Always inject proximal to distal in both subcutaneous and periosteal injections to avoid sharp needle penetration of nonanesthetized tissue.

- For periosteal injection, start the injection at the side where the bone is easily palpable (anterior aspect of tibia).

- Start by injecting at the proximal aspect of the tibial fracture. Do not remove the needle as you need to "walk the bone" to go to the medial and lateral aspects of the tibia. Do this at three or four intervals along the middle and inferior aspects of the tibial fracture.

- Do not rush the injections. The whole process should take about 10 to 30 minutes. Score yourself every time you inject to try to get a hole-in-one every time. (See Chapter 5 for other hints on how to decrease the pain of local anesthesia injection.)

- Inject 30 minutes before incision to allow the epinephrine to take optimal effect and provide adequately dry working field, as outlined in Chapter 4 and Chapter 14.

- Inject your patients (lying down to decrease risk of fainting) in the waiting area before going into the operating room (see ▶ Video 6.1).

TIPS AND TRICKS FOR OPERATIVE REDUCTION OF TIBIA AND FIBULA FRACTURES WITH THE WIDE AWAKE APPROACH

- Wait at least 25 to 30 minutes between injection and incision. It is more efficient to inject them on a stretcher before they come into the operating room.

- Before surgery, test the anesthetic effect by manipulating the fracture site. The pain score should be "0" during manipulation. This is a sign that the local anesthesia has taken effect and it is safe to proceed with the surgery without pain.

- Close the skin with buried intradermal simple interrupted 4-0 Monocryl sutures as shown in detail for carpal tunnel closure in

▶ Video 26.9. Buried simple interrupted sutures of absorbable monofilament Monocryl mean that there are no sutures to remove.

- Do not forget to inject the fibula even though you are not going to fix it. This is to make sure the patient is painless when you manipulate the fracture site for both tibia and fibula.

- After the reconstruction, take down the drape and have patients see and move their limb in all directions. This will be motivation for the patient to start the physiotherapy.

Video 52.3
Plating of the tibial fracture and checking the stability of the fixation with active movement (Ahmad, Malaysia).

Video 52.4
Injection of local anesthesia and screw reduction of tibial plateau fracture (Rafiqi, Morocco).

Video 52.5
Injecting local anesthesia and plating tibia midshaft fracture (Rafiqi, Morocco).

CHAPTER 53

FOOT AND ANKLE FRACTURES AND SURGERY

D. Joshua Mayich, Amir Adham Ahmad, Chris Chun-Yu Chen, Kamal Rafiqi, Luke MacNeill, Egemen Ayhan, and Donald H. Lalonde

ADVANTAGES OF WALANT VERSUS SEDATION AND TOURNIQUET IN FOOT AND ANKLE SURGERY

- All of the general advantages listed in Chapter 2 apply to both the surgeon and the patient (no nausea, no tourniquet pain or let-down bleeding, decreased cost without sedation in minor procedure room, safer surgery without sedation, etc.).

- Significant evidence exists that demonstrates the efficacy and safety of WALANT for forefoot surgery.[1,2,3,4]

- WALANT was the preferred method of anesthesia for forefoot surgery for the first author, and over a 7-year period over 1,000 WALANT forefoot surgeries were successfully completed. Additionally, several procedures involving the midfoot, hindfoot, and ankle were performed with increasing confidence and effect as time went on.

- In the setting of scarce resources, not requiring an anesthesiologist increases operating room access for both surgeons and patients.

- Full active motion of the foot and ankle can be observed. This includes the stability of the fixation with fluoroscopy. This allows greater confidence to give more accurate weightbearing recommendations postoperatively.

- Advantage can be taken of the patient being awake during the procedure to perform patient education interventions around everything from natural history of their diagnosis to required postoperative rehabilitation protocols. In addition, this time with the patient is often used to improve the patient and physician relationship with discussions, etc.

- In patients whose general anesthesia risk is high, and urgent surgery is required, WALANT can allow for effective anesthesia while minimizing/eliminating the risk of more involved general anesthetic techniques (e.g., cardiac event in the past 6 months).

- After reduction and fixation of fractures, the patient who is awake and comfortable can demonstrate the movements of the affected limb and perform simulated weightbearing on the operative table by lowering the foot of the bed and using a sterile footplate. This allows the surgeon to assess the position and stability of the fixation during active motion.[1]

WHERE TO INJECT THE LOCAL ANESTHETIC FOR MAJOR ANKLE SURGERY (FRACTURE, FUSION, ARTHROSCOPY, IRRIGATION AND DEBRIDEMENT, ETC.)

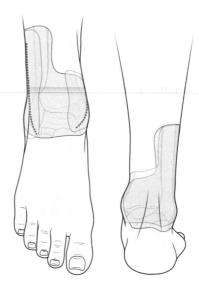

Fig. 53.1 Prepare 105 mL of tumescent local anesthesia with 50 mL of 1% lidocaine with 1:100,000 epinephrine added to 5 mL of 8.4% bicarbonate and 50 mL of saline. Inject 10 to 20 mL of this 0.5% lidocaine with 1:200,000 epinephrine solution subcutaneously (*blue*) along both incision sites using a long 27-gauge needle. Inject an additional 20 to 30 mL of the same solution at the periosteal level covering the proximal, middle, and distal aspects of the fracture site at the lateral malleolus. Inject an additional 20 to 30 mL surrounding the medial malleolus and distal tibia. Inject an additional 10 to 15 mL at the posterior malleolus. *Red dotted lines* are the possible incisions.
If more than 100 mL of tumescent local anesthesia is required for patients with larger and longer legs, dilute the solution even further to 0.3% lidocaine with 1:300,000 epinephrine by adding 50 mL of saline to the solution which will provide a total of 155 mL.

SPECIFICS OF MINIMALLY PAINFUL INJECTION OF LOCAL ANESTHESIA FOR MAJOR ANKLE SURGERY (FRACTURE, FUSION, ARTHROSCOPY, IRRIGATION AND DEBRIDEMENT, ETC.)

- Local anesthetic injection should barely hurt at all if the rules of Chapter 5 for hints to minimize injection pain are followed. Patients will think you are magical if you follow those instructions. For example, inject with a long 27-gauge needle while performing distraction techniques to minimize injection-related pain.

- Always err on the side of too much local anesthesia instead of not enough. The goal is for patients to only feel the small sting of the first local anesthesia needle. They should feel no pain with the rest of the injections or during the subsequent procedure/surgery.

- There are two types of injections for fractures. The first injection is the subcutaneous injection involving the planned incision site(s). The second injection is the periosteal, intra-articular, and fracture hematoma injection to bathe the entire area of bone or joint where dissection or noxious stimuli will occur.

- Start by injecting the first 10 to 20 mL subcutaneously along the incision site(s) and/or the path of the planned intra-articular anesthesia.

- Always inject proximal to distal in both subcutaneous and periosteal injections to avoid sharp needle penetration of nonanesthetized tissue.

- With intra-articular injuries, consider beginning anesthesia by performing an intra-articular ankle joint block. This often will gain rapid pain relief at medial, lateral, and posterior malleolar fracture sites within one to two half-lives of the utilized local anesthetic.

- For intra-articular joint injections in ankle fractures:
  - Always use sufficiently buffered local anesthetic mixture to avoid preventable cartilage injury by acidic local solutions (see Chapter 5 for buffering instructions).
  - Pass a larger bore (22 gauge) needle through anesthetized tissue into the fracture hematoma in the joint. Use a 10-mL syringe filled with a smaller amount of buffered local anesthetic mixture (usually 2–3 mL). Once confirmed to be intra-articular, pass the local anesthetic into the joint. Wait about 1 minute, and then aspirate the joint hematoma. Once this has been done, leave the needle in situ, fill the syringe matching the amount of aspirated fluid, and then replace this with local anesthetic mixture. This will avoid the pressure-related discomfort of the initial joint and maximize anesthesia in the injured joint.
  - Always be patient after administration of the intra-articular ankle block, allowing for 5 to 10 minutes to pass prior to proceeding with the remainder of the injections, as pain relief is usually significant following the block of the associated joint, leaving the patient much more relaxed and comfortable throughout the remainder of the additional required injections.
  - Ensure that both the medial and lateral gutters have been well anesthetized. This may require injection of local anesthetic both anterior

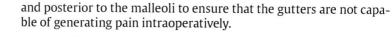
and posterior to the malleoli to ensure that the gutters are not capable of generating pain intraoperatively.

- For periosteal injections (including a fracture hematoma injection):

  - Start proximally at the anterior tibia where the bone is easily palpable. Ensure that you have plenty of tumescent local anesthesia at least 2 cm proximal to the planned area of surgery.
  - Start fibular injections proximal to the lateral malleolus fracture site. Do not remove the needle and "walk along the bone." Go to the medial and lateral aspects of the lateral malleolus. Do this at three or four intervals along the middle and inferior aspect of the lateral malleolus.
  - Drop into the fracture site and draw back. Ensure that any blood vessel has not been entered. Sufficient often darker colored blood return indicates that the fracture hematoma has been entered. Ensure sufficient localized hematoma block has occurred—as should have happened with the intra-articular injection.
  - Pay careful attention to ensure adequate syndesmotic anesthesia. When injecting medially in the syndesmosis, ensure that both sides of the interosseous membrane of the tibia and fibula are well blocked. There is commonly a "pop" felt when this structure is traversed. This indicates the needle is posterior to the intraosseous membrane, allowing for more complete posterior anesthesia.
  - When injecting the buffered local mixture medially and posteriorly, take great care to avoid neurovascular and tendinous structures to ensure safe injection.

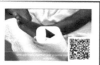

Video 53.1
Local anesthesia injection for WALANT ankle fracture (Amir Ahmad, Malaysia).

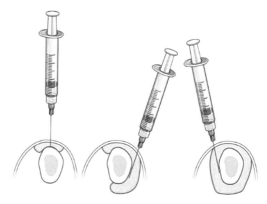

Fig. 53.2 Cross-section of the lateral malleolus (or any other long bone) for injection at the periosteal layer. Only one skin needle entry site is required in each of the three injection sites. The skin can be pushed from side to side with the needle to keep the needle tip at the periosteal level.

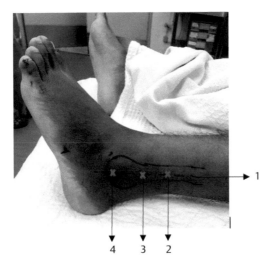

Fig. 53.3 Schematic outline of the injection technique: (1) Inject 10 to 20 mL subcutaneously along the dotted skin incision. (2) Inject 8 to 10 mL periosteally proximal to the fracture site of the lateral malleolus. (3) Inject 8 to 10 mL periosteally at the fracture site. (4) Inject 8 to 10 mL periosteally distal to the fracture site.

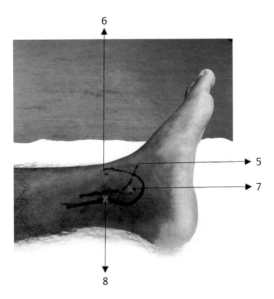

Fig. 53.4 (5) Inject 10 to 20 mL proximally to distally subcutaneously along the dotted skin incision. (6) Inject 10 to 15 mL subperiosteally at the anterior tibia. (7) Inject 10 to 15 mL periosteally at the fracture site and surrounding the medial malleolus. (8) Inject 10 to 15 mL periosteally at the posterior malleolus.

- Do not rush the injections. The whole process should take 15 to 30 minutes. The injecting surgeon should score himself/herself every time, as a means of continuing to learn and improve technique. (See Chapter 5 for this and other hints on how to decrease the pain of local anesthesia injection.)

- Inject 30 minutes before incision to allow the epinephrine to take optimal effect and provide adequately dry working field, as outlined in Chapter 4.

- Patients are blocked (lying down to decrease risk of fainting) in the waiting area before going into the operating room (see ▶ Video 6.1).

SPECIFICS OF MINIMALLY PAINFUL INJECTION OF LOCAL ANESTHETIC IN ELECTIVE ANKLE AND ACHILLES TENDON SURGERY

- A summary of considerations to be given when operating on the ankle and hindfoot is noted in ▶ Table 53.1.

- Local anesthesia injection should cause a small amount of discomfort if at all if the injection pearls noted in Chapter 5 are followed. Directed distraction techniques are often utilized in the foot and ankle, which specifically involve stimulating the injected nerve territory proximal to the injection site with a nonpainful but significant stimulus. Commonly utilized techniques include thumb pressure, gentle pinching or bunching of skin, firm rubbing, etc.

- It is important to understand that complete anesthesia almost always requires large volumes of injection.

- Allow at least 30 minutes between injection and surgery to give the anesthesia enough time to work well, and to permit maximal vasoconstriction with epinephrine.

- Do not rush the injections. The whole process should take 20 to 30 minutes. (See Chapter 5 for additional hints and ideas to improve technique.)

- Inject patients (lying down in a comfortable position, at an agreeable room temperature with the head of the bed not elevated to decrease risk of fainting) in the waiting area, or preferably in a designated injection space with sufficient privacy, before going into the operating room (see ▶ Video 6.1).

Table 53.1   Considerations to keep in mind when performing WALANT on the ankle and Achilles tendon

Ankle joint (fusion, osteotomy, arthroscopy)	Achilles tendon work
Start with 155 mL of 0.33% lidocaine with 1:300,000 epinephrine (commonly required volume) Ensure circumferential periosteal/bony block at least 2 cm above and below joint has been done (including posteriorly) Consider blocking/injecting the subtalar joint Ensure appropriate block of the medial and lateral gutter is done Beware of anatomic variability of neurovascular anatomy about the ankle—carefully drawback and inject slowly; stop if there is resistance In situations with a significantly diseased ankle joint, consider the use of fluoroscopy to inject local anesthetic in ankle (to ensure that ankle is well blocked)	Position patient prone—"like lying on the beach" Ensure appropriate anesthetic is present anterior and posterior to the tendon Fill the sheath Be generous with local anesthetic proximally around the tendon up to the musculotendinous junction, and posteriorly behind the ankle and subtalar joints Be aware of the sural nerve and the tibial nerve and artery when injecting

- See injection of ankle fractures above for more suggestions.

- *For periosteal injections (when doing bony work):*

  - When working on bone (ankle fusion, osteotomy, instrumentation, etc.) start proximally. Ensure at least 2 cm of tumescent local anesthesia above and beyond anywhere dissection is planned or required.
  - Circumferential injection of the periosteum is required when more significant bony work is planned (fusion, osteotomy, insertion of fixation, etc.).
  - Careful attention must be paid to ensure adequate syndesmotic anesthesia. When injecting medially along the fibula or along the lateral border of the tibia ensure that both sides (anterior and posterior) of the interosseous membrane of the tibia and fibula are injected. A palpable "pop" is commonly felt when this structure is traversed with the needle tip.
  - When injecting medially and posteriorly take great care to avoid neurovascular and tendinous structures during the safe injection of the buffered local mixture.

SPECIFICS OF MINIMALLY PAINFUL INJECTION OF LOCAL ANESTHETIC FOR HINDFOOT AND MIDFOOT SURGERY

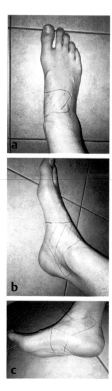

Fig. 53.5 Anesthetic area for a planned talonavicular joint fusion. Note that the joints above and below the planned surgery are included to ensure complete anesthesia of the entire operated bony structures and their associated joints and joint capsular tissue. Prepare 105 mL of tumescent local anesthesia with 50 mL of 1% lidocaine with 1:100,000 epinephrine added to 5 mL of 8.4% bicarbonate and 50 mL of saline. Inject 10 to 20 mL of this 0.5% lidocaine with 1:200,000 epinephrine solution subcutaneously along all planned incision sites using a long 27-gauge needle. Inject an additional 20 to 30 mL of the same solution at the periosteal level covering the proximal, middle, and distal aspects of the fracture site at the lateral malleolus. Inject an additional 20 to 30 mL surrounding the medial malleolus and distal tibia. Inject an additional 10 to 15 mL at the posterior malleolus. If more than 100 mL of tumescent local anesthesia is required (multisite procedures, more significant soft tissue procedures, etc.) or patients have larger feet, dilute the solution even further to 0.3% lidocaine with 1:300,000 epinephrine by adding 50 mL of saline to the solution which will provide a total of 155 mL.

WALANT in hindfoot and midfoot surgery

- Start with 105 mL of 0.5% lidocaine with 1:200,000 epinephrine local mixture (Chapter 4 for commonly required volume).

- Ensure circumferential periosteal/bony block at least 2 cm above and below joint, including plantarly.

- Take great care to not overinsufflate the fat pad of the heel.

- Ensure all joints adjacent to the area of planned surgery are anesthetized.

- Plan out the required surgery with skin markers, including areas of important related procedures (Achilles lengthening, forefoot surgery, etc.). Ensure these areas are anesthetized prior to going to the operating room. In situations where these procedures need to be added intraoperatively: (1) ensure safe doses of anesthetic are still available to the patient and dose appropriately; (2) administer the local anesthesia as soon as possible; and (3) adhere to the 30-minute preincision time post injection.

- Beware of anatomic variability of neurovascular anatomy around the foot and ankle. Carefully draw back and inject slowly. Stop if there is resistance.

- In situations of multiple incisions/procedures or surgeries involving the whole of the calcaneus (specifically calcaneus fractures), "backing up" local field blocks with a proper malleolar level ankle block is a reasonable and often efficient method of achieving reliable anesthesia. It is important to remember that in such cases the use of local anesthesia containing epinephrine in the areas of planned surgery remains critical to obtaining good pain control and maintaining good intraoperative hemostasis and cannot be ignored or forgotten.

- See sections above for more tips on local anesthesia injection in the ankle.

- In the metatarsal pad, more patient and judicious injections are encouraged. A cycle of injecting and then examining for effect is likely the best approach to avoid pressure injury to this sensitive structure.

- Injection is always performed in a proximal to distal fashion in both subcutaneous and periosteal injections to avoid creating multiple painful stimuli.

- *For periosteal injections (when doing bony work)*:
  - When working on bone (calcaneus, navicular, talus, metatarsals, cuneiforms, etc.) start proximally. At least 2 cm of tumescent local anesthesia above and beyond anywhere dissection is planned is required.
  - Circumferential injection of the periosteum is required when more significant bony work is planned (fusion, osteotomy, insertion of fixation, etc.). This must include the injection of adjacent joints.
  - Careful attention must be paid to ensure adequate plantar/inferior anesthesia. This often requires the use of longer needles that can reach the plantar surface of the structures of interest. Once reached,

appropriate volume should be administered to confirm appropriate coverage of the plantar periosteum. Failure to appropriately gain anesthesia on the plantar aspect of the bony surfaces can lead to intraoperative pain.

– Injecting the fat pad of the metatarsals is often required, and in the experience of the authors has not led to any observable complications. It is important to note, however, that observing the injection of a reasonable amount of fluid into this space is an important consideration and should not be overdone.

– When injecting in the areas of the known intermetatarsal neurovascular bundles, take great care to avoid neurovascular and tendinous structures during the safe injection of the buffered local mixture.

– Injecting the fat pad of the heel is often required, and in the experience of the authors has not led to any observable complications. It is important to note, however, that observing the injection of a reasonable amount of fluid into this space is an important consideration and should not be overdone.

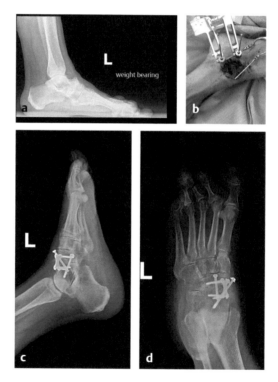

Fig. 53.6 A 58-year-old female with severe rheumatoid arthritis and talonavicular joint disease **(a)** was treated with an isolated talonavicular joint fusion using WALANT **(b)**. Because of contracture a joint distractor had to be used. Despite the instrumentation and bony work, the patient reported 0/10 pain in 15-minute intervals throughout her entire surgery. She went on to a successful result at 2 years with no reported talonavicular joint pain **(c, d)**.

SPECIFICS OF WALANT OF MINIMALLY PAINFUL INJECTION OF LOCAL ANESTHETIC FOR FOREFOOT SURGERY

- Local anesthesia injection should barely hurt at all if the simple rules of Chapter 5 for hints to minimize injection pain are followed.

- See sections above for more tips on local anesthesia injection in the foot and ankle.

- Always err on the side of too much local anesthesia instead of not enough. The goal is for patients to feel a small sting when the first local anesthesia needle is inserted. They should feel no pain for the rest of the injections or during the subsequent surgery.

- Prepare 105 mL of tumescent local anesthesia with 50 mL of 1% lidocaine with 1:100,000 epinephrine added to 5 mL of 8.4% bicarbonate and 50 mL of saline (Chapter 4). Inject 10 to 20 mL of this 0.5% lidocaine with 1:200,000 epinephrine solution subcutaneously along all planned incision and dissection sites using a long 27-gauge needle.

- If the patient requires more than 100 mL of tumescent local anesthesia (multi-site procedures, more significant soft tissue procedures, etc.) or patients with larger feet, dilute the solution even further to 0.3% lidocaine with 1:300,000 epinephrine by adding 50 mL of saline to the solution which will provide a total of 155 mL.

- Ensure circumferential periosteal/bony block at least 2 cm above and below the joint has been done (including plantarly).

- Ensure web spaces of operated toes are injected proximally—at the level of the metatarsal bases—to ensure entire region is blocked.

- Do not overinsufflate the fat pad of the metatarsal heads. Use enough local anesthetic to achieve the required anesthesia.

- Ensure all joints adjacent to the area of planned surgery are anesthetized utilizing fluoroscopy where needed to ensure accuracy of anesthetic injection.

- Plan out the required surgery with skin markers, including areas of important related procedures (adjacent toes, etc.). Ensure these areas are anesthetized prior to going to the operating room. In situations where other procedures need to be added intraoperatively: (1) ensure safe doses of anesthetic are still available to the patient and dose appropriately; (2) administer the local anesthetic as soon as possible; and (3) adhere to the 30-minute preincision time post injection.

- In situations where multiple incisions/procedures or surgeries involving the whole of the forefoot are required, consider doing a "whole forefoot block" (blocking the forefoot at the level of the metatarsal bases). This involves: (1) subcutaneously starting medially, along the medial border of the foot, at the level of the tarsometatarsal (TMT) joints, all the way across to the lateral border—lateral to the fifth metatarsal; (2) injecting each web space as well as medial to the first metatarsal and lateral to the fifth metatarsal; (3) injecting at the periosteal level with a long needle along the plantar aspect of the metatarsals going medial to lateral, and then lateral to medial—to ensure complete anesthesia of all plantar structures; and (4) pausing for 5 to 10 minutes after completing the first

Video 53.2
Local anesthesia injection for metatarsal phalangeal surgery (Mayich, Canada).

three steps. Return and assess the epinepherinized skin and perform a physical examination. Address any areas that have not been blocked with directed local injections. **DO NOT proceed to the operating room until TOTAL anesthesia of the forefoot has been obtained.**

- Perform appropriate vascular examination of each affected toe at the conclusion of the surgery.

- Always have phentolamine available when performing WALANT forefoot surgery.

Managing the "White Toe"

- When in doubt, rescue with phentolamine as described in Chapter 3.

- In cases where ischemia is a result of the epinephrine injection, it always respond to phentolamine. If there is no response to phentolamine and the toe remains ischemic, consider alternative causes for ischemia (reposition toe, examine dissection for vascular injury, etc.).

- Be cautious about injecting epinephrine in toes which show very little capillary refill when squeezed preoperatively. Epinephrine is not required in these cases.

- If there is good capillary refill in the toe nail bed, the circulation will likely recover nicely.

Caution: Revision surgeries, cases with significant preexisting scarring, cases with significant hardware removal, case of active infection, and patients with a high burden or anxiety (either subjectively reported or documented in their clinical history) have been demonstrated to present challenges in achieving anesthesia. WALANT may be difficult in these cases. See ▶ Table 53.2 for contraindications to WALANT in foot and ankle surgery. **It is critical to note that in forefoot surgery contraindications are noted and strictly followed to prevent ischemic insult to the toes.** Toes may not be as well vascularized as fingers because of preexisting vascular disease.

Table 53.2   List of contraindications to the use of WALANT in the foot and ankle

Contraindication	Relative/Absolute	Notes
Documented anxiety disorder + stated significant apprehension to WALANT	Absolute	Poor intraoperative experiences reported
Stated anxiety to WALANT	Relative	Often taking time to discuss and explore reasons can quickly clarify patient concerns and often can be successfully treated with WALANT

Table 53.2 **List of contraindications to the use of WALANT in the foot and ankle (*Cont.*)**

Contraindication	Relative/Absolute	Notes
No palpable pulses and/or documented peripheral vascular disease	Relative	Use local mixture without epinephrine; alter dose appropriately
Significant traumatic scarring, previous circumferential/crushing injury, previous multiple surgeries/incisions/scars	Relative	Poor penetration of local mixture that often results in significant intraoperative pain
Infection	Relative	Can be done successfully if sufficient "halo" of local is injected, including at least 3 to 4 cm of local anesthetic surrounding infected area, with sufficient periosteal local anesthetic administered
Hardware removal	Relative	Intraoperative pain has been reported; counsel patients appropriately
Significant associated comorbidities (diabetes mellitus, Raynaud's disease, etc.)	Relative	In cases with concern, proceed without epinephrine injection, especially in cases with Raynaud's disease; have phentolamine rescue present PRIOR to initiating local anesthetic use and use as required if you choose to use epinephrine

WALANT AS A METHOD OF ANESTHESIA FOR CLOSED REDUCTION OF DISPLACED ANKLE FRACTURES

- WALANT can be a safe and effective means of performing closed reduction of some types of displaced rotational ankle fractures **without evidence of axial instability/significant limb shortening** in the emergency department.

- This allows delivery of effective anesthesia in a busy and often chaotic environment in a method that minimizes the requirements of other clinicians (emergency room physicians and nurses). This can expedite and improve patient care.

- In unfortunate cases where patients do not have access to the resources needed for definitive care, using this technique can also allow the clinician to significantly improve the alignment of the injured ankle at a low cost and with minimal resources, which may in the final analysis allow for a much more functional extremity for the patient.

TIPS AND TRICKS FOR SUCCESSFUL CLOSED REDUCTION OF ANKLE FRACTURES WITH THE WALANT APPROACH

- As is the case with any plan for operative management of diagnosed ankle fractures using WALANT, **ensure with absolute certainty that the presumed rotational ankle fracture does not involve open injury, associated neurovascular injury, any axial instability, or more proximal or distal injuries**. Specifically, a misdiagnosis of a distal tibia-fibula or so-called "pilon" fracture as a simpler rotational "ankle fracture" **must** be avoided. Although this has been successfully done in specific cases, these injuries are rarely amenable to WALANT technique as they require more significant anesthesia for safe performance of a closed reduction with operative stabilization with the management of the more extensive wound, and usually the application of an external fixator.

- A thorough prereduction of peripheral nerve and vascular examination must be performed and documented.

- The fracture site(s) and the planned path for ankle joint intra-articular injection are marked using a washable skin marker.

- Utilizing a small gauge needle (26 gauge or higher) and keeping with standard WALANT technique, the skin overlying the planned needle paths for fracture and joint injection is anesthetized.

- Once completed, the intra-articular ankle injection aspiration and local injection are performed.

- Allow sufficient passage of time following this injection (30 minutes time which can be easily utilized to finish details of the patient's clinical examination, confirm or complete the informed consent process, complete hospital paperwork, answer patient or family questions, etc.).

- Perform periosteal injection around the known fractures, including ensuring adequate hematoma blocks are in place (using a large bore, 22 gauge or lower, needle as often clotting can occur and prevent the passage of anesthetic present in the intra-articular ankle).

- Ensure the posterior fibula and the syndesmosis are adequately injected.

- Following the sufficient passage of time, palpate the area of the ankle fracture and perform a manipulation of the (unstable) ankle.
  - If anesthesia is present, at this point manipulation and a reduction can be easily performed.
  - If anesthesia is NOT present:
    - Confirm suspected diagnosis and rule out the presence of a missed diagnosis (associated unrecognized injury, etc.).
    - Ensure a minimum of 30 minutes has passed. If that has occurred, examine the patient carefully and determine where remaining pain is located.
    - In the setting where the pain is located within the fracture as suspected, address the painful areas examined with a repeat periosteal injection fracture hematoma block.
    - In cases where pain is generalized to the ankle, consider using a larger bore needle (18 gauge) to clinically confirm an intra-articular block of the ankle has been performed. Perform a repeat aspiration of the ankle and subsequent injection of local anesthetic.

- In cases where the patient is uncomfortable, has unremitting anxiety, or is unwilling to proceed consult with an available emergency room or anesthesia clinician to proceed with more generalized anesthetic.

TIPS AND TRICKS FOR OPERATIVE REDUCTION OF ANKLE FRACTURES

- Before surgery, test the anesthetic effect by manipulating the fracture site. The pain score should be "0" during manipulation. This is a sign that the local anesthesia has taken effect and it is safe to proceed with the surgery without pain.

- Do not forget to inject the syndesmosis and posterior malleolus adequately even in cases where there is no initial plan for fixation. This will ensure that in the case of unexpected intraoperative findings of instability of either structure it can be addressed surgically. It will also ensure that the patient is painless when the remainder of the fractured ankle is manipulated in cases where no fixation is required.

- As there is significant anatomic variability of neurovascular structures, as well as a large number of tendons around the foot and ankle, always be very careful to draw back and confirm a needle position outside of a vascular structure; never force in fluid if unexpected resistance is noted (as this may indicate the needle is located in an important anatomic structure like a ligament, tendon, or nerve).

- After the reconstruction, and in the setting where the patient is amenable, take down the drape and have the patients see and move their limb in all directions. Closely observe the fracture(s) as well as the stability of the construct. Pay careful attention to the rotation of the fibula, and always remember to evaluate the syndesmosis for stability. This will provide motivation to the patient during physiotherapy.

- Close the skin with buried intradermal simple interrupted 4-0 Monocryl sutures as shown in detail for carpal tunnel closure in ▶ Video 26.9.

SPECIFIC CONSIDERATIONS BASED ON THE TYPE OF SURGERY

ACHILLES SURGERIES (DEBRIDEMENT, ACUTE AND CHRONIC REPAIR, ADVANCEMENT, LENGTHENING, RELATED TENDON TRANSFERS, ETC.)

- The prone position (lying on their abdomen) is well tolerated in awake patients.

- Awake prone patients are able to comfortably control their position and protect their eyes.

- Achilles tendon repair sufficiency, length and tension, transferred tendon sufficiency, and other key factors such as resultant foot position can be assessed awake on the table in the prone position and with simulated weightbearing.

- Achilles tendon surgeries as an "add on" or required procedure for other operations (i.e., diabetic foot, pes planus and cavus reconstructions, etc.) are also well tolerated.

BONY SURGERIES (FUSION, OSTEOTOMY, ETC.)

- This allows the surgeon to assess both the resultant position of the foot and ankle as a result of the operative intervention. This can be compared to the contralateral side in applicable cases. The other foot can also be prepped and draped to be visible for intraoperative comparison of appearance and active movement.

- The stability of the fixation strategy applied to all foot and ankle bones during active foot motion and simulated weightbearing can be directly assessed clinically and fluoroscopically by lowering the foot of the bed and using a sterile footplate.

- This is of particular interest during first metatarsophalangeal (MTP) fusion and hallux valgus correction as it allows the surgeon to "dial in" rotational alignment (pronation/supination position of the first toe) during weightbearing—a common issue when weightbearing alignment is not assessed intraoperatively.

TENDINOUS PROCEDURES

- In cases of tendon transfer surgeries (peroneal tendon transfers, tibialis anterior transfer/Bridal procedure) the tension of the tendon transfer can be assessed both in the supine position as well as in the position of simulated weightbearing.

- In cases of tendon transfer and repair, the tension of the reconstructed tendon can be assessed in the supine position as well as in the position of simulated weightbearing. In addition, the impact of transferred tendons can also be assessed on the table. (The impact of flexor digitorum longus [FDL] transfer on lesser toe flexion, and on the pes planus reconstruction immediately prior to and following the harvesting of the tendon. This information can be used to assist the surgeon in patient counseling postoperatively.)

- In cases of tendon transfer and repair surgeries such as the Jones procedure, lesser toe transfers, plantar plate repairs, extensor hallucis longus (EHL) repair, etc., the tension of the repaired or transferred tendon and its impact on functional toe position can be assessed both in the prone and supine positions, as well as in the position of simulated weightbearing.

- The resultant active range of motion of the operated joints can be assessed.

- Sufficiency of tendon repair can be assessed and can be ensured, thereby optimizing the technique of the tendon transfer utilized (side-to-side vs. endobutton vs. interference screw vs. suture anchor, combination, etc.). This is of particularly critical importance in patients with poor bone or tendon tissue quality.

- The resultant soft tissue tension and its effect on foot and ankle position can be functionally assessed intraoperatively. As an example, the impact of a peroneus longus to brevis tendon transfer plus or minus Achilles lengthening and a medical column dorsal closing wedge osteotomy for a Silverskjold and Coleman block positive forefoot diabetic ulceration can be assessed for its effectiveness in correcting foot position and alleviating forefoot point pressure. This can help directly inform intraoperative decision-making process for determining which additional procedures are (or are not) required to get the desired clinical effect.

- In the repair of a deformed toe with a more complex underlying cause such as plantar plate rupture, previous surgeries, etc., the reconstruction can be assessed in a weightbearing position intraoperatively. This will allow for a more accurate understanding of the results of the surgical reconstruction immediately on the table.

ARTHROSCOPIC PROCEDURES

- Active range of motion on the table can help inform the results of the procedure, as well as confirm returned functional stability following ligamentous reconstruction procedures.

- In cases of tendinoscopy, particularly peroneal, Achilles, and EHL tendinoscopy, the function stability and action of the tendons can be directly observed, and the resultant functional foot and ankle tension can be directly observed.

- By being aware, alert, and sober in cases where it is desired, the patients can engage in their care by learning and discussing findings with the operating surgeon.

A list of surgeries about the ankle, hindfoot, and midfoot successfully completed by the authors is noted in ▶ Table 53.3 and ▶ Table 53.4. These surgeries can be successfully done when patients are appropriately selected.

Table 53.3   List of procedures of the ankle and Achilles that have been successfully performed by the authors

Procedures

- Tibiotalocalcaneal fusion (minimally invasive/miniopen)
- Tibial osteotomy
- Bridle procedure
- Tibialis posterior to anterior tendon transfer
- Ankle fracture ORIF (single, bimalleolar, and trimalleolar fractures)
- Talus ORIF
- Open ankle fusion
- Achilles tendon debridement, acute and delayed open repair
- Achilles tendon V-Y advancement, w calcaneoplasty + FHL transfer
- Ankle arthroscopy (diagnostic, OCD lesion microfracture and synthetic cartilage insertion, anterior ankle joint debridement for arthritis)
- Ankle arthroscopy and Broström-type lateral ligament reconstruction
- Arthroscopic removal of os trigonum
- Peroneal tendon transfer, open repair +/- staged allograft reconstruction (with Hunter rods), tendinoscopy

---

Abbreviations: FHL, flexor hallucis longus; OCD, osteochondral; ORIF, open reduction internal fixation.

Table 53.4   List of procedures of the hindfoot and midfoot that have been successfully performed by the authors

Procedures

- Triple fusion, isolated subtalar, talonavicular fusions—both primary and revision
- Calcaneocuboid joint replacement (Orthosphere)
- Calcaneus, talus, navicular ORIF—both primary and revision
- Pes planus reconstruction (including calcaneal osteotomy, FDL transfer, spring ligament imbrication, gastrocnemius recession and medial column plantarflexion osteotomy)
- Revision adult clubfoot reconstruction
- Subtalar arthroscopy and debridement, arthroscopic-assisted subtalar fusion
- Charcot realignment surgery (including multiple osteotomies and reconstruction)
- Irrigation and debridement surgery for infection
- Midfoot fusion (multiple forms including for reconstruction, deformity, and trauma)
- Lapidus-type hallux valgus corrections
- Extensor tendon repair, including acute, delayed, and staged (Hunter rod) repairs
- Tibialis anterior tendon transfer + osteotomy and fusion procedures for neuromuscular deformity

Abbreviations: FDL, flexor digitorum longus; ORIF, open reduction internal fixation.

CLOSURE AND POSTOPERATIVE CONSIDERATIONS

- Prior to the application of any covering dressings, examine the foot and ankle for any signs of dysvascularity. If concerned:
  - Wait 5 minutes.
  - Apply sponge soaked in warm saline.
  - Apply phentolamine rescue if concerns persist (Chapter 3).
  - If still ischemic, consider nonanesthetic-related cause (deformity overcorrection, overaggressive dissection resulting in vascular injury, etc.) and address as required.
  - Never leave the operating room with persistent concerns of dysvascularity.
- Apply generous gauze dressings to absorb expected drainage from wound.

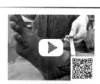

Video 53.3 Check the stability of the fixation after screw fixation of the medial malleolus and plating of the lateral malleolus in active movement (Amir Ahmad, Malaysia).

- Ensure patients are well educated about the expected behavior of the injected anesthetic, and the usual course of postoperative pain. This will ensure that the patients are sufficiently prepared for postoperative pain and understand what is normal and what is abnormal.

- Consider the use of a postoperative information sheet customized for the surgeon, the planned surgeries, and the patients to educate patients as much as possible.

- Maximize the use of non-narcotic pain management postoperatively, including the routine practice of:
  - Elevation.
  - Ibuprofen or equivalent nonsteroidal anti-inflammatory agent.
  - Acetaminophen.

- – Distraction techniques.
- – Support of friends and family.
- • Understand that drainage from WALANT can be significant.
- • Consider postoperative follow-up at 1 week for dressing and splint change.
- • The WALANT approach is also very helpful for fibular plate removal.[6]

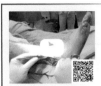

Video 53.4
Injection of local anesthetic and surgery for lateral malleolus fracture plate fixation (Chen, Taiwan).[5]

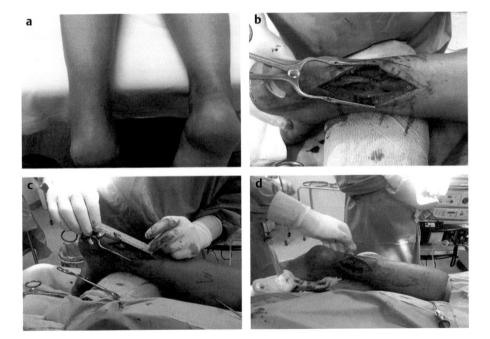

Fig. 53.7 A 38-year-old female presented with a neglected Achilles tendon rupture that was 4 months old, demonstrating an inability to plantar flex her left ankle **(a)**. Following administration of WALANT anesthesia using the described technique with the patient positioned prone, the ruptured Achilles was identified **(b)** and the dead and devitalized tissue was removed, leaving a gap of 4 cm **(c)**. The Achilles was then released and an advancement was performed and a repair was done. The plantaris was utilized as a local graft. **(d)** The patient reported no pain (0/10) throughout the entire surgery, measured at 15-minute intervals, and went on to experience a full recovery of Achilles function at 1 year postoperatively (Mayich, Canada).

Video 53.5
Injection of
local anesthetic
and surgery for
bimalleolar ankle
fracture (Rafiqi,
Morocco).

Video 53.6
Injection of local
anesthetic and
surgery for Achilles
tendon repair
(Rafiqi, Morocco).

Video 53.7
Extensor hallucis
longus repair
(Ayhan, Turkey).

References

1. Bilgetekin YG, Kuzucu Y, Öztürk A, Yüksel S, Atilla HA, Ersan Ö. The use of the wide-awake local anesthesia no tourniquet technique in foot and ankle injuries. Foot Ankle Surg 2020;S1268-7731(20)30141-7. doi:10.1016/j.fas.2020.07.002 [published online ahead of print]
2. MacNeill AL, Mayich DJ. Wide-awake foot and ankle surgery: a retrospective analysis. Foot Ankle Surg 2017;23(4):307–310
3. Wright J, MacNeill AL, Mayich DJ. A prospective comparison of wide-awake local anesthesia and general anesthesia for forefoot surgery. Foot Ankle Surg 2019;25(2):211–214
4. MacNeill AL, Wright J, Mayich DJ. Qualitative aspects of patient pain during surgery with wide-awake local anesthesia. J Orthop 2019;16(1):105–108
5. Li YS, Chen CY, Lin KC, Tarng YW, Hsu CJ, Chang WN. Open reduction and internal fixation of ankle fracture using wide-awake local anaesthesia no tourniquet technique. Injury 2019;50(4):990–994
6. Poggetti A, Del Chiaro A, Nicastro M, Parchi P, Piolanti N, Scaglione M. A local anesthesia without tourniquet for distal fibula hardware removal after open reduction and internal fixation: the safe use of epinephrine in the foot. A randomized clinical study. J Biol Regul Homeost Agents 2018; 32(6, Suppl. 1):57–63

Section V

PENCIL TEST AND RELATIVE MOTION SPLINTING TO
SOLVE HAND PAIN PROBLEMS AND IMPROVE RANGE OF
MOTION IN STIFF FINGERS

CHAPTER 54

PENCIL TEST AND RELATIVE MOTION SPLINTING TO SOLVE HAND PAIN AND STIFFNESS AFTER TRAUMA AND SURGERY

Donald H. Lalonde, Lisa Flewelling, and Amanda Higgins

WHAT IS THE PENCIL TEST AND HOW DOES IT WORK?

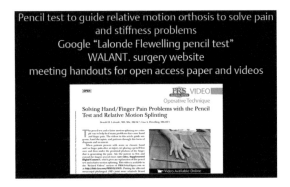

Fig. 54.1 Open access video paper on using the pencil test to solve hand/finger pain and stiffness problems with relative motion splinting.[1] This link[1] takes you to many other video examples of hand and finger pain and stiffness after injury or surgery that we solved with relative motion splinting.

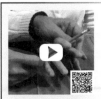

Video 54.1 Video explaining how to do the pencil test, and how you use it to build relative motion splints to solve hand pain problems (Lalonde, Canada).[1]

- The pencil test and relative motion splinting are a simple way to help heal many problems that cause hand and finger pain and stiffness.

- When patients present with acute or chronic hand and/or finger pain after any injury or operation, try placing a pencil first over and then under the proximal phalanx of the finger that is generating the pain. Ask the patient to flex and extend all the fingers several times (see ▶ Video 54.1). Putting the affected metacarpophalangeal (MP) joint more relatively flexed or extended than the other MP joints will often take away the pain with active movement with the pencil in place. When this happens, our hand therapist builds a relative motion splint that simulates the effect of the pencil.

- The relative motion extension splint keeps the MP joint of the injured finger more extended than the other MP joint. This takes the tension off the long extensor forces, even when fingers are actively flexing (▶ Video 54.1).

- The relative motion flexion splint keeps the MP joint of the injured finger more flexed than the other MP joints. This relaxes the intrinsic muscle forces and lets it heal if it is injured (▶ Video 54.1).

PAIN-GUIDED HEALING

- We tell all our patients with hand pain: "We did not spend two billion years evolving pain because it is bad for us. It is our body's only way to tell us: 'Hey, would you stop that? I am trying to heal in here and you are screwing it up! Stop that!' That is a little voice in our ears that we should listen to and we cannot hear it with pain killers in our ears. Stop pain killers and listen to your body and do not do what hurts. This is called pain-guided healing."[2]

- If the pencil test takes the pain away, we have the patients live with a pain-relieving relative motion splint for at least 2 weeks.

- Pain-relieving relative motion splints rebalance the forces so the body can heal.

- Relative motion splints are user friendly. Most patients can continue to work and do most activities while wearing the splints (even surgeons!).

- Patients continue to wear the splint until their pain is gone, which is their best indicator that whatever injury that was causing the pain is now healed.

- Relative motion splints were first introduced to our practice by Wyndell Merritt and Julie Howell.[3]

- Relative motion extension splints are most helpful in early protected movement of extensor tendon laceration, sagittal band tears, proximal interphalangeal (PIP) flexor lag after injury (see ▶ Video 19.TT9), and hand or finger pain of unknown origin. Relative motion flexion splints are most useful in boutonniere, interosseous tear, PIP extension lag after trauma or Dupuytren's release, and hand or finger pain of unknown origin.[1]

HOW TO BUILD RELATIVE MOTION FLEXION AND EXTENSION SPLINTS

- Lisa Flewelling shows how to build relative motion flexion and extension splints (▶ Video 54.2).

- If you do not have access to the materials or a hand therapist to build these splints, you can use tape such as rubber tape or hockey tape as shown in ▶ Video 54.4.

Video 54.2 How to build relative motion splints (Flewelling, Canada).

EXAMPLES OF PAIN PROBLEMS SOLVED WITH THE PENCIL TEST AND RELATIVE MOTION SPLINTING

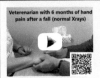

Video 54.3 Hand pain of 6 months of a veterinary surgeon solved with pencil test and relative motion splinting (Lalonde, Canada).

Video 54.4 Acute hand pain and snapping of a house painter solved with pencil test and relative motion splinting (Lalonde/Flewelling, Canada).

Video 54.5 Pain after collateral ligament fracture avulsion of base of fifth proximal phalanx, which had persisted for 7 weeks, was solved with 1 week of relative motion splinting after pencil test (Lalonde, Canada).

Video 54.6 Pain and range of motion improved in a patient with 9-month-old complex regional pain syndrome (Lalonde/Higgins, Canada).

Video 54.7 Small finger pain and abduction deformity for 18 months solved in a patient referred for Dupuytren. She presented with finger pain and abduction deformity after a fall (Lalonde, Canada).

Video 54.8 A pain which persisted for 3 months after minimally displaced fracture of fifth metacarpal was solved with pencil test and relative motion flexion splinting (Lalonde/Flewelling, Canada).

Video 54.9 Hand swelling and pain causing 2 years of hand pain from work injury greatly improved with pencil test and relative motion splinting (Lalonde, Canada).

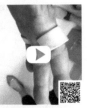

Video 54.10 Pain from boutonniere fracture avulsion injury solved with 7 weeks of relative motion flexion splinting (Lalonde, Canada).

- Relative motion flexion splinting has revolutionized the treatment of boutonniere and extensor tendon injuries. See Chapter 21 for many more examples.

EXAMPLES OF STIFFNESS AND EXTENSOR LAG PROBLEMS SOLVED WITH THE PENCIL TEST AND RELATIVE MOTION SPLINTING

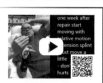

Video 54.11
Relative motion flexion splinting after Dupuytren to improve proximal interphalangeal (PIP) extensor lag (Lalonde, Canada).

Video 54.12
Relative motion flexion splinting after finger fracture to improve proximal interphalangeal (PIP) extensor lag, pain, and swelling (Lalonde, Canada).

Video 54.13
Relative motion flexion splinting after metacarpo-phalangeal (MP) axe injury with two fractured bones and extensor tendon repair. First relative motion extension splint was used to get the extensor tendon repair moving at 7 days. Then we used a relative motion flexion splint to improve proximal interphalangeal (PIP) extensor lag (Lalonde/Higgins, Canada).

- Relative motion flexion splinting has revolutionized the treatment of PIP extensor lag after Dupuytren's surgery or Xiaflex injection. See ▶ Video 32.1 for another great example of this concept.

- Relative motion flexion splinting has revolutionized the treatment of PIP extensor lag after finger fracture. The splint forces patients to use the index finger they have been holding out of the way. The MP extension force is redirected to the PIP joint. Patients exercise while they are living instead of stopping living to exercise (see ▶ Video 54.12).

- Relative motion flexion splinting has revolutionized the treatment of PIP extensor lag after extensor tendon repair, as well as extensor tendon repair itself (see ▶ Video 54.13, Chapter 21, and Chapter 22).

References

1. Lalonde DH, Flewelling LA. Solving hand/finger pain problems with the pencil test and relative motion splinting. Plast Reconstr Surg Glob Open 2017;5(10):e1537
2. Brand P, Yancey P. Pain: The Gift Nobody Wants., Harper Collins Publishers and Zondervan Publishing House, Michigan. 1997
3. Howell JW, Merritt WH, Robinson SJ. Immediate controlled active motion following zone 4-7 extensor tendon repair. J Hand Ther 2005;18(2):182–190

INDEX